W9-AAE-623

GAYLE SCHANTZEN, MD
DEA ███████████
LIC ████████████

PAIN MANAGEMENT AND ANESTHESIOLOGY

DEVELOPMENTS IN
CRITICAL CARE MEDICINE AND ANESTHESIOLOGY

Volume 33

The titles published in this series are listed at the end of this volume.

148 — 188.50

PAIN MANAGEMENT AND ANESTHESIOLOGY

Papers presented at the 43rd Annual Postgraduate Course in Anesthesiology, February 1998

edited by

MICHAEL A. ASHBURN, PERRY G. FINE
AND THEODORE H. STANLEY

Department of Anesthesiology,
The University of Utah Medical School,
Salt Lake City, Utah, U.S.A.

KLUWER ACADEMIC PUBLISHERS
DORDRECHT / BOSTON / LONDON

A C.I.P. Catalogue record for this book is available from the Library of Congress.

ISBN 0-7923-4995-4

Published by Kluwer Academic Publishers,
P.O. Box 17, 3300 AA Dordrecht, The Netherlands.

Sold and distributed in the U.S.A. and Canada
by Kluwer Academic Publishers,
101 Philip Drive, Norwell, MA 02061, U.S.A.

In all other countries, sold and distributed
by Kluwer Academic Publishers,
P.O. Box 322, 3300 AH Dordrecht, The Netherlands.

Printed on acid-free paper

TABLE OF CONTENTS

Preface

Michael A. Ashburn, M.D.

Pain contains the refresher course manuscripts of the 43rd Annual Postgraduate Course in Anesthesiology which took place at the Cliff Conference Center in Snowbird, Utah on February 20-24, 1998. The chapters reflect recent advances in the understanding of the basic science and clinical management of pain. Sections on basic science related to pain processes as well as sections on the clinical management of acute, chronic, cancer-related, and pediatric pain are included. Each chapter represents a focused summary of the salient points pertaining to the subject of interest and has been edited only to the extent necessary to produce a coherent book.

The purposes of this textbook are to 1) act as a reference for the individuals attending the meeting and 2) serve as a concise review of the topic for those unable to participate in the meeting. Each presentation is intended to stand by itself, but the views expressed by the multiple authors offer the reader the opportunity to understand the multifaceted aspect of this field.

This textbook is the sixteenth in a continuing series documenting the proceedings of the postgraduate course in Salt Lake City. We hope that this series continues to serve as a resource to document the continuing evolution of anesthesiology and pain management.

T. H. Stanley et al. (eds.), Pain Management and Anesthesiology, ix.
© 1998 *Kluwer Academic Publishers. Printed in the Netherlands.*

LIST OF CONTRIBUTORS

Allan Basbaum, PhD
Department of Anatomy, University of California, San Francisco, San Francisco, California, U.S.A.

Lynn M. Broadman, M.D.
Departments of Anesthesiology and Pediatrics, West Virginia University, Morgantown, West Virginia, U.S.A.

Daniel B. Carr, MD, PhD
Departments of Anaesthesia and Medicine
Tufts University School of Medicine, New England Medical Center, Boston, Massachusetts, U.S.A.

Michael J. Cousins, AM, MBBS, MD, FRCA, FANZCA
Department of Anesthesia and Pain Management, University of Sydney, Royal North Shore Hospital, St. Leonards, NSW, Australia

Talmage D. Egan, MD
Department of Anesthesiology, University of Utah School of Medicine, Salt Lake City, Utah, U.S.A.

Gerald F. Gebhart, PhD
Department of Pharmacology, The University of Iowa College of Medicine, Iowa City, Iowa, U.S.A.

Henrik Kehlet, MD, PhD
Department of Surgical Gastroenterology, Hvidovre University Hospital, Hvidovre, Denmark

Juri Lindy Pedersen, MD
Department of Surgical Gastroenterology, Hvidovre University Hospital, Hvidovre, Denmark

L. Brian Ready, MD
Acute Pain Service, University of Washington School of Medicine, Seattle, Washington, U.S.A

Linda Jo Rice, MD
Anesthesia Specialists, St. Petersburg, Florida, U.S.A.

Philip J. Siddall, MBBS, PhD, MMed (Pain Management)
Department of Anesthesia and Pain Management, University of Sydney, Royal
North Shore Hospital, St. Leonards, NSW, Australia

David A. Taylor, MA (Hons), MAppliedSc, PhD
Department of Anesthesia and Pain Management, University of Sydney, Royal
North Shore Hospital, St. Leonards, NSW, Australia

Bernadette T. Verring, MD, PhD
Department of Anaesthesiology, University of Leiden, Leiden, The Netherlands

Paul F. White, PhD, MD, FFARACS, FANZCA
Department of Anesthesiology and Pain Management, The University of Texas
Southwestern Medical Center at Dallas, Dallas, Texas, U.S.A.

Suellen M. Walker, MBBS, FANZCA
Department of Anesthesia and Pain Management, University of Sydney
Royal North Shore Hospital, St. Leonards, NSW, Australia

Alon P. Winnie, MD
Department of Anesthesiology and Critical Care, Cook County Hospital,
Chicago, Illinois 60612

MECHANISMS OF OPIOID ANALGESIA AND TOLERANCE

A. Basbaum

Recent studies have clarified important new features about the mechanisms through which opioids exert their analgesic action. Based on a variety of anatomical, pharmacological and electrophysiological studies, it is generally assumed that systemic administration of morphine produces analgesia by a combined action at supraspinal sites, including the midbrain periaqueductal gray (PAG) and at the spinal cord level (1,2). Binding of morphine to opioid receptors in the PAG activates a powerful descending inhibitory control system that blocks the firing of spinal cord dorsal horn nociresponsive neurons. In part the inhibition is mediated by bulbospinal axons that originate in the medullary nucleus raphe magnus (3), the axons of which project to the spinal cord dorsal horn via the spinal cord dorsolateral funiculus (DLF). In fact, lesions of the DLF interrupt the analgesia produced by systemic morphine (4). Although early studies emphasized the contribution of the serotonergic outflow from the raphe magnus, other studies have provided evidence for an important contribution of noradrenergic systems to descending control (5).

In addition to the activation of brainstem inhibitory controls, there is obviously considerable evidence that opioids exert an action directly at the spinal cord. Most important is the demonstration that spinal administration of opioids produces a profound and long lasting analgesia. The anatomical evidence for the presence of opioid receptors on primary afferent terminals and on postsynaptic neurons of the dorsal horn provides the likely target of the spinal opioids (6-11). To what extent opioids act presynaptically to regulate the release of neurotransmitters from primary afferents, however, remains a controversial subject. As noted in our paper on the contribution of substance P to nociceptive processing in the dorsal horn, some laboratories, largely using *in vitro* models, reported that morphine can block the release of substance P from primary afferents (12). The *in vivo* studies of Duggan and colleagues (13), and our own analysis evaluating the central consequences of release of substance P, however, found little evidence that morphine blocks the release of substance P from primary afferents. The latter results argued for a predominant postsynaptic

1

T. H. Stanley et al. (eds.), Pain Management and Anesthesiology, 1–11.
© *1998 Kluwer Academic Publishers. Printed in the Netherlands.*

mechanism through which spinal opioids produce an antinociceptive effect.

Although arguments have been put forth that indicate a greater importance of supraspinal vs. spinal sites in the analgesia produced by systemic injection of morphine, the issue is really irrelevant. Clearly both sites are simultaneously activated, and indeed there is considerable evidence for a synergistic action when the opioid binds receptors at both sites (14).

More recently considerable evidence has been provided that in addition to the brainstem and spinal sites, opioids, including morphine, exert an antinociceptive effect via an action in the periphery, after binding to opioid receptors located both on neuronal and nonneuronal sites (15-17). It has been known for years that opioid receptors (indeed all subtypes) are synthesized by small diameter dorsal root ganglion cells and that the receptor is transported both to the spinal cord dorsal horn and via the peripheral branch of the primary afferent to peripheral terminals. Until recently, however, the functional significance of the peripheral opioid receptor was not clear. Early studies using hydrophilic forms of morphine that do not penetrate the central nervous system demonstrated that peripheral targeting of opioids may be beneficial for pain control, but the mechanism was unclear. Stein and colleagues have provided the most convincing evidence that it is by an action either at the peripheral terminal of the primary afferent nociceptor (particularly in the setting of injury where there appears to be an upregulation of the receptor) or on nonneural, immunocompetent cells that influence inflammatory and healing processes. Several laboratories have also demonstrated that components of the neurogenic inflammatory response (18,19), which depends upon release of peptides from the terminals of small diameter afferents in the periphery, can be significantly reduced by opioids acting locally. Finally, Levine and colleagues have provided evidence that delta and kappa opioid receptor agonists exert on effect on the peripheral terminals of sympathetic postganglionic efferents; the mu receptor appears to predominantly target the primary afferent (20). Of particular importance, of course, is the evidence that intraarticular injection of morphine in postarthroscopy patients can produce significant and relatively prolonged analgesia by a local action in the joint (21).

To follow-up on some of these studies we have been examining the effects of a new highly potent opiate, remifentanil, an analog of fentanyl that is unique because it is broken down by esterases in the blood, resulting in an incredibly short half-life (22). For example, in the rat a single bolus injection can produce profound analgesia but this resolves within a few minutes. This feature provided us with a unique opportunity to address the contribution of injury-evoked central sensitization (the process through which dorsal horn neurons are made hyperexcitable) in a standard model of pain, namely the formalin test (23). The formalin test is characterized by having two phases of pain behavior. The first phase begins soon after hindpaw injection of the formalin and lasts about 5 minutes. This phase is thought to result from direct action of formalin on "pain" fibers; in this respect it is a form of acute pain. The second phase begins about five minutes after the first phase (after a quiescent interphase). It lasts about 40 minutes. There are two hypotheses as to the origin of the second phase. Some groups believe that it arises as a result of a late-developing inflammation secondary to the formalin injection. Others believe that the second phase of the formalin test arises secondary to central sensitization in the spinal cord established by activity during the first phase. In fact, it has been suggested that input during the second phase is minimal; it is hypothesized that activity within the spinal cord drives the second phase. Consistent with the latter hypothesis, some laboratories have reported that when drugs (such as morphine) are administered during the first phase, it is possible to significantly reduce the second phase, even though the drug does not act during the second phase because the morphine was followed at five minutes by naloxone (24).

Since there may be difficulties limiting the drug to the first phases, we took advantage of the very short half-life of remifentanil to reevaluate the contribution of central sensitization to the second phase of the formalin test. We used remifentanil to eliminate the first phase of the formalin test, and then evaluated the extent to which the second phase was modified. We found that complete blockade of the first phase with remifentanil was readily established without altering the magnitude of the second phase. The only effect that we found on the second phase was a delay of its onset and of its termination (22). Indeed as we increased the duration of the remifentanil from 5 to 15 minutes we found a proportional increase in the delay in onset and termination of the second phase. This suggested to us that the first phase does not set up a central sensitization that mediates the second phase but rather that the delay of the second phase is due to an opioid-induced delay in the development of inflammation via an action in the periphery.

To test this hypothesis we repeated the experiment using remifentanil but simultaneously made a continuous infusion of a hydrophilic form of naloxone. This quaternary form of naloxone makes it possible to selectively block the peripheral action of opioids, leaving the central action unchanged, because the antagonist cannot cross the blood brain barrier. With this combination of drugs, we found that the first phase remained blocked, presumably because the analgesia produced in the first phase is due to a CNS action of remifentanil. The delay of onset and termination of the second phase of the formalin test, however, was eliminated when the peripherally acting naloxone was on board. That is, the second phase returned to "normal." Based on these results, we concluded that the delay was due to a remifentanil action in the periphery, probably retarding the development of the inflammation that we believe drives the second phase. We are presently following up on these studies, specifically addressing the target of the peripheral remifentanil. One could imagine a variety of mechanisms, including an action on peripheral afferent nociceptors, on sympathetic efferents, or on blood vessels. Regardless of the mechanism, these studies emphasize that there are profound peripheral effects of opioids that inevitably will come into play when an opiate, such as morphine, is administered systemically.

Of course, establishing that the spinal cord is a target of opioids is just the first step in determining the underlying mechanisms through which the analgesic action at the cord is generated. As noted above, both pre- and postsynaptic inhibitory mechanisms have been proposed. To what extent any given population of neurons must be inhibited in order to produce a behavioral inhibition is, however, unclear. With a view to identifying the populations of spinal cord neurons that are influenced by opioids we turned to an approach that allows monitoring of large populations of neurons and which makes it possible to correlate the pattern of inhibition with the behavior that is produced. In these studies, we used immunocytochemistry to monitor expression of the Fos protein product of the immediate early gene c-fos, which is induced in neurons that are "active."

As expected, based on the known distribution of nociresponsive neurons in the spinal cord gray matter, we found that a noxious stimulus induced Fos expression in large numbers of neurons in laminae I, II, V, and VII (25). Although opioids profoundly inhibited the noxious stimulus induction of Fos expression, we were never able to completely eliminate the induction of this gene. In particular, we found that almost 50% of the neurons in the superficial dorsal horn continued to express the Fos protein, despite the fact that the dose of morphine used produced a profound analgesia (26,27). This suggests that pain behavior can be blocked without completely eliminating the central consequences of a noxious stimulus. We subsequently demonstrated that some of the lamina I neurons that continue to express the Fos protein in the setting of morphine analgesia project to higher centers (28), which indicates that not only is there "activity" and cell biological consequences of the noxious stimulus under conditions of analgesia, but that this information is also transmitted to higher centers.

These studies provided new information on the mechanisms through which acute administration of opioids affects the transmission of nociceptive messages at the level of the spinal cord. More recently, we turned to the question of changes that occur when morphine is administered chronically, i.e., when tolerance develops. This is a controversial subject. In animals there is no question that tolerance to the analgesic actions of opioids can be readily demonstrated. In humans the situation is less clear. There is no doubt that there are clinical cases in which the amount of opioid used to treat pain is increased progressively. However, it is argued by some that this is not a sign of opioid tolerance, but a natural requirement because the pain is increasing (for example, because of tumor progression). This difference highlights the major distinction between the clinical and the laboratory experience. In the laboratory we can control the pain stimulus; in the clinical situation, at least in the case of cancer pain, where opioid use is most common, there is no control. In fact in the clinical situation it may even be difficult to identify the nature of the pain-producing stimulus. This is exacerbated by situations in which there is a combination of nociceptive/inflammatory and neuropathic pains due to concurrent involvement of tissue and nerve. Under some conditions the failure of an opioid could be interpreted as tolerance; in another situation the failure may reflect the fact that a relatively opioid-insensitive pain has developed, namely neuropathic pain.

Of interest to our laboratory are the mechanisms through which tolerance to the analgesic action of opioids develops. The traditional view is relatively straightforward (29). Cells that respond to opioids express the opioid receptor. The receptor in turn is coupled to an inhibitory G protein that transmits the downstream consequences of the opioid, leading to inhibition of cyclic AMP production, inhibition of calcium conductance, and increased potassium conductance and hyperpolarization (inhibition) of the neuron. The prevailing view is that tolerance develops when there is a decoupling of the opioid receptor from the inhibitory G protein. That is, in the setting of opioid tolerance, the opioid binds the receptor but it does not work. Our own view and that of a some laboratories is quite different and is based on observations that have been known for many years. Specifically, if you take an animal or for that matter a patient that has received a chronic infusion of morphine and administer the opioid antagonist naloxone, you will almost certainly precipitate an abstinence or withdrawal syndrome. Naloxone is an opioid antagonist that has no intrinsic activity; i.e., it does nothing by itself. Thus, when naloxone is administered to a naive subject nothing happens. All that naloxone can do is to displace the opioid from the opioid receptor. If the opioid is not "working" in the setting of tolerance then naloxone should be without effect. The fact that it produces a withdrawal syndrome indicates that the "tolerant" state must be one in which the opioid receptor remains coupled to the G protein.

What naloxone does is break the connection, resulting in withdrawal. The result is manifest at the biochemical and behavioral levels. For example, there is a dramatic increase in adenyl cyclase activity and an increase in cyclic AMP levels (30). What accounts for the overshoot? Based on a variety of studies, notably those of Nestler and colleagues (31,32), it has been suggested that chronic use of opioids induces a compensatory response that tries to counteract the inhibitory effects of the drug. According to this formulation, the withdrawal syndrome is a manifestation of the compensatory response being unleashed. Specifically opioids down regulate cyclic AMP; with chronic opioid treatment the cell or the circuits that have been affected counteract the effect of the opioid, by increasing the level of cyclic AMP, returning it to normal, i.e., there is a compensation for the inhibition exerted by the opioids.

How the hyperpolarization is overcome and why cells become spontaneously active during withdrawal is much less clear. There is some evidence that a particular sodium conductance is turned on as part of the compensatory response. The compensated setting therefore is effectively a state of latent sensitization that can be manifest by removal of the opioid or by injection of naloxone. This eliminates the inhibitory effect of the opioid, resulting in an overshoot, i.e., increased cyclic AMP production, increased excitation and spontaneous activity, and the behavioral hyperactivity that characterizes the withdrawal syndrome.

Interestingly, this state of latent sensitization is remarkably similar to the state of central sensitization that is proposed to occur at the level of the spinal cord when noxious stimuli or pain persists (33-36). Thus the threshold for firing of dorsal horn neurons drops, allodynia and hyperalgesia are produced and there is spontaneous pain, thought to result from increased activity of hyperexcitability dorsal horn neurons. Pharmacological evidence provides further evidence for similarities between the central sensitization that occurs following noxious stimulation and the compensatory response that is hypothesized to develop with chronic opioid use. Specifically, antagonists of the NMDA receptor have been shown to prevent the development of long-term changes/central sensitization in dorsal horn neurons (36) and to reduce the development of tolerance to morphine and to almost completely prevent the withdrawal syndrome that is generated when an antagonist is administered (37-39).

Since we have demonstrated that it is possible to monitor the activity of dorsal horn neurons using Fos expression, we reasoned that we could use this approach to identify the locus of the compensatory response by evaluating the distribution of Fos-positive neurons in animals made tolerant to morphine. To this end, we made rats tolerant to morphine and then monitored Fos expression in the spinal cord before and after imposing a noxious stimulus (the formalin injection described above). Consistent with the fact that we are dealing with a *latent* sensitization, there was no induction of the Fos protein in populations of dorsal horn neurons in animals that just received the morphine. However when we evaluated the effect of the noxious stimulus in the tolerant animals we found a very dramatic increase in the distribution of Fos-positive neurons both ipsilateral and contralateral to the stimulus, compared to the numbers of neurons that expressed the gene in animals that did not receive the morphine (40). In other words, the state of tolerance resulted in an exacerbated response of dorsal horns neurons to the noxious stimulus. The change was manifest as an increased Fos expression not only on the contralateral side of the cord but at segments considerably rostral and caudal to the locus of the afferent input from the hind paw. Taken together these results suggest that continued use of opioids does result in altered responses of dorsal horn neurons because of the development of a compensatory, long-term change that may share features with the changes that occur in the setting of persistent injury.

With a view to identifying how these changes are initiated, we next performed a study in which we administered naloxone to tolerant animals to precipitate a withdrawal symptom and evaluate where the Fos was manifest in these animals (41). When the study was performed in animals that were awake, i.e., that underwent a withdrawal syndrome, we not surprisingly found activity/Fos expression in large number of neurons throughout the dorsal and ventral horns. Since much of this activity could have arisen secondary to the heightened behavior that occurs in animals that are withdrawing from morphine, we repeated the experiment in animals that were anesthetized with halothane, i.e., they withdrew under a general anesthetic and thus did not have any motor activity. In these animals we found that naloxone-induced withdrawal evoked a remarkably localized distribution of Fos-immunoreactive neurons in the most superficial lamina of the dorsal horn, lamina I. This of course is precisely the target of primary afferent C-fibers and may be the locus of many neurons that express the opioid receptor. Interestingly, the same neurons undergo central sensitization in response to C-fiber stimulation, leading to a reduction of their threshold for activation, which is presumed to contribute to the allodynia and hyperalgesia that characterize many persistent pain states. Taken together these results raise the possibility that the locus of the chronic morphine induced compensatory response is in lamina I of the spinal cord and that a noxious stimulus evokes enhanced fos expression because of these changes.

We are presently addressing whether the neurons that express Fos during withdrawal under anesthesia are those which synthesize the opioid receptor or whether this response is in neurons that are downstream of the neurons that express the opioid receptor. Although we hypothesize that the compensatory response is focused in lamina I, the compensatory response need not occur in neurons that express the opioid receptor. Rather it could be a manifestation of the circuits in which the opioid receptor-laden neurons are but one element. In this respect, opioid tolerance would be more of a systems response to continued use of than opioids rather than a cellular one. An important study emphasizes this distinction. Roerig and colleagues (42) performed a study in the mouse in which they administered opioids both supraspinally and spinally and evaluated the interaction in a pain response test. As has been reported previously they found a profound synergy in tests of analgesia. That is, when subthreshold doses were administered simultaneously at spinal and supraspinal sites, profound analgesia was produced. However when they repeated the studies in animals made tolerant to systemic, they found that the tolerance did not occur at the individual sites (i.e., the ED_{50} at each site was unchanged). Rather they found that the synergy resulting from an action at the two sites was lost. Thus, in the conditions of their experiment, which in part mimic the injection approach to treating patients, morphine tolerance is manifest as a loss of the circuit interaction between the two sites.

In summary, these studies illustrate several important features of the mechanisms through which opioids exert their analgesic action. First, there are multiple sites, including spinal , supraspinal and peripheral loci. In addition, considerable changes take place when an opioid is administered chronically. These changes will affect not only the subsequent response to the opioid, but may also modify the extent to which injury stimuli (and the pain associated with them) are processed.

REFERENCES

1. Basbaum, AI, Fields, HL: Endogenous pain control systems: Brainstem spinal pathways and endorphin circuitry.   Ann Rev Neurosci 1984;7: 309-338.
2. Basbaum AI, Fields HL: Endogenous pain control mechanisms: Review and hypothesis. Ann Neurol 1978;4: 451-462.
3. Basbaum, AI, Clanton, CH, Fields, HL: Three bulbospinal pathways from the rostral medulla of the cat. An autoradiographic study of pain modulating systems. J Comp Neurol 1978;178: 209-224.

4. Basbaum AI, Marley NJ, O'Keefe J, Clanton CH: Reversal of morphine and stimulus-produced analgesia by subtotal spinal cord lesions. Pain 1977;3: 43-56.

5. West WL, Yeomans DC, Proudfit HK: The function of noradrenergic neurons in mediating antinociception induced by electrical stimulation of the locus coeruleus in two different sources of Sprague-Dawley rats. Brain Res 1993;626: 127-135.

6. Arvidsson U, Dado RJ, Riedl M, et al: Delta-opioid receptor immunoreactivity: Distribution in brainstem and spinal cord, and relationship to biogenic amines and enkephalin. J Neurosci 1995;15: 1215-1235.

7. Arvidsson U, Riedl M, Chakrabarti S, et al: Distribution and targeting of a mu-opioid receptor (MOR1) in brain and spinal cord. J Neurosci 1995;15: 3328-3341.

8. Ji RR, Zhang Q, Law PY, et al: Expression of mu-, delta-, and kappa-opioid receptor-like immunoreactivities in rat dorsal root ganglia after carrageenan-induced inflammation. J Neurosci 1995;15: 8156-8166.

9. Lamotte C, Pert CB, Snyder SH: Opiate receptor binding in primate spinal cord: distribution and changes after dorsal root section. Brain Res 1976;112: 407-412.

10. Mansour A, Fox CA, Akil H, Watson SJ: Opioid-receptor mRNA expression in the rat CNS: Anatomical and functional implications. Trends Neurosci 1995;18: 22-29.

11. Mansour A, Fox CA, Burke S, et al: Mu, delta, and kappa opioid receptor mRNA expression in the rat CNS: An in situ hybridization study. J Comp Neurol 1994;350: 412-438.

12. Jessell TM, Iversen LL: Opiate analgesics inhibit substance P release from rat trigeminal nucleus. Nature (Lond.) 1977;268: 549-551.

13. Morton CR, Hutchison WD, Duggan AW, Hendry IA: Morphine and substance P release in the spinal cord. Exp Brain Res 1990;82: 89-96.

14. Yeung JC, Rudy TA: Multiplicative interaction between narcotic agonisms expressed at spinal and supraspinal sites of antinociceptive action as revealed by concurrent intrathecal and intracerebroventricular injections of morphine. J Pharmacol Exp Ther 1980;215: 633.

15. Czlonkowski A, Stein C, Herz A: Peripheral mechanisms of opioid antinociception in inflammation: Involvement of cytokines. Eur J Pharmacol 1993;242: 229-235.

16. Parsons CG, Czlonkowski A, Stein C, Herz A: Peripheral opioid receptors mediating antinociception in inflammation. Pain 1990;41: 81-93

17. Stein C, Schäfer M, Hassan AHS: Peripheral opioid receptors. Ann Med 1995;27: 219-221.

18. Joris JL, Dubner R, Hargreaves K M: Opioid analgesia at peripheral sites: A target for opioids released during stress and inflammation? Anesth Analg 1987;66: 1277-1281.

19. Levine JD, Taiwo YO: Involvement of the mu-opiate receptor in peripheral analgesia. Neuroscience 1989;32: 571-575.
20. Taiwo YO, Levine JD: Kappa- and delta-opioids block sympathetically dependent hyperalgesia. J Neurosci 1991;11: 928-932.
21. Stein C, Comisel K, Haimerl E, et al: Analgesic effect of intraarticular morphine after arthroscopic knee surgery. New Engl J Med 1991;325: 1123-1126.
22. Taylor BK, Peterson MA, Basbaum AI: Early nociceptive events influence the temporal profile, but not the magnitude of the tonic response to subcutaneous formalin: Effects with remifentanil. J Pharmacol Exp Ther 1997;280: 876-883.
23. Dubuisson D, Dennis S G: The formalin test: A quantitative study of the analgesic effects of morphine, meperidine, and brain stem stimulation in rats and cats. Pain 1977;4: 107-126.
24. Abram SE, Yaksh TL: Morphine, but not inhalation anesthesia, blocks post-injury facilitation. Anesthesiology 1993;78:713-721.
25. Menétrey D, Gannon A, Levine J D, Basbaum A I: Expression of c-fos protein in interneurons and projection neurons of the rat spinal cord in response to noxious somatic, articular, and visceral stimulation. J Comp Neurol 1989;285: 177-195.
26. Gogas KR, Presley RW, Levine JD, Basbaum AI: The antinociceptive action of supraspinal opioids results from an increase in descending inhibitory control: Correlation of nociceptive behavior and c-fos expression. Neuroscience 1991;42: 617-628.
27. Presley RW, Menétrey D, Levine JD, Basbaum AI: Systemic morphine suppresses noxious stimulus-evoked Fos protein-like immunoreactivity in the rat spinal cord. J Neurosci 10: 323-335.
28. Jasmin L, Wang H, Tarczy-Hornoch K, Levine JD, Basbaum AI: Differential effects of morphine on noxious stimulus-evoked Fos-like immunoreactivity in subpopulations of spinoparabrachial neurons. J Neurosci 1994;14: 7252-7260.
29. Cox BM: Molecular and cellular mechanisms in opioid tolerance. Pages 137-156 in A I Basbaum and J-M Besson, Eds., Towards a New Pharmacotherapy of Pain. John Wiley & Sons, Chichester, UK, 1991.
30. Guitart X, Thompson MA, Mirante CK, et al: Regulation of cyclic AMP response element-binding protein (CREB) phosphorylation by acute and chronic morphine in the rat locus coeruleus. J Neurochem 1992;58: 1168-1171.
31. Nestler EJ: Molecular mechanisms of drug addiction. J Neurosci 1992;12: 2439-2450.
32. Nestler EJ, Alreja M, Aghajanian GK: Molecular and cellular mechanisms of opiate action: Studies in the rat locus coeruleus. Brain Res Bull 1994;35: 521-528.
33. Cook AJ, Woolf CJ, Wall PD: Prolonged C-fibre mediated facilitation of the flexion reflex in the rat is not due to changes in afferent terminal or motoneurone excitability. Neurosci Lett 1986;70: 91-96.

34. Dubner R, Basbaum AI: Spinal dorsal horn plasticity following tissue or nerve injury. Pages 225-241 in PD Wall and R Melzack, Eds., The Textbook of Pain. Churchill-Livingstone, London, 1994.

35. Woolf CJ: Evidence for a central component of post-injury pain hypersensitivity. Nature (Lond). 1983;308: 686-688.

36. Woolf CJ, Thompson S: The induction and maintenance of central sensitization is dependent on N-methyl-D-aspartic acid receptor activation; Implications for the treatment of post-injury pain hypersensitivity states. Pain 1991;44: 293-299.

37. Elliott K, Hynansky A, Inturrisi C E: Dextromethorphan attenuates and reverses analgesic tolerance to morphine. Pain 1994;59: 361-368.

38. Elliott K, Kest B, Man A, et al: N-methyl-D-aspartate (NMDA) receptors, mu and kappa opioid tolerance, and perspectives on new analgesic drug development. Neuropsychopharmacol. 1995;13: 347-356.

39. Trujillo K A, Akil H: Inhibition of opiate tolerance by non-competitive N-methyl-D-aspartate receptor antagonists. Brain Res 1994;633: 178-188.

40. Rohde DS, Detweiler DJ, Basbaum AI: Morphine tolerance enhances nociceptive processing in the rat lumbar spinal cord. Brain Res, in press.

41. Rohde DS, Detweiler DJ, Basbaum AI: Spinal cord mechanisms of opioid tolerance and dependence: fos expression increases in subpopulations of spinal cord neurons during withdrawal. Neuroscience, 1996;72: 233-242.

42. Roerig SC, Hoffman RG, Takemori AE, et al: Isobolographic analysis of analgesic interactions between intrathecally and intracerebroventricularly administered fentanyl, morphine and D-Ala$_2$-D-Leu$_5$- enkephalin in morphine-tolerant and nontolerant mice. J Pharmacol Exp Ther 1991;257: 1091-1099.

DESCENDING FACILITATION OF PAIN

G. F. Gebhart

INTRODUCTION

It was first documented in 1969 that electrical stimulation in the midbrain in rats produced an analgesia sufficient to permit laparotomies. Within a few short years, it was documented that electrical stimulation in human brain produced similar potent analgesic effects, subsequently called stimulation-produced analgesia. It was subsequently demonstrated that endogenous opioid peptides are present in the central nervous system and that the opioid receptor antagonist naloxone attenuated the analgesic effects of stimulation-produced analgesia in humans.

Stimulation-produced analgesia has since been widely studied in non-human animals and the descending pathways, spinal neurotransmitters and their receptors, and other characteristics of this phenomenon have been elucidated. It is now clear that there not only exist systems descending from the brainstem that attenuate or inhibit spinal nociceptive transmission, there also exists systems descending from the brainstem that can facilitate (or enhance) spinal nociceptive transmission.

ANATOMY AND NEUROCHEMISTRY OF PAIN MODULATION

The midbrain periaqueductal and periventricular gray matter is the nodal point of the endogenous pain modulatory system. At this anatomical site both exogenously administered opioids like morphine and endogenously released opioid peptides activate inhibitory influences that descend to the spinal cord. There is a critical synapse between the midbrain and spinal cord in the rostral part of the ventral medulla. Thus, descending influences on spinal nociceptive transmission activated in the midbrain are indirect in that there exists a relay between the midbrain and spinal cord. From the medulla, descending influences are direct. Axons of

13

T. H. Stanley et al. (eds.), Pain Management and Anesthesiology, 13–18.
© 1998 *Kluwer Academic Publishers. Printed in the Netherlands.*

neurons in the medulla descend in the spinal cord to terminate on spinal neurons where the nociceptive message from the periphery is received.

An important aspect of descending inhibitory modulation is that the system is tonically active. That is, a moderate brake is applied to spinal neurons by the descending inhibitory system even under normal circumstances. Thus, increases or decreases in spinal nociceptive transmission could be produced by alterations in the activity of this tonic descending system.

The neurotransmitter chemicals that mediate descending inhibition are principally serotonin and norepinephrine. Serotonin is contained in the terminals of neurons descending from the ventral medulla, and norepinephrine is contained in the terminals of neurons descending from the dorsolateral pons such as the locus coeruleus.

Accordingly, drugs that mimic the actions of serotonin and norepinephrine are analgesic when given directly into the spinal epidural or intrathecal space. For example, clonidine is analgesic in humans and has been used to treat cancer pain because it acts in the spinal cord like norepinephrine at the 2-adrenergic receptor. Opioids given exogenously or released endogenously are analgesic because of action at opioid receptors, but at least part of their action is effected indirectly in the spinal cord by the monoamine transmitters serotonin and norepinephrine. This means that pain control by opioids should be enhanced by drugs that mimic or facilitate the actions of serotonin or norepinephrine such as certain antidepressants. Indeed, this has been documented in clinical trials. Consequently, these drugs can be an important adjunct to pain control with the added benefit of reducing the opioid dose requirements and thus slowing the rate of tolerance development.

FACILITATION OF NOCICEPTION

In studies carried out over the past several years, it has been established that either facilitatory or inhibitory effects on spinal nociceptive reflexes or spinal nociceptive transmission can be produced from adjacent sites in the brainstem. The principal area of study has been the rostroventral medulla. Early studies involved the use of electrical stimulation, but subsequent studies established that descending facilitatory and inhibitory effects could be produced by selective activation of cell bodies in the brainstem. Accordingly, bulbospinal neurons in the rostroventral medulla are considered the final common pathway for descending inhibitory as well as descending facilitatory influences on spinal pain transmission. That is, either inhibition or facilitation can be produced from the same sites in the brainstem, depending upon input. Full understanding of how the inputs may differ has not yet been attained. It is clear, however, that axons mediating facilitatory influences descend from the brainstem in different spinal tracts and contain neurotransmitters different from those described above for inhibitory modulation. These neurotransmitters act at cholinergic, cholecystokinin, and kappa opioid receptors and can contribute to the facilitation of nociceptive transmission.

Certain neurotransmitters in the brainstem can similarly mediate either facilitatory or inhibitory effects. For example, neurotensin is contained in nerve pathways from the midbrain to the medulla where, when released, neurotensin can either facilitate or inhibit nociception at the level of the lumbar spinal cord. It has also been shown that γ-aminobutyric acid (GABA) receptors can influence descending effects from the brainstem. Interestingly, it has been established that the putative anti-opioid peptide, cholecystokinin (CCK), mediates the facilitatory effects produced in the brainstem. Accordingly, strategies that might be useful in enhancing analgesia include inhibition of CCK receptors at the level of the spinal cord.

ACTIVATION OF ENDOGENOUS PAIN MODULATION

A wide variety of influences can activate endogenous pain modulation, both inhibitory and facilitatory. Stress, fear, and pain itself can activate descending systems that inhibit pain. An injured animal's escape from a predator, even in the presence of pain, has been cited as an example of the survival role of pain-activated endogenous modulation. In less life-threatening circumstances, pain can inhibit pain by activation of the same endogenous mechanisms, a phenomenon referred to as counterirritation. Pathophysiology such as hypertension can also contribute to activation of descending inhibitory systems and attenuation of pain. Documentation shows that both experimental increases in blood pressure and preexisting hypertension lessen sensitivity to noxious stimuli.

Anxiety and apprehension can lead to enhancement of pain; however, descending facilitation of pain may play a particularly large role in unusual chronic pain states. It is possible but not yet proven that the pain facilitating system can be activated and subsequently not turned off by normal mechanisms, thus contributing to tonic facilitation, rather than tonic inhibition, of spinal neuron activity. Obviously, there are circumstances in which facilitation of nociceptive information is protective, such as during tissue repair, yet if such a system remains inappropriately activated after tissue repair is complete, normal, nonnociceptive inputs could conceivably acquire nociceptive character. Because the mechanisms of chronic pain are poorly understood, there is considerable interest and potential importance in better understanding endogenous systems that can enhance pain.

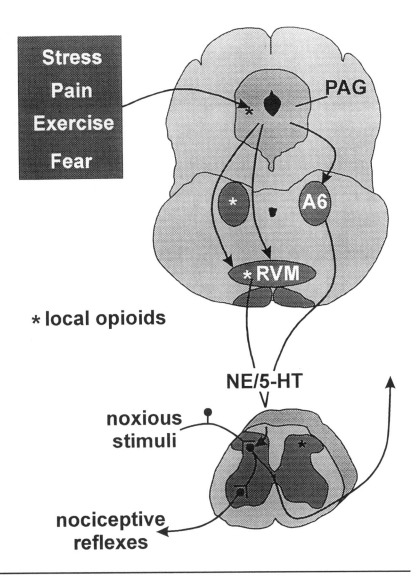

Figure 1. (Schematic diagram illustrating the principal components of descending pain inhibition. External inputs such as stress, exercise, fear and pain itself can activate the neuraxis and contribute to pain inhibition. the midbrain periaqueductal gray matter (PAG) is considered the nodal point in the descending inhibitory system; the descending pathways to the spinal cord (and brainstem nucleus caudalis), however, are indirect. Interposed between the PAG and the sites of inhibition of nociception are the locus coeruleus(A6) and rostral ventromedial medulla (RVM). Spinopetal projections from these areas are noradrenergic (NE, from the A6)and serotonergic (5-HT, from RVM). Local control by NE and/or 5-HT, acting at alpha-adrenoceptors and serotonergic receptors, can be either or both presynaptic (acting on the terminals of primary afferent nociceptors) or postsynaptic (acting on second order spinal neurons in the dorsal horn of the spinal cord). Note also that the 'system' is associated with endogenous opioid peptides. That is, opioid receptors are present and opioids such as morphine act at all levels of the system (indicated by *).

DESCENDING FACILITATION

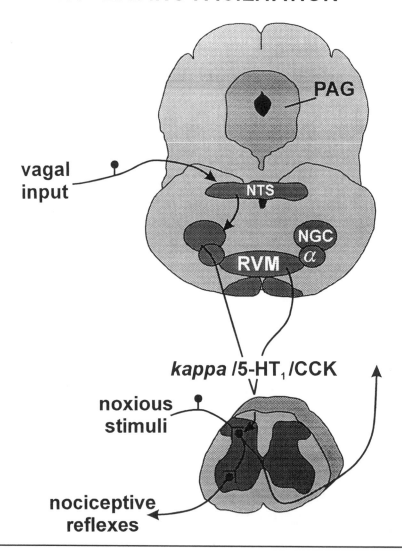

Figure 2.   Schematic diagram illustrating the principal components of descending pain facilitation. A variety of inputs, principally conveyed by vagal afferent fibers, can lead to an enhanced response to a noxious stimulus (termed hyperalgesia) or conceivably give rise to pain in the absence of a peripheral noxious stimulus. The first central synapse is the nucleus of the solitary tract (NTS), with projections to the RVM (see figure 1) and areas adjacent (nucleus gigantocellularis, NGC, and NGC pars alpha), which contribute descending influences to the spinal dorsal horn mediated by kappa opioid receptors, serotonin type 1 receptors and/or cholecystokinin (CCK) type B receptors. Whereas the descending inhibitory influences described in figure 1 descend the spinal cord in the dorsal/dorsolateral funiculus, the descending facilitatory influences are contained in ventral/ventrolateral funiculi.

THE CONTRIBUTION OF NMDA AND SECOND MESSENGERS TO THE PERSISTENT PAIN STATES PRODUCED BY TISSUE AND NERVE INJURY

A. Basbaum

There are two major categories of pain: nociceptive/inflammatory pain produced by tissue injury and neuropathic pain produced by nerve injury. The latter can occur after injury in the peripheral or central nervous system. Recent studies have established that the persistence of the pain in these two conditions results not only from changes that occur at the site of the injury but also from the development of long-term changes in the spinal cord and secondarily in the brainstem and thalamus (9). These secondary changes reflect a reorganization at the molecular level, i.e., the induction of specific genes as well as biochemical changes and even structural remodeling of neuronal circuits.

A very dramatic example of the evidence that normal afferent input can interact with altered central circuits to produce a neuropathic pain state will illustrate the problem. Gracely and colleagues described a patient with an injury to the ulnar nerve who presented with allodynia, hyperalgesia and spontaneous pain (11). Non-noxious stimuli were particularly painful in this patient. The traditional view is that the non-noxious stimulus produced pain because it was activating "pain" producing C-fibers whose threshold had dropped as a result of the injury. Their studies, however, demonstrated otherwise. Specifically, they demonstrated that local anesthetic injection of the injury site completely resolved the pain problem, *without* eliminating all afferent input. What the anesthetic did was normalize the response produced by the non-noxious stimulus. Apparently the local anesthetic had reduced the input that maintained the central abnormal state so that non-noxious stimuli (transmitted as in the normal patient by large A-ß fibers) now produced the normal touch sensation. Many such examples have been demonstrated in other situations. Most notably it has been reported that compression block of large diameter fibers can eliminate the allodynia and hyperalgesia in patients with reflex sympathetic dystrophy/causalgia (4).

T. H. Stanley et al. (eds.), Pain Management and Anesthesiology, 19–27.
© 1998 *Kluwer Academic Publishers. Printed in the Netherlands.*

On the other hand the spontaneous burning pain often persists probably because it arises from hyperactivity of unmyelinated C-fibers.

To appreciate how such long-term changes can be generated at the level of the spinal cord, it is important to understand the mechanism through which glutamate, the major excitatory neurotransmitter activates dorsal horn neurons. Glutamate acts on a variety of receptor subtypes, but two are most important. The AMPA receptor (named after a synthetic compound that mimics action at this receptor) mediates a depolarization of the postsynaptic terminal via influx of sodium and efflux of potassium. A second glutamate target, the NMDA receptor (again named for a synthetic compound) in the normal or resting condition, is blocked by a magnesium ion that sits in the channel. When glutamate is released by a noxious stimulus it can bind the NMDA receptor, but nothing happens. However, when the postsynaptic terminal is depolarized by influx of sodium ions through the AMPA receptor the magnesium ion is kicked out of the NMDA receptor channel and this allows current to flow through the NMDA receptor (22-24).

The most important feature of the NMDA receptor is that, unlike the AMPA receptor which gates Na and K ions, the NMDA receptor allows Ca ions to enter the cell. Calcium entry triggers long-term changes in the postsynaptic neuron including activation of enzymes, genes and establishment of a prolonged hyperexcitable state in the postsynaptic neuron. The heightened sensitivity/facilitation of the postsynaptic neuron can enhance subsequent inputs, thus increasing nociceptive transmission and possibly exacerbating pain (32). This mechanism provides the rationale for the use of NMDA receptor antagonists to treat pain conditions in patients (8). Unfortunately the majority of NMDA receptor antagonists available (with the exception of the relatively weak antitussive compound, dextromethorphan (25)) has side effects that probably make them unacceptable for general use (21).

This model of NMDA receptor contribution to long-term changes argues for a predominate postsynaptic mechanism. To specifically address the location of the NMDA receptor in the spinal cord dorsal horn our laboratory has performed studies using antisera directed against the NMDA receptor (17). Although we confirmed that there is a dense distribution of the receptor in postsynaptic neurons, to our surprise we found a very high concentration located on axon terminals, specifically those in the superficial dorsal horn, in the region that receives a large input from unmyelinated primary afferent fibers. Double-label studies with antisera directed against primary afferent neurotransmitter compounds, such as glutamate or substance P, confirmed that the NMDA receptor is located on the presynaptic terminal, where it can regulate release of transmitter from the primary afferent. In a related study we, in fact, demonstrated that activity at this NMDA receptor can augment the release of substance P from the primary afferent, thus enhancing the postsynaptic effects produced by primary afferent inputs (18). This circuitry establishes a positive feedback which is obviously pathophysiological and may contribute to the abnormal long-term persistent pain states associated with allodynia and hyperalgesia. Thus there are two major targets at which the NMDA receptor can be acted upon to counteract the injury-induced long-term hyperexcitability changes, the postsynaptic neuron and the presynaptic terminal. Although the latter is somewhat inaccessible (one would have to use intrathecal injections to target it) the former conceivably can be targeted with approaches that bring molecular probes into the dorsal root ganglion to affect transcription and translation of the NMDA receptor.

Although the evidence for the contribution of the NMDA receptor is clear, an important question relates to the downstream consequences of the increased calcium that enters through NMDA channel. Among the many possible downstream targets are a host of second messenger systems. Our own laboratory has taken a molecular genetic approach to understanding which second messenger systems are critical and how they contribute to the persistent pain associated with inflammation/tissue injury and with nerve injury. We specifically addressed two second messenger systems (19, 20). The first is the cyclic AMP-dependent protein kinase A (PKA) second messenger system which phosphorylates proteins via the enzyme, PKA. The second is a calcium-dependent system through which enzymes are phosphorylated via the enzyme protein kinase C (PKC). In our studies we evaluated pain behavior in mice in which there has was a specific gene deletion of either protein kinase A (the RIβ regulatory subunit) or the gamma isoform of protein kinase C. We studied PKCγ for two reasons. First although there are at least ten different isoforms of PKC, the gamma isoform is not expressed developmentally. Thus, there is little likelihood that any phenotype attributed to this deletion would be secondary to a compensatory response that occurred during development. Second the gamma isoform is of particular interest because it is found exclusively in a small population of neurons in the inner part of the substantia gelatinosa (lamina II) of the superficial dorsal horn, which limits the possible spinal cord neuronal mechanisms through which this enzyme could act.

Both the PKA-RIβ and the PKCγ mutant mice were created by homologous recombination that substitutes the endogenous gene that transcribes these molecules with an inactive gene. Both mutant strains of mice are viable and otherwise behaviorally normal (13, 14). In all tests of acute pain, including tail flick, hot plate, and mechanical nociceptive tests we found that the mutant mice were completely normal. This is consistent with the view that acute pain is mediated by activity of primary afferents leading to release of glutamate which in turn acts on the AMPA receptor, without a requirement of second messenger-mediated long-term changes.

To test the integrity of the mutant mice in models of tissue injury that are associated with inflammation (i.e., a nociceptive pain model) we used the formalin test which is produced by dilute injection of formalin into the hindpaw of the mouse. This test was developed in the rat (10) and is particularly useful not only because it produces a very reliable pain behavior but also because the behavior is quantifiable. Pain behavior appears in two phases, a first phase thought to reflect direct activation of the primary afferents by the formalin and a second phase that we believe results from a delayed inflammation secondary to the injection (28). In the mice with the deletion of PKA we found absolutely no change in phase one pain behavior. This is consistent with the view that the first phase is an acute pain phase, which as noted above is normal in these animals. On the other hand we recorded a significant decrease in the magnitude of phase two pain behavior indicating that there is a significant decrease in persistent, nociceptive pain.

Since this phase is mediated by the development of inflammation we next used tests that examined the ability of the animal to develop an inflammatory response. In these studies we monitored neurogenic inflammation, the process whereby activity generated in peripheral C-fibers leads to the release of neuropeptides that drive the peripheral inflammatory process. We made an injection of capsaicin into the hindpaw and then monitored one of the major components of neurogenic inflammation, namely plasma extravasation. In our studies we followed the extravasation (i.e., leakage) of a substance (Evan's Blue dye) that normally binds to albumin and does not escape blood vessels. When there is neurogenic inflammation, the vasculature is "open" and the proteinated Evan's Blue dye can escape and be measured. We found that there was a significant decrease in plasma extravasationin the animals with a gene deletion of PKA-RIβ. Since our anatomical studies established that this regulatory subunit is expressed in small diameter primary afferents and since plasma extravasation involves activation of the peripheral terminals of primary afferent fibers, this result indicates that this particular second messenger exerts its effect in the periphery. Importantly, the enzyme was not expressed in sympathetic efferents, which also contribute to plasma extravasation (6).

We also showed that these animals have a defect in the sensitization (allodynia) produced by hindpaw injection of PGE$_2$. Most importantly the reduced sensitization was manifest not only when the drug was injected in the periphery but also when we made intrathecal injections. This suggests that PKA not only exerts an effect in the periphery but also in the central nervous system. We conclude that PKA (or at least the RIβ regulatory subunit that was deleted) contributes both to development of inflammation and to the central sensitization of dorsal horn neurons in the spinal cord that is produced by persistent and/or intense noxious inputs.

What about the response of the animals in tests of nerve injury induced pain? There are a variety of neuropathic pain models that have been developed in the rat, including the sciatic nerve constriction model of Bennett and Xie (3), the spinal nerve section model of Chung and colleagues (15) and the partial sciatic nerve ligation model of Seltzer and colleagues (27). We adapted the latter in the mouse by ligating from one-third to one-half of the sciatic nerve. This produces a very profound thermal and mechanical allodynia that appears within 24 hours after the nerve injury. Otherwise the animals appear completely normal. In the PKA knockout we found that there was normal development of the neuropathic pain state. That is an allodynic state was established and it persisted in the mutant mice, as it did in the normals, for a prolonged period. We found that the thermal allodynia persisted for at least seven weeks. Interestingly, the mechanical allodynia persisted for the duration of the experiment (at least 12 weeks). Taken together these results indicate that the PKA RIβ subunit is necessary for the full expression of tissue injury-evoked persistent pain and inflammation, but that it is not required for the expression of this nerve injury-evoked persistent neuropathic pain condition.

When we examined the mice with the specific deletion of the gamma isoform of PKC, we not only found a defect in the inflammatory models, but we also found a very profound reduction in the neuropathic pain model. Specifically animals with a deletion of PKCγ developed at most a very mild thermal and mechanical allodynia after nerve injury. This indicates that this enzyme is absolutely necessary for the development and maintenance of nerve injury-evoked pain behavior produced by partial nerve injury of the sciatic nerve. In contrast to PKA, PKCγ is not expressed in dorsal root ganglion cells. This indicates that the circuitry through which PKCγ contributes to the development of nerve injury-evoked pain must involve connections in the spinal cord dorsal horn.

Not only does peripheral nerve injury produce a significant neuropathic pain behavior, but it is also produces significant changes in the neurochemistry of the dorsal root ganglion and of neurons in the dorsal horn (12). For example, peripheral nerve injury leads to a decrease in the messenger RNA for the neuropeptide substance P in dorsal root ganglia (DRG) and a decrease in the amount of peptide. Concomitantly there is a dramatic increase in message and peptide of neuropeptide Y (NPY) (29). In fact, in normal animals NPY cannot be detected in DRG cells. Nerve injury also leads to an increase in the expression of the neuropeptides, galanin and VIP in dorsal root ganglia and in dorsal horn (30). Neurotransmitter receptors are also modified after nerve injury. We and others have shown that there is an increase in the expression of the receptor targeted by substance P, namely the neurokinin-1 receptor (1, 26). The latter is found only in neurons of the dorsal horn; it is not present in the primary afferent.

As in the rat, we found that there were significant nerve injury-evoked peptide transmitter and receptor changes in the wild type mice. Although the same was true in the PKA mutant mice we found only minimal changes in the PKCγ mutant mice, i.e., in the animals where we found almost no neuropathic pain behavior after nerve injury. Importantly, although other isoforms of PKC are found in dorsal root ganglia, PKCγ is neither found in the DRG nor in the sympathetic post-ganglionic neurons. Thus the behavioral and anatomical phenotype to which PKCγ contributes must result from influences exerted by PKCγ in the spinal cord. As noted above it is of particular interest that unlike other PKC isoforms, the gamma isoform is restricted to a small population of interneurons of the inner part of the substantia gelatinosa. This region is unique in that it is associated with a unique subset of small diameter primary afferents that expresses the P2X3 subtype of ATP receptor (5) as well as a fluoride resistant acid phosphatase (FRAP (7)) and because neurons of the inner part of the substantia gelatinosa respond primarily to non-noxious stimuli (2,16,31). These results suggest that regulation of non-noxious inputs to the superficial dorsal horn is important in the generation of the neuropathic pain state. PKCγ in the interneuron of the inner part of lamina II must phosphorylate as yet unknown proteins that contribute to the behavioral and anatomical phenotype produced by nerve injury. We are now directing attention at the proteins that are clearly critical in the establishment of these long-term changes as they provide therapeutic targets for the treatment of nerve injury-induced pain states.

In summary, our studies demonstrate that discrete biochemical changes occur in the setting of injury and that these occur in subpopulations of neurons. By characterizing the nature of these changes it is hoped that new therapeutic targets can be identified and that they can be accessed by drugs with fewer side effects. This is possible if the drugs can be administered at the level of the spinal cord. A better understanding of other contributors to the long-term consequences of tissue and nerve injury will no doubt identify additional approaches to treating the persistent pain associated with these conditions.

REFERENCES

1. Abbadie C, Brown JL, Manty PW, Basbaum AI: Spinal cord substance P receptor immunoreactivity increases in both inflammatory and nerve injury models of persistent pain. Neuroscience 1996;70:201-209.
2. Bennett GJ, Abdelmoumene M, Hayashi H, Dubner R: Physiology and morphology of substantia gelatinosa neurons intracellularly stained with horseradish peroxidase. J Comp Neurol 1980;194:809-827.
3. Bennett GJ, Xie Y-K: A peripheral mononeuropathy in rat that produces disorders of pain sensation like those seen in man. Pain 1988;33:87-107.
4. Campbell JN, Raja SN, Meyer RA, Mackinnon SE: Myelinated afferents signal the hyperalgesia associated with nerve injury. Pain 1988;32 :89-94.
5. Chen CC, Akopian AN, Sivilotti L, Coquhoun D, Burnstock G, Wood JN: A P2X purinoceptor expressed by a subset of sensory neurons. Nature (Lond.) 1995;377:428-431.
6. Coderre TJ, Basbaum AI, Levine JD: Neural control of vascular permeability: Interactions between primary afferents, mast cells, and sympathetic efferents. J Neurophysiol 1989;62:48-58.
7. Devor M, Claman D: Mapping and plasticity of acid phosphatase afferents in the rat dorsal horn. Brain Res 1980;190:17-28.
8. Dickenson AH: A cure for wind up; NMDA receptor antagonists as potential analgesics. TIPS 1990;11:307-309.
9. Dubner R, Basbaum AI: Spinal dorsal horn plasticity following tissue or nerve injury. Pages 225-241 in P. D. Wall and R. Melzack, Eds., The Textbook of Pain. Churchill-Livingstone, London, 1994

10. Dubuisson D, Dennis SG: The formalin test: A quantitative study of the analgesic effects of morphine, meperidine, and brain stem stimulation in rats and cats. Pain 1977;4:107-126.

11. Gracely RH, Lynch SA, Bennett GJ: Painful neuropathy: Altered central processing maintained dynamically by peripheral input. Pain 1992;51:175-194.

12. Hökfelt T, Zhang X, Wiesenfeld HZ: Messenger plasticity in primary sensory neurons following axotomy and its functional implications. Trends Neurosci 1994;17:22-30.

13. Huang Y-Y, Kandel ER, Varshavsky L, et al: A genetic test of the effects of mutations in PKA on mossy fiber LTP and its relation to spatial and contextual learning. Cell 1995;83:1211-1222.

14. Kano M, Hashimoto K, Chen C, et al: Impaired synapse elimination during cerebellar development in PKCγ mutant mice. Cell 1995; 83:1223-1231.

15. Kim SH, Chung JM: An experimental model for peripheral neuropathy produced by segmental spinal nerve ligation in the rat. Pain 1992;50:355-363.

16. Light AR, Trevino DL, Perl ER: Morphological features of functionally identified neurons in the marginal zone and substantia gelatinosa of the spinal dorsal horn. J Comp Neurol 1979;186:325-330.

17. Liu H, Wang H, Sheng M, et al: Evidence for presynaptic N-methyl-D-aspartate autoreceptors in the spinal cord dorsal horn. Proc Natl Acad Sci (USA) 1994;91:8383-8387.

18. Liu HT, Mantyh PW, Basbaum AI: NMDA-receptor regulation of substance P release from primary afferent nociceptors. Nature (Lond.) 1997;386:721-724.

19. Malmberg AB, Brandon EP, Idzerda RL, et al: Diminished inflammation and nociceptive pain with preservation of neuropathic pain in mice with a targeted mutation of the RIß subunit of PKA. J Neuroscience, in press.

20. Malmberg AB, Chen C, Tonegawa S, Basbaum AI: Preserved acute pain and reduced neuropathic pain in mice lacking PKCγ. Science, in press.

21. Max MB, Byas-Smith MG, Gracely RH, Bennett GJ: Intravenous infusion of the NMDA antagonist, ketamine, in chronic posttraumatic pain with allodynia: A double-blind comparison to alfentanil and placebo. Clin Neuropharmacol 1885;18:360-368.

22. Mayer ML, Westbrook GL: Permeation and block of N-methyl-D-aspartic acid receptor channels by divalent cations in mouse cultured central neurones. J Physiol 1987;394:501-527.

23. Mayer ML, Westbrook GL: The physiology of excitatory amino acids in the vertebrate central nervous system. Prog Neurobiol 1987;28:197-276.

24. Mayer ML, Westbrook GL, Guthrie PB: Voltage-dependent block by Mg^{2+} of NMDA receptors in spinal cord neurons. Nature (Lond.) 1984;309:261-263.

25. Price DD, Mao J, Frenk H, Mayer DJ: The N-methyl-D-aspartate receptor antagonist dextromethorphan selectively reduces temporal summation of second pain in man. Pain 1994;59:165-174.

26. Schäfer MKH, Nohr D, Krause JE, Weihe E: Inflammation-induced upregulation of NK1 receptor mRNA in dorsal horn neurons. Neuro Report 1993;4:1007-1010.

27. Seltzer Z, Dubner R, Shir Y: A novel behavioral model of neuropathic pain disorders produced in rats by partial sciatic nerve injury. Pain 1990;43:205-218.

28. Taylor BK, Peterson MA, Basbaum AI: Persistent cardiovascular and behavioral nociceptive responses to subcutaneous formalin require peripheral nerve input. J Neurosci 1995;15:7575-7584.

29. Wakisaka S, Kajander KC, Bennett GJ: Increased neuropeptide Y (NPY)-like immunoreactivity in rat sensory neurons following peripheral axotomy. Neurosci Lett 1991;124:200-203.

30. Wiesenfeld HZ, Xu XJ, Langel U, et al: Galanin-mediated control of pain: Enhanced role after nerve injury. Proc Natl Acad Sci (USA) 1992;89:3334-3337.

31. Woolf CJ, Fitzgerald M: The properties of neurones recorded in the superficial dorsal horn of the rat spinal cord. J Comp Neurol 1993;221:313-328.

32. Woolf CJ, Thompson S: The induction and maintenance of central sensitization is dependent on N-methyl-D-aspartic acid receptor activation; Implications for the treatment of post-injury pain hypersensitivity states. Pain 1991;44:293-299.

NEW CLINICAL PHARMACOLOGY CONCEPTS
IN PAIN MANAGEMENT

T. D. Egan

INTRODUCTION

The scientific foundation of clinical pharmacology has advanced remarkably in the last few decades, particularly in anesthesiology and pain management. While it is still not possible to account adequately for all sources of pharmacologic variability, modern pharmacokinetic-pharmacodynamic modeling techniques have enabled physicians to predict drug response with a quantitative exactness that was unimaginable in the early days of modern medicine.

Largely because of advances in drug assay and computer technologies, it is now possible to construct combined kinetic-dynamic models that describe drug behavior in quantitative terms. These models can be used to predict a host of important components of drug response, including latency to peak effect, duration of effect and relative potency. In addition, the influence of common patient covariates on the kinetic or dynamic profile of a drug is often incorporated into these models. Thus, changes in therapy that are necessary because of patient characteristics or disease states such as obesity, the extremes of age, renal failure or hepatic dysfunction can often be anticipated accurately.

These new clinical pharmacology concepts and modeling techniques have important implications for pain management physicians. The aim of this chapter is to review briefly these new concepts and apply them to the use of opioids and other analgesics in pain management, both acute and chronic.

THE VARIABILITY OF HUMAN DRUG RESPONSE

To the chagrin of clinicians, humans exhibit substantial intersubject variability in drug response. In general terms, this variability is at least three- to five-fold and is a function of both pharmacokinetic and pharmacodynamic parameters. In other words, a single dosage regimen cannot be

29

T. H. Stanley et al. (eds.), Pain Management and Anesthesiology, 29–54.
© 1998 *Kluwer Academic Publishers. Printed in the Netherlands.*

expected to be appropriate for all patients, yielding subtherapeutic drug effect in some and toxicity in others. Yet the success of pharmacologic pain management is dependent upon administration of the right agent in the proper dose at the appropriate time.

As is typical with other drug classes, opioids are well known to exhibit substantial pharmacokinetic and pharmacodynamic variability when used for the treatment of postoperative pain (1,2). This variability problem is at least partially responsible for what was until recently the generally dismal effectiveness of postoperative pain management in the eyes of patients (3). Pharmacologic variability has also no doubt contributed to the enthusiasm in the United States for the formation of acute pain management programs (4). The absence of a "one size fits all" condition in the clinical pharmacology of pain management mandates that clinicians develop a practical understanding of pharmacologic variability and a method of dealing with it in the clinical setting.

The sources of this variability for all drugs including opioids are extremely diverse and can be a function of factors both external or internal to the patient (5). Variability can arise from external factors such as drug formulation and administration, or internal factors such as patient pharmacokinetics and pharmacodynamics. Figure 1 illustrates the way in which all these component sources of variability culminate in a widely varying observation of net drug effect for intravenous anesthetics, including opioids.

The large variability in human drug response has spawned the development of pharmacologic modeling techniques. Combined pharmacokinetic-dynamic models can help identify the sources of pharmacologic variability and thereby lead to appropriate changes in therapy that decrease the variability of drug response. The utility of kinetic-dynamic models in precisely describing drug behavior is reflected by the fact that regulatory agencies in the United States now encourage pharmacologic modeling early in the drug development process (6).

PHARMACOLOGIC MODELING

Prior to the days of pharmacokinetic-dynamic modeling, drug behavior was described by simple phenomenologic experiments in which a dose was administered to an experimental subject and the effects were observed. From gross observations made in straightforward experiments like these, a dose-response relationship was established. While such experiments could provide general guidelines for safe and efficacious drug administration, they could not specifically identify the mechanisms responsible for the variability of drug response. Because drug behavior

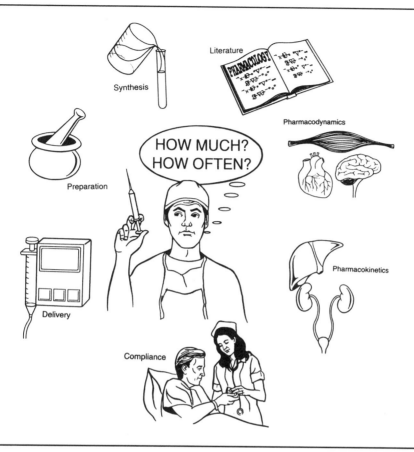

Figure 1. Sources of variability in drug response for all drugs, including opioids. Dosage regimes begin with leterature recommendations, although the study of studies on which the recommendations are based may not apply to the clinical setting or clinical population targeted. Patient external factors such as drug synthesis, preparation and delivery may introduce substantial variability. Patient internal variability in pharmacokinetics and pharmacodynamics may also impact the ultimate level of drug effect. Finally, compliance with the prescribed regimen by patients and nursing staff also introduces variability. (From MA Ashburn and LJ Rice (ed): The Management of Pain, Churchill Livingston, New York, New York, 1998, with permission)

was not separated into pharmacokinetic and pharmacodynamic components, it was not possible to determine whether altered drug response was a function of altered drug levels (pharmacokinetics) or a change in sensitivity to a given drug level (pharmacodynamics). Furthermore, because these more primitive experiments did not produce estimates of pharmacokinetic-dynamic parameters, it was not possible to predict drug response under varying patient conditions and administration regimens through computer simulation.

With the advent of modern drug assay technology and the widespread availability of computers over the last several decades, it has become possible to move beyond simple phenomenologic experiments. It is now commonplace for clinical pharmacologists to analyze their data by constructing combined pharmacokinetic-dynamic models. This high resolution modeling process can separate drug response into pharmacokinetic and pharmacodynamic components. The mechanisms responsible for altered drug response can thus be identified by determining whether an observed alteration is linked to the pharmacokinetic or pharmacodynamic parameters. In addition, because the modeling process results in mathematically defined pharmacokinetic-dynamic parameters, it is possible to predict drug response in a variety of settings through the use of computer simulation.

DISTINGUISHING BETWEEN DRUG LEVELS AND DRUG EFFECT

Separating drug response into pharmacokinetic and pharmacodynamic components is a key feature of the modeling process. Pharmacokinetics, defined broadly as "what the body does to the drug," combined with pharmacodynamics, defined generically as "what the drug does to the body," make up the scientific foundation of drug administration in pain management. Pharmacokinetic parameters govern the relationship between drug dose and drug concentration in the body. Similarly, pharmacodynamic parameters describe the relationship between drug concentration in the body and drug effect. Expectations regarding drug effect, including latency to peak, magnitude and duration are made possible by careful analysis of these pharmacokinetic-dynamic parameters.

Parameters from combined pharmacokinetic-dynamic models interact in a surprisingly complex way. This complex interaction, along with the often puzzling mathematical manipulations involved in estimating them has made pharmacologic modeling a distinctly unpopular discipline among anesthesiologists and pain management physicians. This unpopularity is ironic in view of pharmacologic modeling's immense impact on rational drug use in anesthesiology and pain management. Perhaps no other specialty in medicine is more dependent upon accurate prediction of a drug's behavior than is anesthesiology.

Most settings in clinical medicine do not require immediate onset and rapid offset of pharmacologic effect. When an internist prescribes an oral medication for treatment of diabetes, for example, the fact that several days may be required for the development of a steady state level of drug effect is of little consequence. The anesthesiologist, on the contrary, must rely on drugs with rapid onset and predictable offset of effect in order to ensure maintenance of an anesthetic state intraoperatively with return of consciousness and other vital functions at the appropriate time. Likewise, the pain management specialist must be capable of reliably providing adequate analgesia without producing potentially life threatening side effects such a severe respiratory depression. Thus, accurate prediction of both the temporal and qualitative profile of drug effect, while admittedly not as critical in chronic pain management as in operative anesthesia and acute pain management, is an important part of the clinician's knowledge base.

Pharmacologic modeling concepts are also important in understanding the literature of pain management. The number of clinical pharmacology articles employing modern methods of pharmacologic modeling has mushroomed in the pain management literature in the last decade. Sophisticated pharmacokinetic analysis techniques have become an essential part of clinical pharmacology research in pain management. This surge of interest in combined kinetic-dynamic modeling is in part due to the recognition that, although investigators are primarily interested in a drug's pharmacodynamics, it is necessary to pay attention to pharmacokinetic issues in order to study reliably a drug's pharmacodynamic properties. It is impossible to make meaningful pharmacodynamic observations without controlling the pharmacokinetic aspects of an experiment. Pharmacokinetic-dynamic modeling techniques are important in describing the clinical pharmacology of new analgesic agents, in analyzing the effect of patient coexisting disease or demographic factors on drug disposition and action, and in characterizing drug interactions. Without a working knowledge of basic pharmacologic modeling concepts, many clinical pharmacology articles from the anesthesia and pain management literature that employ advanced analysis techniques are difficult to understand and apply to clinical practice.

PHARMACOKINETIC CONSIDERATIONS

THE IMPORTANCE OF SIMULATIONS IN UNDERSTANDING PHARMACOKINETICS

Table 1 is a listing of important pharmacokinetic parameters for some of the currently available potent opioids (fentanyl congeners). Because these parameters interact in a complex way, it is difficult to draw conclusions based on simple inspection of the parameters.

Recognizing that little insight into a drug's pharmacokinetic profile can be gleaned from simple inspection of its multicompartment pharmacokinetic parameters, computer simulation of the expected rise and fall of drug concentrations utilizing a drug's pharmacokinetic parameters has

34

Table 1. Representative pharmacokinetic parameters for the potent opioids.

	Fentanyl	Alfentanil	Sufentanil
Half-lives (min)			
α	1.0	0.67	1.4
β	19	13	23
γ	475	111	562
Volumes (L)			
Central	1.3	2.2	18[a]
Peripheral			
Rapid	50	6.7	47[a]
Slow	295	15	476[a]
Steady State	358	23	541[a]
Clearances (L/min)			
Central	0.42	0.20	1.2[a]
Intercompartmental			
Rapid	4.8	1.4	4.8[a]
Slow	2.3	0.25	1.3[a]

[a]Normalized to a 70-kg patient.
[Adapted from Shafer (9), with permission.]

assumed an important role in modern pharmacokinetic research and analysis. Making use of population pharmacokinetic parameters estimated in research studies, computers can be programmed to simulate the concentration versus time profile that results from any type of drug input (e.g., various routes, doses, etc.). Although such simulations are subject to certain limitations, they are intuitively comprehensible, graphic representations of the time course of drug concentration (7). Combined with knowledge about the concentration effect relationship (i.e., potency of a drug), this specific information regarding the expected course of drug concentration can aid the clinician in predicting magnitude of and recovery from drug effect (8). Without the aid of a computer it would be very difficult to draw such specific conclusions regarding the time course of drug effect.

HALF-LIVES ARE ONLY HALF THE STORY

After drug entrance into the central circulation either by intravenous administration or absorption from a nonintravenous site, elimination and distribution processes begin to lower the drug concentration in the blood. After intravenous injection most drugs exhibit two discrete phases on the concentration versus time profile. The initial rapid drop in concentration is due largely to drug redistribution and is known as the distribution phase. The second phase, often referred to as the elimination phase, is a slower process and is primarily a function of drug elimination.

These processes follow "first-order" kinetics in that a constant fraction of drug is involved per unit of time.

Half-life, perhaps the most familiar and widely used concept in pharmacokinetics, is the parameter employed to describe the rate at which drug concentrations decline. Defined conceptually as the time required for drug concentration to decrease by 50%, half-life is often relied upon by clinicians as the parameter that best indicates the expected duration of drug effect. Because with each half-life the drug concentration decreases by 50%, after five half-lives have elapsed only about 3% of the original concentration of drug remains.

A common mathematical representation of elimination half-life is:

$$T_{1/2} = \frac{0.693 \bullet Vd}{Cl}.$$

Where Vd is volume of distribution and Cl is clearance.

Half-life is expressed in terms of volume of distribution and clearance, the two fundamental pharmacokinetic parameters. Inspection of the equation reveals that half-life varies directly with volume of distribution and inversely with clearance. The greater the clearance, the shorter the half-life. Similarly, a larger volume of distribution lengthens the half-life. The relationship between half-life and the two fundamental parameters volume of distribution and clearance is one of the most basic ideas of pharmacokinetics.

Half-life is important clinically in predicting the rapidity with which drug concentrations will decrease with time. However, unlike clearance and volume of distribution, half-life is not a fundamental pharmacokinetic parameter. It is, instead, a derived or calculated parameter. Because the value of half-life is dependent upon the primary pharmacokinetic parameters volume of distribution and clearance, half-life is not independently influenced by changes in patient physiology. Alterations in volume of distribution, clearance or both these parameters that come about as a result of changes in patient physiology affect the value of half-life secondarily.

When a change in patient physiology such as coexisting disease mandates a change in a dosing regimen, it is important to know whether the altered patient physiology has impacted clearance or distribution volume. Without this knowledge it is impossible to know whether to modify initial loading dose, maintenance infusion rate or intermittent bolus size and interval. Simply knowing that the half-life has changed does not provide the necessary information for proper dosing strategy because various combinations of altered clearance and volume of distribution can result in an identical half-life. Thus, while half-life is no doubt the most commonly used pharmacokinetic parameter, it is not a fundamental parameter and is therefore not as clinically useful as volume of distribution and clearance.

The clinical relevance of half-life is even more obscure when dealing with multicompartmental models because there are as many half-lives as there are compartments. While the terminal half-life from multicompartmental models has traditionally been the pharmacokinetic parameter relied upon for predictions regarding the duration of drug effect, it can be grossly misleading. Distribution volumes and clearances can be similarly confusing to apply clinically. This confusion relates primarily to the complex way in which these multiple pharmacokinetic parameters interact.

A drug whose pharmacokinetics are described by a three compartment model, for example, will have three half-lives, three clearances and four distribution volumes (the steady state distribution volume is the sum of the 3 compartment volumes). Which of these multiple parameters is important? How do they interact? To the dismay of clinicians and pharmacokineticists alike, the interaction of these parameters is not easily predicted. In fact, in most cases, it is virtually impossible to predict without the aid of computers.

No single parameter from a multicompartmental model can be relied upon to make predictions about the overall pharmacokinetic profile. The terminal elimination half-life is often used clinically as if it constituted the only pharmacokinetic parameter of importance in predicting the duration of drug effect. In fact, for drugs described by multicompartmental models, there are numerous half-lives that must be considered, along with a host of other parameters. Each half-life, or other parameter, contributes variably to the prediction of drug concentration at a given time after drug administration. For some drugs, the terminal elimination half-life has very minimal impact on the overall decline in drug concentration within the range of clinical significance because most of the concentration decrease is accounted for by other components of the model. The popularity of the terminal elimination half-life as an indicator of drug duration of effect, given its lack of usefulness, is a clinical tradition that requires reexamination. While half-lives are important, they are only a part of the overall pharmacokinetic model and can mislead if not viewed in relation to all of the pharmacokinetic parameters comprising the model.

The primary shortcoming of half-lives is that they fail to account for the important influence of distribution processes on drug disposition. Distribution processes refer to the net transfer of drug between the central compartment and the peripheral compartments. Depending on the size of the peripheral compartment and the rate at which drug transfer occurs, distribution into or out of the peripheral compartments can have a major impact on the concentration versus time profile.

Figure 2, a hydraulic representation of a typical pharmacokinetic compartmental model, illustrates how distribution processes influence the concentration versus time profile. If a peripheral compartment volume is large and the rate of transfer into it from the central compartment is slow, the concentrations in the two compartments come to equilibrium very slowly. If equilibrium has not been reached when an infusion of drug is terminated, both elimination from the central compartment and distribution into the slowly equilibrating peripheral compartment can combine to lower central drug concentration. Conversely, a large volume, rapidly equilibrating peripheral compartment serves as a reservoir of drug that floods back into the central compartment after termination of an infusion,

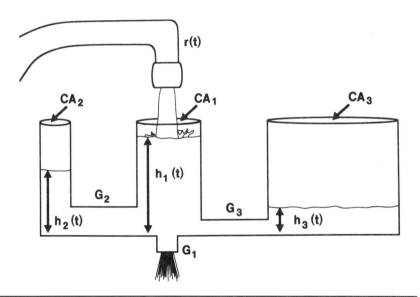

Figure 2. A hydraulic representation of a three-compartment model in which drug administration and elimination occur in the central compartment. The model is composed of three cylindrical areas (CA_i) representing the volume of the pharmacokinetic compartments (or buckets using this hydraulic analogy). The height (h_i) of the water level in each compartment represents drug concentration. The pipes connecting the compartments transfer drug from one compartment to another and to the outside at a rate characterized by the conductance (G_i), denoted by the diameter of the pipe. The water entering the system at a specified rate ($r(t)$) represents drug administration (see text for complete explanation). [From Hughes (10), with permission.]

impeding the decrease in drug concentration produced by elimination from the central compartment. Elimination half-lives are of limited value in predicting the rate of concentration decrease after stopping a continuous infusion because they fail to account adequately for these distribution processes.

CONTEXT SENSITIVE HALF-TIMES: A NEW PHARMACOKINETIC CONCEPT

A recently introduced computer simulation illustrates how conclusions about drug concentration based on terminal half-lives can be misleading. This new simulation technique predicts the time necessary to achieve a 50% decrease in drug concentration after termination of a variable length continuous infusion to a steady state drug level. Using concepts developed by Shafer and Varvel (9), these simulations are an attempt to provide "context sensitive half times" ($CST_{1/2}$) as proposed by Hughes, et al (10). In this case the "context" is the duration of a continuous infusion. The $CST_{1/2}$ has also been referred to as the 50% decrement time (11). Such simulations are intended to provide more clinically relevant meaning to pharmacokinetic parameters.

Figure 3 is a graphical representation of the context sensitive half-times of the fentanyl family of opioids using parameters from the literature (9). Perhaps contrary to contemporary established notions, alfentanil

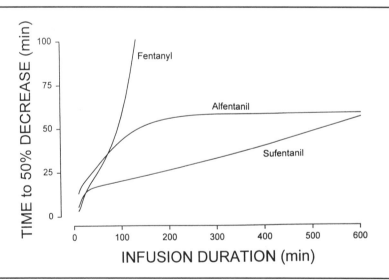

Figure 3. A simulation of the time required for a 50% decrease in plasma concentration of the fentanyl congeners after termination of a continuous infusion (i.e., the context sensitive half-times or 50% decrement times). [From Shafer (9), with permission.]

does not exhibit the most rapid 50% decrease in plasma concentration after termination of a continuous infusion until after approximately 8 hours of infusion. Thus, sufentanil appears to have more favorable pharmacokinetics for infusions lasting less than 8 hours when the goal is to achieve a rapid 50% decrease in concentration. In terms of pharmacokinetic theory, this surprising difference between alfentanil and sufentanil can be explained by the fact that sufentanil's pharmacokinetic model has a large, slowly equilibrating peripheral compartment that continues to fill after termination of an infusion, thus contributing to the faster decrease in sufentanil central compartment concentration. In other words, central compartment sufentanil concentrations fall rapidly after an infusion of less than 8 hours is stopped because of continued elimination and distribution.

Unlike sufentanil and alfentanil, fentanyl exhibits an early time dependent increase in the context sensitive half-time. While fentanyl would be a poor choice for clinical situations in which a rapid decrease in concentration after infusion termination is desirable, in clinical scenarios in which prolonged opioid effect is the goal, fentanyl might well be the drug of choice. For example, fentanyl is well suited for cases after which the patient's trachea will remain intubated for a period of time after the procedure in order to promote a gradual emergence from anesthesia and a long lasting level of significant analgesia.

Note that for cases of very brief duration, the context sensitive half-time for sufentanil, alfentanil and fentanyl are nearly identical. Thus, for brief cases, when the opioid is administered by infusion, there would not be any substantial differences among the three drugs in the time to a 50% drop in concentration after stopping a continuous infusion. Also note that the shapes of these curves vary depending on the percentage decrease in concentration required (9).

PARENT COMPOUNDS VERSUS METABOLITES

While it is possible through computer simulation to predict accurately the time course of drug concentration in the plasma, it is important to recognize that many drugs have metabolites of the parent compound that have either therapeutic or toxic pharmacodynamic activity. Thus, drawing conclusions about drug effect based on predicted drug levels and knowledge of therapeutic windows can be misleading if there are metabolites with significant pharmacologic activity. This issue is further complicated by the fact that the active metabolites of course have pharmacokinetic profiles that are different from the parent compound.

Morphine is a prototypical example of an opioid with active metabolites. Morphine is principally metabolized by conjugation in the liver for later excretion of these water soluble glucuronides by the kidney (12). Although the actions of morphine 3-glucuronide poorly understood, morphine-6-glucuronide is a μ agonist with a potency exceeding that of morphine (13). Despite the fact that because of lower lipid solubility morphine-6-glucuronide is found at lower concentrations in the cerebrospinal fluid than the parent compound (14), it is clear that the metabolite has significant analgesic activity in normal patients (15). In fact, there is data to suggest that morphine-6-glucuronide is the molecule responsible for most of the clinical effect when morphine is given orally (16). This issue is of special relevance in patients with altered renal clearance mechanisms because they can develop dangerously high levels of morphine 6-glucuronide, leading to potentially severe respiratory depression (17,18).

Meperidine is another example of how the time course of drug concentration of the parent compound predicted by a pharmacokinetic model is not very useful in predicting the activity of an active metabolite. Like morphine, meperidine is metabolized in the liver to several metabolites which are subsequently made water soluble by glucuronidation and are eventually excreted by the kidney (19). Normeperidine, the chief metabolite, has not only analgesic activity but also substantial central nervous system excitatory effects (20). These excitatory effects can range from anxiety and tremulousness to multifocal myoclonus and frank seizures (21). As with morphine, because the active metabolites are subject to renal excretion, this potential central nervous system toxicity secondary to normeperidine accumulation is especially a concern in renal failure patients (22).

PHARMACODYNAMIC CONSIDERATIONS

THE SLOPE OF THE CONCENTRATION-EFFECT RELATIONSHIP & PREDICTION OF CLINICAL RESPONSE

While clinicians have traditionally relied upon pharmacokinetic parameters in predicting the time course of drug effect, the duration of drug effect is a function of both pharmacokinetic and pharmacodynamic parameters. Recent computer modeling research has focused attention on the steepness of the concentration-effect relationship as an important parameter in predicting duration of drug effect (23).

For analgesics, the concentration-effect relationship is usually described graphically by a sigmoidal maximum-effect curve in which drug concentration in the site of action is plotted against drug effect. This sigmoid curve is represented mathematically by the equation:

$$E = E_0 + \frac{E_{max} \bullet Ce^{\gamma}}{EC_{50}{}^{\gamma} + Ce^{\gamma}}$$

where E is the predicted effect, E_0 is the baseline effect level, Emax is maximal effect, Ce is effect site concentration, γ is a measure of curve steepness, and EC_{50} is the effect site concentration that produces 50% of maximal effect. EC_{50} is the measure of drug potency, which can be compared to other drugs of the same class.

This mathematical representation of the concentration-effect relationship is appealing not only because it is harmonious with experimental observations but also because it is consistent with the receptor concept of drug action. Many drugs exert pharmacologic effect by binding with specific cellular receptors, activating a series of chemical changes in the cell that culminate in drug action. When all the receptors are occupied by drug, the maximal possible effect is achieved; that is, biologic systems are not capable of an infinite response. Thus, the concentration-effect relationship is well described by a sigmoidal maximum-effect curve in which a plateau in drug effect is eventually observed despite enormous increases in drug concentration.

The γ parameter of the sigmoidal maximum-effect equation is a measure of curve steepness. When γ is large, the concentration-effect relationship is steep. For drugs with a steep concentration-effect relationship, small changes in drug concentration produce large changes in drug effect. For drugs that exhibit a concentration-effect relationships in which γ is small, a small change in concentration does not result in such obvious changes in the magnitude of drug effect.

For drugs that have a steep concentration-effect relationship, the correlation of effect with concentration is often observed to be binary in nature. In other words, the degree of drug effect is either substantial or it is negligible. This is because when drug concentration drops much below the EC_{50}, the probability of substantial drug effect is minimal, whereas when concentrations are much above EC_{50} the probability of near maximal drug effect is high. When the concentration-effect relationship is less steep, the correlation of concentration with effect is more continuous in nature.

The practical application of this concept is that pharmacokinetic parameters cannot be interpreted in isolation in predicting the duration of drug effect. While knowledge of the predicted decline in drug concentration based on pharmacokinetic parameters is helpful, it must be interpreted with knowledge about the drug potency and steepness of the concentration-effect relationship.

For example, in Figure 4, the predicted decline in fentanyl concentration after a steady state infusion is terminated is plotted versus time. The probability of drug effect is also plotted for two different theoretical concentration-effect relationships; one that is steep ($\gamma = 10$) and another that is not steep ($\gamma = 2$). When the concentration-effect relationship is steep, there is a rapid dissipation in the probability of drug effect with declining drug concentration, whereas when the concentration-effect relationship is not steep, there is a much more gradual decline in the probability of drug effect with falling drug concentration. This notion has recently been quantified mathematically and has been designated the mean effect time (MET) (23).

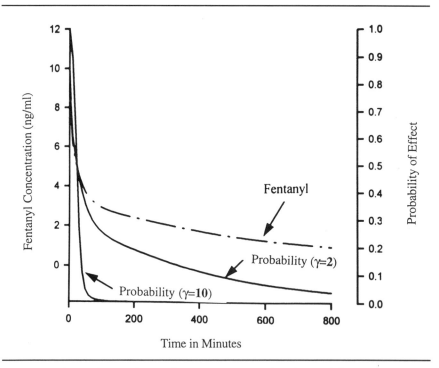

Figure 4. The decline in fentanyl concentration in the plasma (after stopping a 60 minute infusion targeting a concentration of 10 ng/ml) versus the probability of drug effect for 2 concentration-effect relationships, one steep (γ=10), the other less steep (γ=2). Note that when the slope of the concentration-effect relationship is steep the probability of substantial drug effect as a function of concentration is nearly a binary response (see text for complete explanation). [Modified from Bailey (23), with permission.]

The implications of context sensitive half-time (or 50% decrement time) must thus be interpreted in concert with knowledge of the concentration-effect relationship. Duration of drug effect as predicted by the context sensitive half-time closely parallels that predicted by the mean effect time when the concentration effect relationship is steep. When the concentration effect relationship is less steep, the context sensitive half-time may be less useful in predicting the time course of drug effect. For alfentanil, a drug whose concentration-effect relationship is steep, the MET and $CST_{1/2}$ predict a similar time course of drug effect. Conversely, for midazolam, a drug whose concentration-effect relationship is less steep, the MET and $CST_{1/2}$ predict a different time course of drug effect after termination of an infusion.

The clinical application of these concepts with regard to pain management relates to the steepness of the concentration-effect relationship of opioids. Opioids are known to be drugs of relatively steep concentration-effect relationships; that is, the γ parameter is relatively large (24). Thus, very small changes in opioid concentration can produce large changes in the degree of drug effect. This means that for patients who fail a typical analgesic regimen, sometimes very small increases in dosage can result in adequate analgesia. Patient response to opioids is often binary in nature. Analgesia is either adequate or it is not.

THE BIOPHASE CONCEPT AND LATENCY TO PEAK EFFECT

Equilibration delay between peak drug concentration in the blood or plasma and peak drug effect must also be considered in understanding the implications of pharmacokinetic simulations. For many drugs, there is a significant time lag between peak concentration in the plasma and peak drug effect (25). This time lag, or hysteresis, is a function of drug movement into and action within the effect site, or biophase. The hysteresis is a summation of all the events that can conceivably impact the onset of pharmacologic effect such as drug diffusion to the effect site, receptor binding and post receptor binding processes. Because effect-site concentrations lag behind plasma or blood concentrations, pharmacologic effect will also lag behind plasma or blood concentrations. In short, most drugs do not act in the plasma or blood. Thus, this lag time must be considered when using plasma or blood simulations of drug concentration in forecasting drug effect. The time lag is particularly important when giving drugs by bolus administration such as during patient controlled analgesia therapy, whereas for long infusions the time lag assumes less importance because the biophase and plasma are generally much closer to equilibrium.

For many drugs used in pain management, the equilibration delay between peak concentration in the plasma and peak effect has been characterized. Flow of drug to the effect compartment is a first order process and can be elucidated by estimating k_{e0}, a first order rate constant for elimination of drug from the effect compartment (26). When the k_{e0} parameter is available for a drug, theoretical effect compartment concentrations can be simulated along with plasma or blood concentrations, thus making the effect of the time lag easily appreciated. Figure 5 is a simulation of fentanyl administration, showing both the plasma and effect site concentrations based on parameters from the literature (7). Recognizing that drug effect best correlates with effect site concentration, the simulation in Figure 5 is quite revealing, illustrating that the time course of drug concentration in the effect site is much smoother than in the plasma. In general, the fentanyl congeners (especially alfentanil and remifentanil), have short $T_{1/2}k_{e0}$, while morphine's blood-brain equilibration time is much longer. Hence, when administered in "equipotent" doses, the fentanyl congeners reach peak effect considerably faster than morphine.

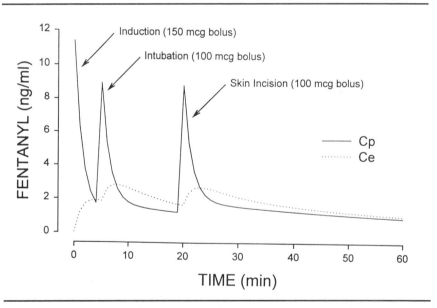

Figure 5: A simulation of plasma and effect site concentrations after intravenous fentanyl administration during a typical anesthetic. In such cases the fentanyl is used as a component of the anesthetic intraoperatively and as an analgesic in the early postoperative period. [From Egan (7), with permission.]

FUTURE CONSIDERATIONS

THE PHARMACOLOGIC AMBIGUITIES OF CHIRALITY

Taken from the Greek word chier (meaning hand), chiral is the term used to designate a molecule that has a center (or centers) of three dimensional asymmetry. The appropriateness of the term's Greek origin is clear when considering that our hands are perhaps the most common example of chirality. While they are mirror images of one another, our hands cannot be superimposed. Similarly, chirality in molecular structure results in a set of mirror image molecular twins that cannot be superimposed. This kind of molecular handedness in biologic systems is ubiquitous in nature and is almost always of function of the unique, tetrahedral bonding characteristics of the carbon atom (27,28).

Chirality is thus the structural basis of enantiomerism. Enantiomers are a pair of molecules that exist in two forms that are mirror images of one another but cannot be superimposed one upon the other (29). Enantiomers are in every other respect chemically identical. A pair of enantiomers is distinguished by the direction in which, when dissolved in solution, they rotate polarized light, either dextro (d or +) or levo (l or -) rotatory; hence, the term optical isomers. When two enantiomers are present in equal proportions they are collectively referred to as a racemic mixture, a mixture that does not rotate polarized light because the optical activity of each enantiomer is canceled by the other.

Chirality is an important issue in clinical pharmacology because the molecular interactions that are the mechanistic foundation of drug action and disposition occur in three dimensions and therefore can be altered by stereochemical asymmetry (30). The schematic "lock and key" hypothesis of enzyme-substrate interplay implies that biologic systems are inherently chiral. As shown in Figure 6, the pharmacologic extension of this notion is that drugs can be expected to interact with the body's pharmacologic proteins in a geometrically specific way. Thus, pharmacologically, not all enantiomers are created equal! Drug-cellular receptor, drug-metabolic enzyme and drug-protein binding interactions are virtually always three dimensionally exacting.

The implications of chirality thus span the entire pharmacokinetic-pharmacodynamic spectrum. Enantiomers can exhibit differences in absorption and bioavailability, distribution and clearance, potency and toxicology (31-35). Enantiomers can even antagonize one another across this pharmacologic spectrum (36). Adding additional complexity, some enantiomers can undergo chiral inversion to the other enantiomer, and drug interactions can also be stereoselective (37-39).

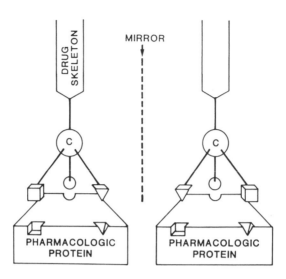

Figure 6: A schematic summarizing the implications of chirality on drug-pharmacologic protein interplay. One enantiomer of the racemic pair may be more effective than the other at binding and interacting with a pharmacologic protein (i.e., a metabolic enzyme, a cellular receptor or a binding protein). [From MA Ashburn and LJ Rice (ed): The Management of Pain, Churchill Livingston, New York, New York, 1998, with permission.]

When a pharmacologic process discriminates in a relative fashion between enantiomers (e.g., such as one enantiomer being metabolized more rapidly than the other), it is termed stereoselective. If the discrimination is absolute (e.g., such as one enantiomer being completely incapable of producing drug effect), the process is termed stereospecific.

The fact that many pharmacologic processes are stereoselective has recently attracted a great deal of interest and controversy. When stereoselective properties are demonstrated for a chiral drug administered as a racemic mixture, it becomes necessary to view the enantiomers as two separate drugs with distinct pharmacokinetic and pharmacodynamic characteristics (40). This means that some of the earlier clinical pharmacology research on racemic mixture drugs may eventually require refinement to account for enantiomeric differences.

Fortunately, the scientific ambiguities associated with chirality do not apply by and large to the clinical pharmacology of opioids. The fentanyl congeners have no chiral center and thus exist in a single form. Morphine, on the other hand, does have a center of molecular asymmetry. As a naturally occurring molecule synthesized by nature's stereospecific machinery, however, it is present in pharmacologic preparations in its pure, active form (l-morphine). On the contrary, some of the synthetic opioids, such as methadone, do exist as racemates and thus the complexities of enantiomer chemistry apply. Similarly, many of the nonopioid analgesics, such as the nonsteroidal antiinflammatory drugs, such as ibuprofen and ketorolac, also have chiral centers and are a mixture of two or more enantiomers.

As in other medical disciplines, enantiomer specific clinical pharmacology research in anesthesia and pain management is proliferating (41). Future research may change the way that some chiral drugs currently administered as racemates are used. Some of the clinical pharmacology database upon which clinicians currently rely requires re-examination to explore the possibility of important enantiomeric differences. Naturally, analgesics and anesthetics that are developed in the future are more likely to be non-chiral molecules or single enantiomers so that the scientific ambiguities associated with chirality can be avoided (42). Remifentanil, sevoflurane, ropivacaine and cis-atracurium are all examples of this trend.

THE ROLE OF REMIFENTANIL IN PAIN MANAGEMENT

Remifentanil (Glaxo), is a synthetic opioid that has recently been released for clinical use in the United States (43). It is unique because of its unusual pharmacokinetic characteristics. As an ester, it is subject to hydrolysis by nonspecific blood and tissue esterases, resulting in extremely rapid metabolism to inactive compounds as shown in Figure 7. Compared to the currently marketed fentanyl congeners, remifentanil's $CST_{1/2}$ is short, on the order of about 5 minutes (44). Pharmacologically, remifentanil exhibits a latency to peak effect similar to alfentanil and a potency slightly less than fentanyl (45).

As a very short acting drug, remifentanil may offer a number of potential advantages in certain pain management applications. For example, remifentanil may be useful in determining whether or not an outpatient undergoing an initial chronic pain evaluation has pain that is opioid sensitive. This could be achieved with a gradually increasing infusion to target concentrations without lasting residual effects at the end of the outpatient visit. Another conceivable application for remifentanil would be for treatment of short periods of "break-through" pain (such as bed to chair transfers in an acutely injured patient).

In addition to the familiar adverse effects associated with the other fentanyl congeners, an obvious drawback of remifentanil is the fact that for sustained effect it must be administered by infusion. Many practitioners may also find the necessity to reconstitute the drug and administer it by

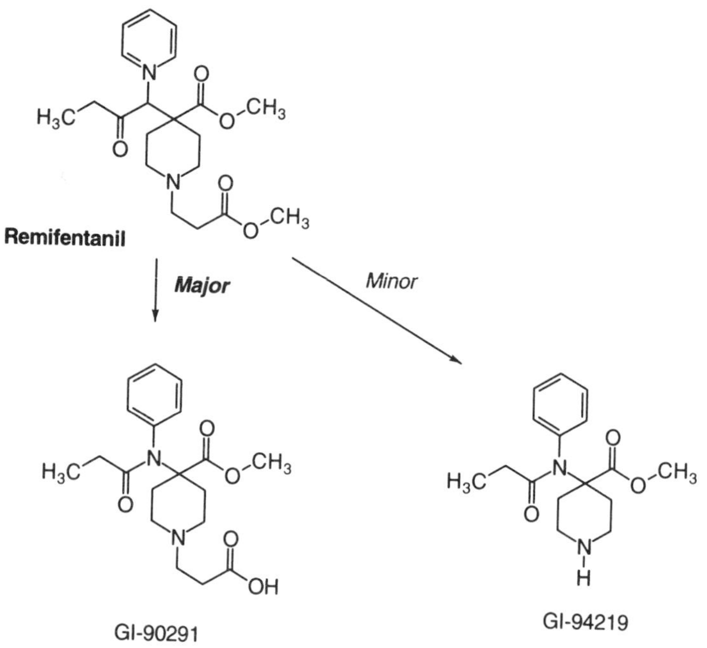

Figure 7: Remifentanil's metabolic pathway. De-esterification by nonspecific
plasma and tissue esterases to form a carboxylic acid metabolite (GI90291)
that has only 1/300th-1/1000th the potency of the parent compound is the
primary metabolic pathway. N-dealkylation of remifentanil to GI94219 is a
minor metabolic pathway. [From Egan (43), with permission.]

infusion as a significant inconvenience. A unique problem associated
with remifentanil is the real possibility of an unwanted, ill-timed dissipation of opioid effect that could occur with an inadvertent, accidental
termination of a remifentanil infusion such as an infusion pump
malfunction (43).

Hence, while by no means is remifentanil the ideal analgesic, its
unique pharmacokinetic properties and its familiar, fentanyl-like pharmacodynamic characteristics may be exploitable when applied to certain clinical challenges in acute and chronic pain management. Further research in
this domain will determine whether the theoretical advantages of a very
short acting opioid are clinically realized.

COMPUTERIZED DRUG DELIVERY METHODS

Until recently, the most sophisticated delivery device for the administration of opioids was the calculator pump, a device that enabled an accurate and precise delivery of fluid per unit of time. Used in both clinical and research settings, the physician operator of these devices simply specifies a delivery rate in terms of mg/hr or µg/kg/min, etc. The patient controlled analgesia machine is a hybrid of the calculator pump that permits patient control of opioid administration within physician constrained parameters. The primary limitation of these calculator pumps is that they do not achieve the pharmacokinetic exactness possible with more advanced methods of administration.

Advances in pharmacologic modeling and infusion pump technology have now made it possible to administer opioids (and other drugs) via a computer controlled infusion pump (46). By coding a pharmacokinetic model into a computer program and linking it to an electronic pump modified to accept computerized commands, delivery according to a drug's specific pharmacokinetics parameters can be achieved. The physician operating a computer controlled infusion pump (CCIP) designates a target concentration to achieve rather than specifying an infusion rate. The CCIP then calculates the necessary infusion rates to achieve the targeted concentration. This is somewhat akin to delivering inhaled anesthetic through the lungs using a vaporizer.

Administering volatile anesthetic through the lung via a calibrated vaporizer affords several fundamental advantages. These advantages are a function of gaining access to the circulation indirectly through the lung. Because uptake of inhaled anesthetic progressively diminishes as equilibrium between the alveolar and pulmonary capillary partial pressures is approached, the setting on the vaporizer is a proportional reflection of the concentration in the blood and the site of drug action. In other words, because of this equilibration process, the partial pressure in the blood cannot rise beyond the partial pressure of the inhaled gas. This enables relatively accurate administration. Moreover, the expired concentration can be measured and confirmed with modern respiratory gas monitoring, ensuring pharmacokinetic exactness. Finally, the clinical meaning of the measured concentration is well described and standardized in terms of minimum alveolar concentration (i.e., MAC), providing pharmacodynamic exactness.

In contrast, when access to the circulation is gained directly, there is nothing to prevent the indefinite uptake of drug. Thus, without the aid of a computer model, the infusion rate of an intravenous anesthetic agent (such as an opioid) does not reveal much about the resulting concentration in the blood, preventing entirely accurate administration. Furthermore, there is as yet no capability to measure the concentration of intravenous anesthetics in real time, preventing equivalent pharmacokinetic exactness. Finally, even if concentrations of intravenous agents were measurable in the clinical setting, the meaning of a given concentration is not yet well understood; that is, a thoroughly researched and widely appreciated analogue of MAC for the intravenous agents is not yet fully developed so that pharmacodynamic exactness equivalent to the volatile anesthetics is not possible.

Borrowing from inhalation anesthesia concepts, computer controlled infusion pumps (CCIPs) make progress toward the concept of a "vaporizer" for intravenous drugs because they address the fundamental limitation associated with delivering drugs directly into the circulation. Constant rate infusions result in continuous drug uptake. CCIPs, in contrast, gradually decrease the rate of infusion based on the drug's pharmacokinetics. Known in its general form as the BET method (i.e., bolus, elimination and transfer) (47), the dosing scheme determined by a CCIP accounts for the initial concentration after a bolus dose and the subsequent drug distribution and clearance while an infusion is ongoing.

Delivery of drug via a CCIP requires a different knowledge base of the pain management physician. Rather than setting an infusion rate based on clinical experience and literature recommendations, the physician using a CCIP designates a target concentration and the CCIP calculates the infusion rates necessary to achieve the concentration over time. The CCIP changes the infusion rates at frequent intervals, sometimes as often as every 10 seconds. Successful use of a CCIP thus requires knowledge of the therapeutic concentrations appropriate for the specific pain management problem.

Computer controlled drug delivery is an exciting area with promising potential in pain management. Available CCIP prototypes typically perform quite well, as exemplified by Figure 8, a fentanyl CCIP application (48). Pharmacokinetic model based patient controlled analgesia is also being developed with optimism (49). This application of CCIP methodology requires the patient to specify whether pain relief is adequate or not. The CCIP raises or lowers the target concentration accordingly.

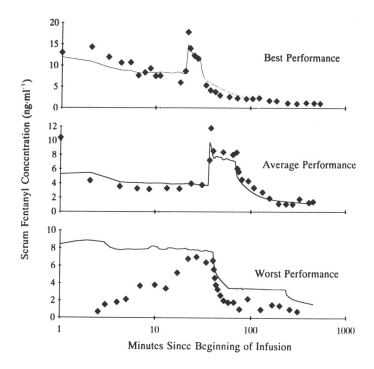

Figure 8: The best, median and worst performance of Stanpump when used to administer fentanyl to 21 patients. The line represents the predicted concentration, the diamonds represent the measured concentrations. [From Shafer (48), with permission.]

REFERENCES

1   Gourlay GK, Kowalski SR, Plummer JL, Cousins MJ, Armstrong PJ: Fentanyl blood concentration-analgesic response relationship in the treatment of postoperative pain. Anesth Analg 1988;67:329-337.

2.   Reilly CS, Wood AJJ, Wood M: Variability of fentanyl pharmaco-kinetics in man: computer predicted plasma concentrations for three intravenous dosage regimens. Anaesthesia 1984;40:837-843.

3.   Owen H, McMillan V, Rogowski D: Postoperative pain therapy: A survey of patients' expectations and their experiences. Pain 1990;41:303-307.

4.   Warfield CA, Kahn CH: Acute pain management: programs in U.S. hospitals and experiences and attitudes among U.S. adults. Anesthesiology 1995; 83:1090-1094.

5. Crankshaw DP: Variability and anaesthetic agents. Anaesthetic Pharmacology Review 1994;2:271-279.
6. Peck CC, Barr WH, Benet LZ et al: Opportunities for integration of pharmacokinetics, pharmacodynamics and toxicokinetics in rational drug development. Clin Pharmacol Ther 1992;51:465-473.
7. Egan TD: Pharmacokinetics and rational intravenous drug selection and administration in anesthesia. Advances in Anesthesia 1995;12:363-388.
8. Ebling WF, Lee EN, Stanski DR: Understanding pharmacokinetics and pharmacodynamics through computer simulation: I. The comparative clinical profiles of fentanyl and alfentanil. Anesthesiology 1990; 72:650-658.
9. Shafer SL, Varvel JR: Pharmacokinetics, pharmacodynamics and rational opioid selection. Anesthesiology 1991;74:53-63.
10. Hughes MA, Glass PSA, Jacobs JR: Context-sensitive half-time in multicompartment pharmacokinetic models for intravenous anesthetic drugs. Anesthesiology 1992;76:334-341.
11. Youngs EJ, Shafer SL: Pharmacokinetic parameters relevant to recovery from opioids. Anesthesiology 1994; 81:833-842.
12. Brunk SF, Delle M: Morphine metabolism in man. Clin Pharmacol Ther 1974;16:51-57.
13. Pasternak GW, Bodnar RJ, Clark JA, Inturrisi CE: Morphine 6-glucuronide is a potent mu agonist. Life Sci 1987;41:2845-2849.
14. Portenoy RK, Khan E, Layman M, et al: Chronic morphine therapy for cancer pain: plasma and cerebrospinal fluid morphine and morphine 6-glucuronide concentrations. Neurology 1991;41:1457-1461.
15. Portenoy RK, Howard TT, Inturrisi CE, Friedlander-Klar H, Foley KM: The metabolite morphine-6-glucuronide contributes to the analgesia produced by morphine infusion in patients with pain and normal renal function. Clin Pharmacol Ther 1992;51:422-431.
16. Osborne R, Joel S, Trew D, Slevin M: Morphine and metabolite behavior after different routes of morphine administration: demonstration of the importance of the active metabolite morphine-6-glucuronide. Clin Pharmacol Ther 1990;47:12-19.
17. Osborne RJ, Joel SP, Slevin ML: Morphine intoxication in renal failure: the role of morphine-6-glucuronide. Br Med J 1986;292:1548-1549.
18. D'Honneur G, Gilton A, Sandouk P, Scherrmann JM, et al: Plasma and cerebrospinal fluid concentrations of morphine and morphine glucuronides after oral morphine: the influence of renal failure. Anesthesiology 1994;81:87-93.
19. Asatoor AM, London DR, Milne MD, Simenhoff ML: The excretion of pethidine and its derivatives. Br J Pharmacol 1963;20:285-298.
20. Shochet RB, Murray GB: Neuropsychiatric toxicity of meperidine. J Intensive Care Med 1988;3:246-252.

21. Kaiko RF, Foley KM, Grabinski PY, Heidrich G, Rogers AG, Inturrisi CE, Reidenberg MM: Central nervous system excitatory effects of meperidine in cancer patients. Ann Neurol 1983;13:180-185.

22. Szeto HH, Inturrisi CE, Houde R, et al. Accumulation of normeperidine, an active metabolite of meperidine, in patients with renal failure or cancer. Ann Intern Med 1977;86:738-741.

23. Bailey JM: Technique for quantifying the duration of intravenous anesthetic effect. Anesthesiology 1995;83:1095-1103.

24. Mather LE: Pharmacokinetic and pharmacodynamic profiles of opioid analgesics: a sameness amongst equals? Pain 1990; 43:3-6.

25. Jacobs JR, Reves JG: Effect site equilibration time is a determinant of induction dose requirement. Anesth Analg 1993; 76:1-6.

26. Verotta D, Sheiner LB: Simultaneous modeling of pharmacokinetics and pharmacodynamics: an improved algorithm. CABIOS 1987; 3:345-349.

27. Mason S: The origin of chirality in nature. Trends Pharmacol Sci 1986;7:20-23.

28. Hegstrom RA, Konderpudi DK: The handedness of the universe. Sci American 1990;262:98-105.

29. Morrison RT, Boyd RN. Organic chemistry. 3rd Edition. Boston: Allyn and Bacon, 1973.

30. Testa B: Mechanisms of chiral recognition in xenobiotic metabolism and drug-receptor interaction. Chirality 1989;1:7-9.

31. Ariens EJ: Chirality in bioactive agents and its pitfalls. Trends Pharmacol Sci 1986;7:200-205.

32. Tucker GT, Lennard MS: Enantiomer specific pharmacokinetics. Pharmac Ther 1990;45:309-329.

33. Williams KM: Chirality: pharmacokinetics and pharmacodynamics in 3 dimensions. Clin Exp Pharmacol Physiol 1989:16:465-470.

34. Drayer DE: Pharmacodynamic and pharmacokinetic differences between drug enantiomers in humans: an overview. Clin Pharmacol Ther 1986;40:125-133.

35. Lee EJD, Williams KM: Chirality. Clinical pharmacokinetic and pharmacodynamic considerations. Clin Pharmacokinet 1990;18:339-345.

36. Wahlstrom G, Norberg L: A comparative investigation in the rat of the anesthetic effects of the isomers of two barbiturates. Brain Res 1984;310:261-267.

37. Kaiser DG, van Geissen GJ, Reisher RJ, Wechter WJ. Isomeric inversion of ibuprofen (R)-enantiomer in humans. J Pharma Sci 1976;65:269-273.

38. O'Reilly RA, Trager WF, Rettie AE, Goulart DA: Interaction of amiodarone with racemic warfarin and its separated enantiomorphs in humans. Clin Pharmacol Ther 1987;42:290-294.

39. Whelan E, Wood AJ, Koshakji R, Shay S, Wood M: Halothane inhibition in propranolol metabolism is stereoselective. Anesthesiology 1989;71:561-564.

40. Ariens EJ: Stereochemistry, a basis for sophisticated nonsense in pharmacokinetics and clinical pharmacology. Eur J Clin Pharmacol 1984;26:663-668.
41. Egan TD: Chirality and anesthetic pharmacology: joining hands with the medicinal chemists. Anesth Analg (in press)
42. Nation RL: Chirality in new drug development-clinical pharmacokinetic considerations. Clin Pharmacokinet 1994;27:249-255.
43. Egan TD: Remifentanil pharmacokinetics and pharmacodynamics: a preliminary appraisal. Clin Pharmacokinet 1995;29:80-94.
44. Egan TD, Lemmens HJM, Fiset P, Hermann DJ, Muir KT, Stanski DR, Shafer SL: The pharmacokinetics of the new short acting opioid remifentanil (GI87084B) in healthy adult male volunteers. Anesthesiology 1993;79:881-892.
45. Egan TD, Minto CF, Hermann DJ, Barr J, Muir KT, Shafer SL: remifentanil versus alfentanil: comparative pharmacokinetics and pharmacodynamics in healthy adult male volunteers. Anesthesiology 1996;4:821-833.
46. Egan TD: Intravenous drug delivery systems: toward an intravenous vaporizer. J Clin Anesth 8:8S-14S, 1996.
47. Schwilden H: A general method for calculating the dosage scheme in linear pharmacokinetics. Eur J Clin Pharmacol 1981;20:379-386.
48. Shafer SL, Varvel JR, Aziz N, Scott JC: Pharmacokinetics of fentanyl administered by computer controlled infusion pump. Anesthesiology 1990;73:1091-1102.
49. van den Nieuwenhuyzen MCO, Engbers FHM, Burm AGL, Vletter AA, van Kleef JW, Bovill JG: Computer controlled infusion of alfentanil versus patient controlled administration of morphine for postoperative analgesia: a double blind randomized trail. Anesth Analg 1995;81:671-679.

THE CONTRIBUTION OF SUBSTANCE P TO LONG-TERM CHANGES IN THE SPINAL CORD DORSAL HORN: REORGANIZATION IN THE SETTING OF PERSISTENT INJURY

A. Basbaum

The traditional view of pain processing illustrates an unmyelinated primary afferent C-fiber making a synapse upon a dorsal horn projection neuron that in turn activates cells in the thalamus and cortex. This relatively hard-wired system ignores or at least does not illustrate the long-term changes that occur when injury inputs are processed at the level of the spinal cord (6). The changes are manifest at the anatomical, molecular and biochemical levels and produce a hyperexcitable state that enhances pain transmission. In another chapter in this book I describe how glutamate, the major excitatory neurotransmitter of primary afferent fibers, can induce long-term changes via an action at the NMDA receptor. As noted in that chapter, in the absence of injury, or intense stimulation, the NMDA receptor is blocked by a magnesium ion that sits in the channel. When the postsynaptic neuron is depolarized, as would occur with persistent stimulation, the magnesium is kicked out of the channel. This allows calcium to enter the cell. Calcium in turn activates a variety of second messenger systems that lead to prolonged changes that establish a sensitized state in the dorsal horn neurons. In the present chapter I will describe other studies that provide a new perspective on the contribution of one of the major neuropeptides found in primary afferents, namely substance P.

If one takes an antibody directed against substance P and uses immunocytochemistry to localize it in the dorsal horn one finds that the peptide is concentrated in the superficial dorsal horn, laminae I and II (11). To a great extent substance P derives from unmyelinated primary afferent fibers whose cell bodies are in the dorsal root ganglion. Since substance P is located in unmyelinated primary afferents it is not surprising to find that substance P is released into the CSF in spinal cord by high intensity, pain producing stimulation (8, 27). Moreover, iontophoresis of substance P in the region of the dorsal horn neurons will activate those neurons which are naturally stimulated by noxious stimulation (5, 10); substance P does

T. H. Stanley et al. (eds.), Pain Management and Anesthesiology, 55–63.
© 1998 *Kluwer Academic Publishers. Printed in the Netherlands.*

not activate cells that do not respond to noxious stimulation. This strongly implicates substance P in the transmission of "pain messages."

A paradox, however, arises when one examines the distribution of the receptors targeted by substance P. Substance P is a member of the tachykinin family of peptides, which target a family of receptors, called neurokinin receptors (9). Substance P preferentially targets the neurokinin 1 (NK-1) receptor. Using an antibody directed against the NK-1 receptor, it is thus possible to identify the cells in the dorsal horn that express the receptor targeted by substance P (26). When we performed these studies we found, not surprisingly, that many neurons in lamina I, the most super-ficial layer of the dorsal horn, express the NK-1 receptor (3). On the other hand we found very few, if any, neurons in lamina II that express the NK-1 receptor. This was true despite the fact that this region contains large numbers of substance P terminals. In general, the only neuronal elements in lamina II that express the NK 1 receptor are dendrites of neurons located deeper, in lamina III. The latter neurons have dendrites that course through lamina II and end in lamina I. These could obviously be targeted by substance P in the substantia gelatinosa (lamina II) but the fact is that the majority of the substance P terminals make no contact with NK-1 receptor positive neurons (17). Our ultrastructural studies established this and demonstrated that there is a significant mismatch between the peptide and its receptor. Finally, there are many neurons in deeper parts of dorsal horn, in laminae V and VI and around the central canal, which express the NK-1 receptor but are not surrounded by or perhaps even con-tacted by substance P-containing terminals. What then is the relationship of substance P and the NK-1 receptor and under what condition does sub-stance P activate these neurons that express the receptor?

What is needed is a method to monitor the interaction between substance P and its receptor. Based on *in vitro* studies in other receptor systems it has been established that when a ligand, such as substance P, binds its receptor, the ligand receptor complex is often internalized into the cell. Under normal conditions the receptor is found on the plasma membrane, but when its binds the transmitter it internalizes into the cytoplasm where it is either processed and degraded or recycled back to the membrane, without the neurotransmitter. Our first studies tested whether this also occurs in case of the substance P and NK-1 receptors in the central nervous system. We performed studies in the striatum which contains a relatively uniform population of neurons that express the NK-1 receptor (18). In these studies, in the anesthetized rat, we injected substance P directly into the striatum on one side and injected the vehicle solution into the other side. We let the animals survive from five minutes to one hour at which time the animals were perfused for immunohistochemistry.

Using confocal microscopy, which allows very detailed, high resolution analysis of the distribution of the receptors to be performed, we found that within five minutes of exposure to substance P there is massive internalization of the NK-1 receptor from the membrane to the cytoplasm. Note that this occurred over the entire surface of neurons, whether or not the receptors were apposed by substance P terminals. Based on these results we concluded not only that there is internalization of the NK-1, or substance P receptors, in response to binding with substance P, but also that substance P induces internalization of "nonsynaptic receptors", which are located distant from sites of synaptic contact. The latter conclusion derived from the fact that although greater than 80% of the plasma membrane receptor is "non-synaptic", almost the entire surface receptor was internalized in these studies. Importantly within one hour of the injection of substance P, the NK-1 receptor recycled back to the membrane, suggesting that the re-sensitization of neurons can be regulated by the time its takes to return the receptor to the plasma membrane.

This somewhat artificial system encouraged us to evaluate the NK-1 receptor in dorsal horn neurons and particularly to determine whether natural stimuli that release substance P can induce internalization of the NK-1 receptor in dorsal horn neurons. Our first studies used capsaicin injection into the hindpaw of the rat (19). We found that within five minutes of capsaicin injection there was massive internalization of the receptor in the cell bodies and dendrites of lamina I neurons that express the NK-1 receptor. In addition, we found internalization of the receptor in the most distal dendrites of neurons that arise from lamina III. On the other hand the receptor that was located on the cell body and proximal dendrites of the lamina III neurons remained on the membrane.

This result is important as it establishes several important features of the substance P-neurokinin-1 receptor interaction that were necessary for our subsequent analysis. First this study demonstrated that we can use internalization of the receptor to monitor cells that respond to substance P release. Second, since there is a great mismatch of the receptor and the substance P terminals in the superficial dorsal horn, our results indicate that there must be some diffusion of the peptide from its site of release to act on nonsynaptic receptors in the neighborhood of the release. In this respect substance P is quite different from glutamate which appears to act at receptors that immediately appose its site of release, in a fashion similar to the release of acetylcholine, which acts at nicotinic receptors at the neuromuscular junction.

In subsequent studies we evaluated the effect of other types of noxious stimuli, including noxious mechanical and thermal stimuli (2). Interestingly we found that noxious mechanical stimuli were the most effective in inducing internalization of the receptor, but again all of the changes that we recorded in the normal animal were in cells of the superficial dorsal horn, lamina I and the distal dendrites of deeper cells. Noxious thermal stimuli interestingly only evoked internalization when the temperatures were greater than 48°C, a temperature that probably initiates an inflammatory reaction at the site of injury. This is of interest because traditionally 45°C is the threshold for activation of C-fibers. This preferential effect of mechanical stimuli on the release of substance P (in our case documented by the postsynaptic receptor internalization) is consistent with a report demonstrating that noxious thermal stimuli preferentially evoke the release of somatostatin while noxious mechanical stimuli evoke the release of substance P (14).

In further studies we asked whether the distribution and threshold for evoking internalization of the substance P receptor changed in the setting of injury. Our first studies evaluated the consequences of persistent inflammation of a single hindpaw of the rat. We used injection of Complete Freunds's Adjuvant, which induces a profound inflammation that develops over a period of one to three days. Our first studies demonstrated that there are significant changes in the distribution of the neurokinin-1/substance P receptor under these conditions (1). In particular, we found an upregulation of the receptor in neurons of the superficial dorsal horn. Interestingly, the changes were not only found in the medial part of the dorsal horn, which receives input from the hindpaw but also rostral and caudal to that region. There also were increases of the receptor in the lateral parts of the dorsal horn. This result suggests that in the setting of persistent injury there is a activation of large regions of spinal cord, outside the normal topographic representation of the site that was injured. Presumably this can contribute to spread of sensitivity that occurs with persistent injury.

Although there was significant upregulation of the receptor in the setting of inflammation, the receptor, in the absence of stimulation, remained on the plasma membrane. This suggests that the peptide-receptor interaction only comes into play when a stimulus is superimposed upon the inflamed paw, and that there is minimal ongoing activity in the absence of stimulation. Thus, in the next series of studies we addressed the effect stimulating the inflamed paw. When we applied the noxious stimulus to the hindpaw of the animals with persistent inflammation we found a dramatic change in the distribution of neurons that internalized the NK-1 receptor. With mechanical stimuli, we found that there was an almost 100% response of neurons in the superficial dorsal horn as well as a significant response of neurons in lamina III, V, and VI. In other words, in the setting of inflammation where there is upregulation of neurokinin-1 receptor (1, 24) and increased concentration of substance P (16), the population of neurons that "responds" to the noxious stimulus, as evidenced by internalization of the receptor, increased dramatically. This again was not only found at the input zone, L4 and L5 of the rat lumbar spinal cord, but also more rostrally and caudally. Importantly, we also found that the threshold for inducing internalization changed. Specifically in the normal animal only a noxious pinch stimulus was effective in inducing internalizing in the cells in lamina I. A brush stimulus was totally ineffective. However in the animals with persistent inflammation we found that even light brushing of the paw for two minutes induced NK-1 receptor internalization, not only in lamina I but also in a significant percentage of neurons in the neck of the dorsal horn. Whether the brush stimulus induced the internalization because it activated C-fibers whose threshold had dropped (as a result of a cyclo-oxygenase dependent sensitization of the peripheral terminals) or whether it was secondary to activation of large diameter afferents is unclear. The latter hypothesis is of particular interest in light of recent studies that demonstrated not only that dorsal horn neurons can be driven by large diameter afferents in the setting of injury, but that large diameter afferents begin to express substance P when there is inflammation (22).

There is an interesting aside to these studies. All of the animals in these studies were deeply anesthetized with pentobarbital, i.e., the animals were not in a behaving state. Nevertheless receptor internalization was induced, and the size of the population of neurons in which we recorded these changes increased in the setting of inflammation. This indicates that significant cellular changes occur at the level of the spinal cord even under conditions in which the animal is anesthetized. This, of course, brings to mind studies that have emphasized the significance of preemptive analgesic approaches in the operative setting (20). That is, even though the animals were anesthetized, the noxious stimulus activated, i.e., induced receptor internalization, in neurons of the spinal cord. If this internalization is part of a signaling system that can generate long-term changes, it follows that the anesthetic is not sufficient to prevent them. If a local anesthetic were used to prevent the afferent drive to the spinal cord, then the long-term changes could be prevented.

Taken together these results indicate that substance P can induce internalization of the receptor in neurons of the deep dorsal horn only in conditions in which there is persistent injury. Since there is minimal primary afferent projection of substance P-containing afferents to these neurons, the possibility must be raised that in the setting of injury substance P diffuses from its site of release in the superficial dorsal horn to act on receptors located ventrally. Comparable conclusions have, in fact, been previously drawn based on studies using antibody-coated microelectrodes that can detect the release of substance P. In the setting of arthritis in the cat (after injection of inflammatory mediators in the knee joint) there is considerable spread of substance P ventrally (25). Interestingly, the authors found evidence that diffusion of substance P could be enhanced by intrathecal injection of calcitonin-gene related peptide, (CGRP; (7)) a peptide that is co-stored with substance P in dense core vesicles of primary afferent terminals (4). Interestingly, CGRP has been shown by many authors to do little by itself; rather CGRP enhances the effects produced by substance P. Thus, the primary afferent terminal appears to contain peptides that are co-released and may regulate the endopeptidases that degrade substance P. Note that substance P differs considerably from amino acids and monoamines whose action at the synapse is terminated by a reuptake mechanism. In the case of peptides, termination of action can only occur by diffusion or degradation. This suggests that drugs directed at the endopeptidases that degrade substance P could significantly influence the population of neurons that are acted upon by this peptide when it is released from primary afferents.

It is clearly of interest to understand the factors that activate neurons by these peptides and to evaluate mechanisms to block these effects. Our first studies used opiate analgesics. Early reports found that morphine can block the release of substance P from primary afferents (13). These studies were based largely on *in vitro* analysis of the effects of morphine on the release of substance P produced by potassium depolarization of slices of the dorsal horn. Although one *in vivo* study confirmed the claim that morphine can block the release of substance P, Duggan and colleagues (15, 21) failed to reproduce these results using the antibody-coated microelectrode technique. In our studies we evaluated the effect of morphine and other opiate analogs (injected either systemically or intrathecally) on the internalization of the receptor induced by noxious stimulation. Despite using doses of analgesics that in the awake freely moving animal produced profound analgesia in a variety of pain tests, we never found significant inhibition of internalization of the receptor. In other words, despite the fact that the animals were made profoundly analgesic, substance P interacted with postsynaptic receptors and could conceivably induce long-term changes.

These results are reminiscent of our previous studies that evaluated the effect of morphine on the noxious stimulus-evoked induction of the immediate early gene c-fos, a marker of neuronal activity. In those studies, we found that despite using doses of opiates that produce profound analgesia, approximately 50% of the neurons in lamina I continued to express the Fos protein (23). Moreover the persistent Fos protein was expressed in a population of lamina I neurons that sent an axon to the brain (12), indicating that there may be information processing from the periphery to the brain even under conditions in which there is complete analgesia. To what extent such changes contribute to the central sensitization process that exacerbates the transmission of nociceptive messages remains to be determined. Regardless, since such long-term changes appear to be exclusively deleterious (i.e., they make pain worse), it is clearly important to identify molecules that can interfere with the process. As noted above, the idea of preemptive analgesia is based on the assumption that long-term changes induced by noxious stimuli at the level of the spinal cord contribute to increased postoperative pain and that intervening in the development of that process is valuable. Apparently opiate analgesics are not a satisfactory approach to preventing these long-term changes. Rather our studies and those of others emphasize that it may be necessary to block the afferent input to the cord, e.g., with local anesthetics.

In summary, these studies provide important new information on the contribution of the peptide substance P which is costored with glutamate, in primary afferent nociceptors. Our results illustrate the conditions under which substance P comes into play when noxious stimuli are presented and provide evidence that the different populations of neurons are "activated" by substance P release in the normal state and in the setting of inflammation. The consequences of internalization of the receptor in these different populations of neurons remains to be determined.

REFERENCES

1. Abbadie C, Brown JL, Mantyh PW, Basbaum AI: . Spinal cord substance P receptor immunoreactivity increases in both inflammatory and nerve injury models of persistent pain. Neuroscience 1996;70:201-209.
2. Abbadie C, Liu H, Trafton J, et al: Inflammation increases the distribution of dorsal horn neurons that internalize the neurokinin-1 receptor in response to noxious and non-noxious stimulation of the hindpaw. J Neurosci, in press.
3. Brown JL, Liu H, Maggio JE, et al: Morphological characterization of substance P receptor-immunoreactive neurons in the rat spinal cord and trigeminal nucleus caudalis. J Comp Neurol 1995;356:327-344.
4. De Biasi S, Rustioni A: Glutamate and substance P coexist in primary afferent terminals in the superficial laminae of spinal cord. Proc Natl Acad Sci (USA) 1988;85:7820-7824.

5. De Koninck Y, Henry JL: Substance P-mediated slow excitatory postsynaptic potential elicited in dorsal horn neurons in vivo by noxious stimulation. Proc Natl Acad Sci (USA) 1991;88:1344-11348.

6. Dubner R, Basbaum AI: Spinal dorsal horn plasticity following tissue or nerve injury. Pages 225-241 in P. D. Wall and R. Melzack, Eds., The Textbook of Pain. Churchill-Livingstone, London, 1994.

7. Duggan AW, Furmidge LJ: Probing the brain and spinal cord with neuropeptides in pathways related to pain and other functions. Front. Neuroendocrin 1994;15: 275-300.

8. Duggan AW, Morton CR, Zhao ZQ, Hendry IA: Noxious heating of the skin releases immunoreactive substance P in the substantia gelatinosa of the cat: a study with antibody microprobes. Brain Res 1987;403: 345-349.

9. Helke CJ, Krause JE, Mantyh PW, et al: Diversity in mammalian tachykinin peptidergic neurons: multiple peptides, receptors, and regulatory mechanisms. FASEB J 1990;4:1606-1615.

10. Henry JL: Effects of substance P on functionally identified units in cat spinal cord. Brain Res 1976;114: 439-451.

11. Hökfelt T, Kellerth J, Nilsson G, Pernow B: Experimental immunohistochemical studies on the localization and distribution of substance P in cat primary sensory neurons. Brain Res 1975;100: 235-252.

12. Jasmin L, Wang H, Tarczy-Hornoch K, et al: Differential effects of morphine on noxious stimulus-evoked Fos-like immunoreactivity in subpopulations of spinoparabrachial neurons. J Neurosci 1994;14: 7252-7260.

13. Jessell TM, Iversen LL: Opiate analgesics inhibit substance P release from rat trigeminal nucleus. Nature (Lond.) 1977;268: 549-551.

14. Kuraishi Y, Hirota N, Sato Y, et al: Evidence that substance P and somatostatin transmit separate information related to pain in the spinal dorsal horn. Brain Res 1985;325: 294-298.

15. Lang CW, Duggan AW, Hope PJ: Analgesic doses of morphine do not reduce noxious stimulus-evoked release of immunoreactive neurokinins in the dorsal horn of the spinal cat. Br J Pharmacol 1991;103:1871-1876.

16. Lembeck F, Donnerer J, Colpaert FC: Increase of substance P in primary afferent nerves during chronic pain. Neuropeptides 1981;1:175-180.

17. Liu H, Brown JL, Jasmin L, et al: Synaptic relationship between substance P and the substance P receptor: Light and electron microscopic characterization of the mismatch between neuropeptides and their receptors. Proc Natl Acad Sci (USA) 1994;91:1009-1013.

18. Mantyh, PW, Allen CJ, Ghilardi JR, et al: Rapid endocytosis of a G protein-coupled receptor: Substance P-evoked internalization of its receptor in the rat striatum in vivo. Proc Natl Acad Sci (USA) 1995; 92:2622-2626.

19. Mantyh PW, DeMaster E, Malhotra A, et al: Receptor endocytosis and dendrite reshaping in spinal neurons after somatosensory stimulation. Science 1995;268: 1629-1632.

20. McQuay HJ: Pre-emptive analgesia: A systematic review of clinical studies. Ann Med 1995;27:249-256.

21. Morton CR, Hutchison WD, Duggan AW, Hendry IA: Morphine and substance P release in the spinal cord. Exp Brain Res 1990;82:89-96.

22. Neumann S, Doubell TP, Leslie T, Woolf, CJ: Inflammatory pain hypersensitivity mediated by phenotypic switch in myelinated primary sensory neurons. Nature (Lond.) 1996;384: 360-364.

23. Presley RW, Menétrey D, Levine JD, Basbaum AI: Systemic morphine suppresses noxious stimulus-evoked Fos protein-like immunoreactivity in the rat spinal cord. J Neurosci 1990;10: 323-335.

24. Schäfer MKH, Nohr D, Krause JE, Weihe E: Inflammation-induced upregulation of NK1 receptor mRNA in dorsal horn neurons. Neuro Report 1993;4:1007-1010.

25. Schaible HG, Jarrott B, Hope PJ, Duggan AW: Release of immunoreactive substance P in the spinal cord during development of acute arthritis in the knee joint of the cat: A study with antibody microprobes. Brain Res 1990;529:214-223.

26. Vigna SR, Bowden JJ, McDonald DM, et al: Characterization of antibodies to the rat substance P (NK-1) receptor and to a chimeric substance P receptor expressed in mammalian cells. J Neurosci 1994;14:834-845.

27. Yaksh TL, Jessell TM, Gamse R, et al: Intrathecal morphine inhibits substance P release from mammalian spinal cord in vivo. Nature (Lond.) 1980;286:155-157.

PAIN AND THE SURGICAL STRESS RESPONSE

H. Kehlet

Surgical injury leads to profound changes in body homeostasis characterized by a catabolic state with increased secretion of catabolically acting hormones, decreased secretion and/or effect of anabolically acting hormones and additional alterations in various humoral cascade systems, coagulation and fibrinolysis and immune function. Other important sequelae for the surgical patient are pain, increased demands on the heart, impaired pulmonary function, nausea, vomiting and ileus and loss of muscle tissue contributing to postoperative fatigue. Since pain-induced reflex responses may adversely influence body organ functions and enhance the stress responses to surgical injury, pain relieving techniques may modify these responses and ultimately influence surgical outcome.

In this chapter the effect of pain relieving techniques on endocrine metabolic and inflammatory responses are shortly reviewed and updated. Specific references are only provided for the most recent literature, since the topic has been thoroughly reviewed recently (1,2).

PAIN RELIEF BY ANTAGONIZING PERIPHERAL MEDIATORS OF PAIN

NSAID's have been demonstrated to attenuate the endocrine metabolic response to endotoxin administration in human volunteers, but in most surgical studies NSAID's have had no or only a slight inhibitory effect on the classical catabolic stress hormones, acute phase protein responses or leukocytic responses (1-3). In patients with sepsis ibuprofen reduced levels of prostacyclin and thromboxane and decreased fever, tachycardia and oxygen consumption, but without positive effects on pulmonary complications or survival (4).

There are no data on the modifying effect of substance P-antagonists, antihistamines, serotonin antagonists or peripheral opioids on the surgical stress response.

Incisional local anesthetics reduce pain and the classical endocrine metabolic response to surgery in most studies (1,5), but without effects on acute phase protein or leukocytic responses (1,5). Intravenous, intraperi-

T. H. Stanley et al. (eds.), Pain Management and Anesthesiology, 65–73.

toneal or intrapleural local anesthetics have no important effects on surgical stress responses (1).

Systemic administration of high-dose glucocorticoids may improve pain relief and alter several of the responses mediated by various cascade systems (arachidonic cascade metabolites, cytokines, etc.) Thus, hyperthermia, acute phase protein responses and IL-6 and PGE2 changes are inhibited as well as pulmonary function may be improved (1,6). Intraarticular glucocorticoid may improve pain relief and reduce the postarthroscopic inflammatory response (7). On the negative side glucocorticoids may enhance postoperative immunosuppression (6), but without impairment in wound collagen synthesis (6). There are no data on other potential side effects or on nitrogen economy following perioperative glucocorticoid administration.

TRANSCUTANEOUS ELECTRIC NERVE STIMULATION

In accordance with the lack of significant analgesic effects in the postoperative period, no significant intra- and postoperative changes in the usual endocrine-metabolic response have been observed following application of transcutaneous electric nerve stimulation (1).

SYSTEMIC AND EPIDURAL OPIOID ADMINISTRATION

Opioids administered systemically in conventional dosages in patient-controlled analgesia or intermittently have only very slight or no stress-reducing effects (1,8). In contrast, high-dose opioid anesthesia may reduce intraoperative, but not postoperative endocrine metabolic changes (1,9),unless the opioid treatment is continued postoperatively (1).

Epidural analgesia with opioids may have some inhibitory effects on the catecholamine responses to surgery, but the results are not consistent in the literature (1). In general, the effects are relatively small, especially in major operations (1,2,10,11). In some studies the inhibitory effects of an initial intraoperative epidural local anesthetic block combined with epidural opioid, persisted into the postoperative period (1,10). So far, no differential effects have been demonstrated between various opioids on the surgical stress responses (1).

SYSTEMIC, EPIDURAL AND INTRATHECAL ALPHA-2 AGONISTS AND NEOSTIGMINE

The pain relieving effect of clonidine administered at various sites is well-documented (12), but overall the effect on endocrine metabolic changes are relatively minor (1,12,13), except for the decrease in the cardiovascular response to surgery. There are no data on the effect of intrathecal neostigmine on postoperative stress responses.

NEURAL BLOCKADE WITH LOCAL ANESTHETICS

Since the activation of the peripheral and central nervous system plays a key role in initiating the hormonal and metabolic responses to surgical injury (1,2) a neural block with local anesthetics may profoundly alter most hormonal and metabolic changes, but with smaller or no influence on humoral cascade systems (1,2). In lower abdominal (gynecologic) procedures and operations in the lower extremities lumbar epidural anesthesia will provide an effective afferent blockade as assessed by evoked potentials (1), and at the same time block pituitary hormonal responses, adrenocortical and sympathetic responses and glucagon, and adrenergic inhibition of insulin secretion. In contrast, the neural block has no effect on thyroid or sex hormone changes and no information is available on gastrointestinal hormones. Some responses such as catecholamines seem to be easier to inhibit by neural blockade than pituitary responses (1,10). Metabolism is profoundly changed by neural blockade and concomitant hormonal inhibition, since hyperglycemia is prevented and glucose tolerance improved (1,2). Similarly fat metabolism with increased lipolysis is reduced as well as conventional increases in lactate and ketones are reduced. Of most clinical relevance, postoperative protein economy is improved with lower increase in nitrogen excretion parallel to inhibition of the catabolic hormonal responses (table 1). In this context a single dose block has no important effect on protein economy, while a 24 hour block improves nitrogen economy with a further improvement by a 48 hours block (table 1). The effect of epidural local anesthetic blockade on protein economy is more pronounced than pain relief with epidural opioids (table 1). Also, the usual postoperative shift in amino acid composition in skeletal muscle is inhibited and the overall postoperative protein synthesis rate is less decreased with a continuous epidural blockade.

Although a neural block with local anesthetics may modify several hormonal responses that may influence renal function (cortisol, catecholamines, aldosterone, renin, ADH) no clinically important effect on postoperative fluid and electrolyte balance has been demonstrated except for reduced potassium excretion parallel with reduced catabolism (1). Oxygen consumption is reduced in accordance with sympathetic block and reduced catabolism (1).

The modifying effects of neural blockade with local anesthetics on surgical stress responses are most pronounced in lower body procedures

68

Table 1.   Effect of epidural and spinal analgesia on postoperative nitrogen economy (ref. 1,19,20).

	Surgery	Comment	Author
Lumbar epidural local	Hysterectomy	24-h block with inhibition of cortisol and glucose response and improvement in nitrogen balance	Brandt(1)
anesthetic	Colonic	44-h block. Postoperative nitrogen balance improved and 3-methylhistidine excretion reduced	Vedrinne(1)
	Hip surgery	No effect of single-dose epidural bupivacaine on urinary nitrogen and 3-methylhistidine excretion	Carli(1)
	Hip surgery	24-h block with reduction of cortisol and glucose response as well as usual 72-h postoperative shifts in amino acid composition in skeletal muscle	Christensen(1)
Thoracic epidural local anesthetic	Colonic	24-h block with reduction of urinary excretion of catecholamines, but not cortisol, Urinary nitrogen excretion and whole body protein turnover (leucine oxidation) reduced.	Carli(1)
	Gastric	48-h block with reduced plasma cortisol and glucagon response and decreased urinary catecholamine excretion; urinary nitrogen excretion reduced compared to pain relief with systemic opioids and epidural opioids	Tsuji(1)
	Aortic	24-h block with reduced plasma cortisol and urinary catecholamine excretion; no effect on urinary nitrogen and cortisol excretion (n=2 x 5).	Smeets(1)
	Abdominal	Single-dose postoperative block (-6 h duration) with slightly reduced plasma catecholamines, glucagon, and cortisol levels, isotope study with decrease in glucose and urea turnover rates	Shaw(1)

(Continued)

Table 1.   Continued.

	Surgery	Comment	Author
	Abdominal and thoracic	24-h block with no influence on plasma glucose, free fatty acids, and lactate except at the end of operation, and no effects on postoperative nitrogen urea or 3-methylhistidine excretion	Seeling(1)
	Abdominal	Single-dose epidural analgesia: no effect on plasma cortisol, glucose prolactin, or nitrogen balance	De Lalande(1)
	Abdominal	24-h block, but without effects on plasma cortisol, glucose, or prolactin, but improved nitrogen balance	De Lalande(1)
	Colonic	A 24-h continuous epidural block reduced postoperative protein break down more effectively than a 24-h block	Carli(19)
	Colonic	A 48-h continuous epidural block improved postoperative protein synthesis rate compared with general anesthesia and systemic opioids	Carli(20)
Lumbar epidural opioid	Colonic	48-h treatment (epi.meperidine); no effect on nitrogen and 3-methylhistidine excretion	Vedrinne(1)
Lumbar or thoracic local + anesthetic + opioid	Gastric	Intraoperative epidural local anesthetic + 72-h postoperative epidural morphine; Reduced plasma cortisol and glucagon and urinary excretion of catecholamines and nitrogen	Tsuji(1)
	Abdominal	24-h intermittent local anesthetic and 72-h epidural morphine with insignificant reduction in urinary catecholamines and cortisol, but unchanged 4-day nitrogen excretion	Hjortsø(1)
	Hysterectomy	24-h block with improved glucose homeostasis and insignificant reduction in urinary nitrogen excretion	Licker(1)

and with less effects in upper abdominal and thoracic operations. The explanation for this discrepancy is most probably an insufficient afferent blockade in the somatic and visceral nervous system with thoracic epidural analgesia. This is supported by less inhibition of evoked potentials following peripheral electrical stimulation, as well as the finding that an additional splanchnic block may further reduce the stress response during thoracic epidural analgesia (1). Also, continuous spinal anesthesia with or without additional epidural analgesia may reduce the stress response more effectively than epidural analgesia alone in major abdominal surgery, although the data are not consistent (1,14). Recently, the role of the phrenic nerves in the stress response to upper abdominal surgery has been evaluated by differential blocks, where a high cervical epidural block reduced ACTH and arginine vasopressin responses more effectively than a high thoracic epidural block (15).

The use of multimodal, balanced epidural analgesia has been demonstrated to improve pain relief. However, so far effective analgesic combinations of epidural local anesthetic and opioid combinations have not been demonstrated to block the classical hormonal responses to upper abdominal or thoracic surgery, indicating than pain relief per se may not necessarily be followed by blockade of these responses (1,16). The stress modifying effect of a neural blockade technique is not altered by additional general anesthesia (1).

INFLUENCE OF TIMING OF ANALGESIA ON POSTOPERATIVE STRESS RESPONSES

It has been hypothesized that a preemptive neural block may have a greater effect than a postinjury block on neuroplastic spinal cord changes and pain behavior. However, this has not been firmly established from clinical controlled studies comparing identical pre- and postoperative pain treatments. The limited data available to compare the effects of identical pre- and postoperative neural blocks or opioid analgesia, suggest that endocrine metabolic responses may be more difficult to modify after the nociceptive stimulus has been initiated compared with a block before skin incision (1). However, there seems to be no difference between a single dose block given pre- versus postoperatively (1,17). Nevertheless, post-surgery epidural blockade with local anesthetics may provide a considerable attenuation of catecholamine and thermogenic responses (18). The timing of neural blockade may be important in our future understanding of and development of measures to modify postinjury metabolism.

EFFECT OF TYPE AND DURATION OF BLOCK

As mentioned above lumbar epidural techniques are more effective than thoracic blocks, probably because of more effective afferent blockade and because of the use of more local anesthetics (1,2). The optimal duration of the afferent block has not been firmly established in systematic studies, but single-dose blocks lasting for 2-4 hours have no prolonged endocrine metabolic effects (1,2,17). In contrast, studies using continuous epidural blocks with local anesthetics for 24-72 hours have demonstrated metabolic effects extending for several days, including changes in protein economy (table 1). However, further investigations on the optimal duration and composition of the neural blockade in individual procedures are needed to provide final and procedure-oriented conclusions. Since we have an imperfect knowledge on equipotent dosages of the various local anesthetics, the few existing studies comparing the stress-reducing effects of different local anesthetics do not allow final conclusions (1).

CONCLUSIONS

It is apparent from the large amount of data on the effect of various pain relieving techniques on surgical endocrine metabolic changes that afferent blockade with local anesthetics is the most effective technique, followed by high-dose opioids, epidural opioids and clonidine, PCA opioid and NSAID, in that order. A prolonged pain treatment is necessary to provide effective inhibition of the stress responses. Effects of humoral cascade systems are usually not influenced by the various pain relieving techniques except for effective inhibition when glucocorticoids are added. Further studies of various pain relieving techniques combining of neural block with humoral cascade system modification are warranted, based upon the hypothesis that such modification may ultimately have a positive effect on surgical outcome (1).

REFERENCES

1. Kehlet H. Modification of responses to surgery and anesthesia by neural blockade: clinical implications. In: Cousins MJ., Bridenbaugh, PO (eds). Neural Blockade in Clinical Anesthesia and Management of Pain. Third ed., Philadelphia, Lippincott 1998 (in press).
2. Liu S, Carpenter RL, Neal JM. Epidural anesthesia and analgesia: Their role in postoperative outcome. Anesthesiology 1995;82:1474-1506.

3. Chambrier C, Chassard D, Bienvenu J, et al. Cytokine and hormonal changes after cholecystectomy. Ann Surg 1996;224:178-182.

4. Bernard GR, Arthur PW, Russell JA, et al. The effects of ibuprofen on the physiology and survival of patients with sepsis. N Engl J Med 1997;336:912-919.

5. Eriksson-Mjöberg M, Kristiansson M, Carlström K, et al. Preoperative infiltration of bupivacaine - effects on pain relief and trauma response (cortisol and interleukin-6). Acta Anaesthesiol Scand 1997;41:466-472.

6. Schulze S, Andersen J, Overgaard H, et al. Effect of prednisolone on the systemic response and wound healing after colonic surgery. Arch Surg 1997;132:129-135.

7. Rasmussen S, Larsen AS, Thomsen ST, et al. Intraarticular glucocorticoid reduces pain, inflammatory response and convalescence after arthroscopic meniscectomy (submitted).

8. Mangano DT, Siliciano D, Hollenberg M, et al. Postoperative myocardial ischemia: therapeutic trials using intensive analgesia following surgery. Anesthesiology 1992;76:342-353.

9. Tayler NM, Lacoumenta S, Hall GM, et al. Fentanyl and the inter-leukin-6 response to surgery. Anaesthesia 1997;52:112-115.

10. Breslow MJ, Parker SD, Frank SM, et al. Determinants of cate-cholamine and cortisol responses to lower extremity revasculariza-tion. Anesthesiology 1993;79:1202-1209.

11. Chaney MA, Smith KR, Barclay JC, et al. Large-dose intrathecal mor-phine for coronary artery bypass grafting. Anesth Analg 1996;83:215-222.

12. Eisenach JC, de Kock M, Klimscha W. Alpha-2 adrenergic agonists for regional anesthesia - a clinical review of clonidine. Anesthesiology 1996;85:655-674.

13. Lyons FM, Bew S, Sheeran P et al. Effects of clonidine on the pituitary hormonal response to pelvic surgery. Br J Anaesth 1997;78:134-137.

14. Scott NB, James K, Murphy M, et al. Continuous thoracic epidural analgesia versus combined spinal/thoracic epidural analgesia on pain, pulmonary function and the metabolic response following colonic resection. Acta Anaesthesiol Scand 1996;40:691-696.

15. Segawa H, Mori K, Kasai K, et al. The role of the phrenic nerves in stress response in upper abdominal surgery. Anesth Analg 1996;82:1215-24.

16. Moore CM, Cross MH, Desborough JP, et al. Hormonal effects of thoracic extradural analgesia for cardiac surgery. Br J Anaesth 1995;75:387-393.

17. Katz J, Clairoux M, Kavanagh BP. Pre-emptive lumbar epidural anaesthesia reduces postoperative pain and patient-controlled morphine consumption after lower abdominal surgery. Pain 1994; 59;395-403.

18. Carli F, Kulkarni P, Webster JD, et al. Post-surgery epidural blockade with local anaesthetics attenuates the catecholamine and thermo-

genic response to perioperative hypothermia. Acta Anaesthesiol Scand 1995;39;1041-1047.

19. Carli F, Phil M, Halliday D. Modulation of protein metabolism in the surgical patient. Reg Anesth 1996;21:430-435.

20. Carli F, Phil M, Halliday D. Continuous epidural blockade arrests the postoperative decrease in muscle protein fractional synthetic rate in surgical patients. Anesthesiology 1997;86:1033-1040.

VISCERAL PAIN AND VISCERAL HYPERALGESIA

G. F. Gebhart

INTRODUCTION

It is widely appreciated that visceral pain differs in several important ways from more commonly experienced and better understood pain arising from cutaneous structures. Visceral pain is diffuse in nature, poorly localized and typically referred to cutaneous and/or other somatic structures. Most importantly, visceral pain is not linked to tissue injury as is cutaneous pain. Because few clinical or basic scientists have in the past focused on the study of visceral pain, knowledge specific to visceral pain (as opposed to cutaneous pain, for which models were readily available) was slow to accumulate. However, recent developments have led to better understanding of visceral pain (see chapters in 1).

VISCERAL HYPERALGESIA

As they usually do, clinical observations led the way to changes in the way in which visceral pain is considered today. In 1973, Ritchie documented that irritable bowel syndrome patients reported pain at lower volumes of balloon distention of the colon than did normal subjects (see Figure 1). Less than 10% of normal subjects reported pain at a distending volume of about 60ml whereas greater than 50% of irritable bowel patients reported pain at the same distending volume. It has also been documented that the areas of referred sensation in irritable bowel patients are significantly greater in size than in normal patients when the colon is distended. Results such as these were subsequently confirmed by others and also extended to other hollow viscera in patients with other of the so-called functional bowel disorders (non-cardiac chest pain, non-ulcer dyspepsia, and irritable bowel syndrome). Similar outcomes would likely be obtained in other circumstances such as associated with interstitial cystitis. Currently, it is considered that the altered sensations, principally

T. H. Stanley et al. (eds.), Pain Management and Anesthesiology, 75–79.

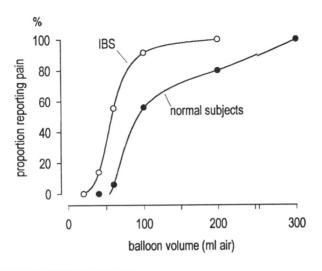

Figure 1. Illustration of human visceral hyperalgesia. In 1973, Ritchie reported that balloon distention of the colon in irritable bowel syndrome (IBS) patients produced pain in a greater proportion of patients, at any volume of distention tested, than the same volumes of distention in normal subjects.

discomfort and pain, associated with these disorders represent visceral hyperalgesia (2,3). If this hypothesis is correct, then visceral afferent fibers should exhibit sensitization and the spinal neurons on which they terminate should undergo a change in excitability.

BASIC ANATOMY

The viscera are innervated by vagal and spinal afferent pathways comprised principally of thinly myelinated Ad-fibers and unmyelinated C-fibers. Although the focus of this presentation is on visceral pain, it should be understood that most activity in visceral afferent fibers, whether in vagal afferent fibers or spinal afferent fibers, does not reach consciousness. For example, there is regularly input into the central nervous system from gastric and hepatic chemoreceptors, aortic baroreceptors, etc. that are not perceived. Visceral afferent fibers innervate mucosa, muscle and serosa layers of viscera and exhibit chemosensitivity, thermosensitivity and mechanosensitivity. It has become clear in recent years that visceral afferent fibers are generally polymodal in character and thus may represent a phylogenetically older sensory apparatus than the well defined receptors associated with cutaneous structures. The cell bodies of visceral afferent neurons, like the cell bodies of cutaneous afferent neurons, are located in dorsal root ganglia. However, the route visceral afferent neurons take to the spinal cord typically involves passage through or near pre-vertebral ganglia (where they can give off collateral axons to influence autonomic ganglion cell bodies and, accordingly, secretory and motor function and para-vertebral ganglia. In contrast to afferent fibers arising from somatic structures, the number of spinal visceral afferent fibers is estimated to be only 2-10% of the total spinal afferent input from all sources. Some compensation for this low number is provided by the significantly greater rostral-caudal intraspinal spread of visceral afferent fiber terminals (relative to cutaneous afferent fiber terminals). Finally, the spinal neurons upon which visceral afferent fibers terminate typically also receive convergent cutaneous and/or other deep input (e.g., from muscle or other viscera).

VISCERAL NOCICEPTION

Experimentally, balloon distention is the most reliable stimulus for hollow visceral organs and is the most widely used stimulus in both human and non-human animal experiments. Accordingly, we know most about the response properties for mechanosensitive visceral afferent fibers, usually those innervating the muscle layer. The past decade has documented that the hollow viscera are innervated by two populations of mechanosensitive afferent fibers: a larger group (70-80%) of fibers have low thresholds for response and a smaller group (20-30%) of afferent fibers have high thresholds for response (e.g., >30 mmHg distending pressure). It was long argued that the viscera were innervated by a homogenous population of afferent fibers and that pain was encoded in the discharge frequency of the afferent neurons. We now know that almost hollow viscera studied (esophagus, gall bladder, stomach, urinary bladder, colon, uterus) in a number of different species that have been studied are innervated by a population of afferents that do not begin to respond until the distending stimulus intensity is in the range of pressures associated with production of pain. Whether these afferent fibers are nociceptors, which are best studied in skin, is currently a matter of debate.

SENSITIZATION AND SILENT NEURONS

Cutaneous nociceptors, but not non-nociceptors, are characterized by their ability to be sensitized. By sensitization is meant an increase in response magnitude to a noxious stimulus or a reduction in the threshold at which an afferent neuron responds. Sensitization is also typically associated with induction of spontaneous activity of afferent fibers. Sensitization, which is a key component in the development of primary hyperalgesia, is produced by the wide variety of chemical mediators that are released at the site of tissue injury, synthesized at the site of tissue injury, or attracted to the site of injury and include prostaglandins, histamine, serotonin, cytokines, peptides such as substance P, neurotrophins, etc. It has recently been documented that visceral afferent fibers can also be sensitized experimentally (Figure 2).

visceral afferent fibers sensitize

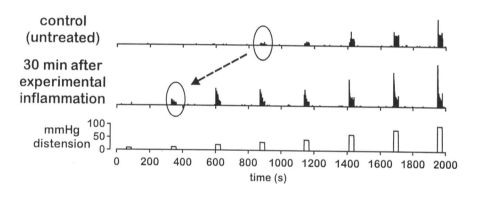

Figure 2. Illustration of sensitization of a pelvic nerve afferent fiber after experimental inflammation of the colon in the rat. In skin, nociceptors are characterized by their ability to sensitize when tissue is injured. When nociceptors sensitize, they typically exhibit a reduced threshold for activation and often also acquire spontaneous activity. In this example, the response threshold of the fiber is shown to be significantly reduced after inflammation of the colon. In addition, response magnitude to colonic distention is increased. Accordingly, visceral afferent fibers will respond to stimuli that are in the normal physiologic range and the afferent barrage arriving in the spinal cord will be greater than normal.

Because low threshold and high threshold mechanosensitive visceral afferent fibers can become sensitized during experimental visceral inflammation, there is debate whether the viscera are innervated by nociceptors and non-nociceptors (as opposed to the concept that all afferent fibers that innervate the viscera can convey nociceptive information).

Regardless, sensitization of visceral afferent fibers results in increased afferent input to the spinal cord and contributes to altered sensation. Tissue injury or visceral inflammation can also contribute to increased afferent input to the spinal cord by activation of previously silent or "sleeping" afferent fibers. It has been shown that mechanically insensitive cutaneous or visceral afferent fibers acquire spontaneous activity and mechanical sensitivity after tissue injury or inflammation. Activity in these newly discovered afferent fibers adds to the total afferent barrage entering the spinal cord.

CENTRAL SENSITIZATION

One consequence of the increased afferent barrage is increased release in the spinal cord of neurotransmitters such as glutamate and substance P. The increased release of glutamate and substance P from visceral afferent fiber terminals in the spinal cord increases the excitability of second order spinal neurons. These spinal neurons become more easily excitable, including from a wider area in the periphery (which likely explains the increased area of referral associated with balloon distention in irritable bowel patients). In addition to the increase in size of peripheral receptive fields, there is likely also an increased sensitivity to previously sub-threshold intensities of stimulation. This phenomenon has been termed "central sensitization" and can lead to altered sensations that may outlive the period of increased afferent barrage.

Thus, visceral afferent fibers and the spinal neurons upon which they terminate undergo similar changes in sensitivity that have been better documented to date in models of cutaneous nociception. It would appear that visceral hyperalgesia is analogous to cutaneous hyperalgesia and is mediated by similar, if not the same mechanisms.

REFERENCES

1   Gebhart GF: Visceral Pain Mechanisms. In: Current Emerging Issues in Cancer Pain: Research Practice (Chapman and Foley, eds.), Raven Press, New York, 1993, pp. 99-111.

2. Gebhart GF (ed.): Visceral Pain, IASP Press, Seattle, 1995, pp. 516.

3. Mayer EA, Gebhart GF: Basic and Clinical Aspects of Visceral Hyperalgesia. Gastroenterology 1994;107:271-293.

POSTOPERATIVE PAIN: ASSESSMENT AND CHOICE OF METHODS OF TREATMENT

L. B. Ready

MEASUREMENT OF ACUTE PAIN

Sound approaches to acute pain treatment must include appropriate assessment. A number of instruments that can be used at the bedside to evaluate pain and thereby gauge the success or failure of a particular treatment plan (see Appendix). These include subjective reports from patients, both qualitative and quantitative, as well as objective observations by the pain therapist including the effect of therapy on important functions such as the ability to breathe deeply, cough, move in bed, or ambulate. Additional insight can be gained by asking the simple question: "Are you satisfied with the treatment of your pain?" It is important that any measurement scale be applied both before and after treatment so that the effects of treatment (success or failure) can be measured.

THERAPEUTIC PRINCIPLES

Any treatment plan should include consideration of the natural history of acute pain, and should be flexible with regard to changing needs. The following four principles of therapy for acute pain should be identified and applied to all treatment plans:
1. Determine the source and magnitude of nociception.
2. Understand the relationship between ongoing nociception and other components of suffering (anxiety, ethnocultural components, meaning of pain, etc.) and provide therapy for these components as necessary.
3. Establish adequate drug levels to achieve and maintain analgesia.
4. Reevaluate and refine therapy regularly based on the needs of individual patients.

T. H. Stanley et al. (eds.), Pain Management and Anesthesiology, 81–94.

OPTIONS FOR THE TREATMENT OF ACUTE PAIN

SYSTEMIC OPIOIDS

Opioids produce analgesia as a result of their agonist effects on opiate receptors in the central nervous system. Effective doses of appropriate drugs can be administered by the oral, rectal, transdermal, or sublingual route, or by subcutaneous, intramuscular, or intravenous injection or infusion. Because intramuscular opioid injection is such an unpredictable delivery system, effective and safe analgesia requires careful ongoing assessment of patients, with adjustments in doses and frequency of administration until individual care is optimized. Intravenous opioid infusions can abolish wide swings in drug concentration and permit prompt titration to the needs of individual patients.

Oral opioids in appropriate doses are remarkably effective. Frequently they can be used in place of parenteral drugs 12-24 hours after superficial surgery, and after some intra-abdominal procedures as soon as oral intake is established. Placing oral analgesics at the bedside can improve analgesia by permitting patients to choose the dose and frequency of administration best suited to their individual needs.

Transdermal delivery of fentanyl, a synthetic opioid, after surgery has been demonstrated to be effective (1-4). This method of opioid administration avoids the discomfort of injections and offers a useful alternative for patients unable or unwilling to swallow oral medications. Therapeutic blood levels are achieved, and the usual side effects associated with opioid administration are seen.

PATIENT-CONTROLLED ANALGESIA

Over the past decade, intravenous patient controlled analgesia (PCA) using opioids rapidly achieved widespread use for the treatment of postoperative and other forms of acute pain. Most hospitals in the United States now make PCA available (5). Like many innovations which initially appear to be quite simple, PCA has produced interesting and unexpected questions in the areas of science, clinical practice, economics, politics, and the law.

Advantages of patient-controlled analgesia have been documented in numerous studies and are obvious to all therapists who listen to their patients. They include no waiting when pain relief is needed, no painful IM injections, the ability to match drug delivery to times of need, and the confidence felt when "control" of medicating decisions resides with patients themselves. Clearly, PCA addresses the large interpatient variability in opioid need found in any population of patient in pain.

There are a number of publications reporting the incidence of respiratory depression using PCA at academic centers with anesthesiology-based pain services (6-9). In reviewing these reports, it is noted that the commonest identifiable cause of respiratory depression is pump programming errors, particularly when the continuous mode is used.

REGIONAL ANESTHETIC TECHNIQUES

A variety of neural blockade techniques continued into the post-operative period can result in effective and safe analgesia. These include topical application, local infiltration of incisions with long-acting local anesthetics (10-12), blockade of peripheral nerves or plexuses, and continuous block techniques at various sites in the periphery or neuraxis. Postoperative local anesthetic infusions into the brachial plexus sheath (13), femoral sheath (14), lumbar plexus, and sciatic nerve have been used to maintain analgesia and sympathetic blockade after a variety of surgical procedures. Spinal anesthesia can provide analgesia for several hours after the completion of surgery if long-acting agents are used. Continuous epidural anesthesia through a catheter offers several options for postoperative analgesia. Local anesthetic boluses or infusions can provide profound analgesia, improved bowel function, higher arterial oxygen tension, and fewer pulmonary complications. Many regional anesthetic techniques can be adapted for use in infants and children.

EPIDURAL ANALGESIA

Following initial reports in 1979 of the clinical efficacy of intrathecal and epidural opioids, they have been used to control pain following a wide variety of surgical procedures (15). Intrathecal opioids have the appeal of ease of administration, either at the time of intrathecal local anesthetic injection for surgical anesthesia, or as a separate technique when general anesthesia is administered. Many patients will remain comfortable for 24 hours or more after a single injection of intrathecal morphine.

The epidural route has been used much more extensively for postoperative pain control. Every opioid that is available has been used in the epidural space. In the United States the commonest agents are morphine, fentanyl, sufentanil, hydromorphone and meperidine. The features of epidural analgesia mediated by opioids include potent analgesia (with improved outcomes in some patients), absence of sympathetic, sensory, or motor block, and little chance of masking serious postoperative complications.

Hydrophilic opioids such as morphine and hydromorphone produce effective analgesia at a fraction of the equipotent systemic dose (16). In the case of morphine, a single dose of 3-5 mg will be effective within 45 minutes and will last 6-12 hours. Such a profile is well suited to a bolus dosing schedule.

A lipophilic agent such as fentanyl can be useful when rapid onset of analgesia and/or short duration of effect is needed. Intermittent epidural boluses of 50-100 micrograms can achieve analgesia that begins in 5-10 minutes and last 60-120 minutes. Fentanyl's short duration of action makes it unsuitable for bolus administration but it can be used as a continuous infusion of 25-100 micrograms per hour (17,18). The predominant site of analgesic action using such infusions of fentanyl is likely systemic in most clinical situations and current evidence favors the position that epidural fentanyl has little, if any advantage over the same dose given systemically. Sufentanil has no clinical advantages over other lipid-soluble opioids for epidural administration.

Epidural opioids used alone are imperfect. They commonly cause a variety of side effects, they have not been as effective as hoped in patients with opioid tolerance, and they do not consistently block the metabolic-endocrine stress response. The side effects seen most commonly are itching, nausea and vomiting, urinary retention, and sedation (especially with lipid-soluble opioids). Delayed respiratory depression in patients receiving intraspinal opioids has been attributed to the rostral spread of drug in cerebrospinal fluid. The target site is thought to be the respiratory center located superficially in the floor of the fourth ventricle. The actual incidence of this event is not known. Current estimates are dependent on a number of factors including the populations studied, how they are monitored, and the definitions of respiratory depression used. In a large, multi-institutional Swedish questionnaire survey in 1987, the incidence of events defined as "requiring treatment with naloxone" was 0.09% (19). It has been assumed that the risk of severe respiratory depression is greater after intraspinal opioids than following opioid administration by more conventional routes. In 860 hospitalized patients receiving morphine orally or parenterally (IV, IM, SC), a 0.9% incidence of "life-threatening respiratory depression" was seen (20)—that is, ten times higher that in the Swedish survey! Respiratory depression can certainly occur but it should be a rare event in modern practice. It is now well established that the regular bedside evaluation of respiratory rate and level of sedation can be a reliable approach to identifying impending respiratory depression. By using appropriate guidelines, epidural opioids can be used safely throughout an institution (21). These guidelines apply within or outside the ICU setting:

1. Careful patient selection with modification of opioid doses for patient age and physical status.
2. Regular follow-up by skilled and knowledgeable physicians.
3. Sound education of all nursing personnel regarding use and risks of intraspinal opioids including instruction in bedside monitoring techniques which ensure early detection of respiratory depression.
4. Provision of periodic nursing education updates.
5. The use of printed protocols and standard orders developed jointly by physicians and nurses to govern the use of epidural opioids, including those permitting immediate intervention by nurses, if necessary.
6. Provision of a support system within the hospital which is capable of providing immediate airway management and ventilatory support at all times.
7. Continuing quality assurance review of all problems.

Epidural local anesthetics used alone can obviously provide excellent postoperative analgesia. Since their mechanism of action does not depend on a responsive opioid receptor, they will usually remain effective in the presence of underlying opioid tolerance. Epidural local anesthetics can at least partially block the metabolic-endocrine stress response including the undesirable catabolic events associated with major surgery (22).

Epidural local anesthetics are also imperfect. An infusion of a local anesthetic can lead to accumulation and subsequent toxicity. Further, the block produced not only involves nociception, but also causes dose-related effects on sympathetic, sensory, and motor nerve fibers, and associated problems for the recovering surgical patient (Table 1). Although tachyphylaxis would logically be expected to occur, this has usually not been problematic when long-acting amide local anesthetics are employed. Monitoring strategies for patients receiving an epidural local anesthetic must incorporate methods of early detection of these effects.

The rationale for combining epidural opioids and local anesthetics is to use lower doses of each drug, preserve effective analgesia, and reduce the side effects and problems associated with the use of the individual drugs. Some degree of blunting of the stress response may also be possible. While the opioid molecules in the mixture act by inhibiting the release of

Table 1. Possible problems with epidural local anesthetic techniques.

Function Blocked	Possible Problem
Sympathetic	Hypotension (thoracic > lumbar)
Proprioception	Difficulty ambulating
Sensory	Pressure injury Mask a complication
Motor	Loss of function (cough, ambulation)

substance P in the dorsal horn of the spinal cord, the local anesthetic molecules block transmission of impulses at the nerve axonal membrane level. These two distinctive actions may contribute to the synergy of analgesic effect that has been demonstrated with opioid/local anesthetic mixtures.

Bupivacaine is the most widely used local anesthetic for postoperative analgesia because of its tendency to preferentially block sensory fibers with relative sparing of motor fibers. Dilute bupivacaine solutions can therefore provide analgesia while preserving the ability of some patient to ambulate. Figure 1 shows the frequency of motor block limiting ambulation using either lumbar or thoracic epidural catheters at the University of

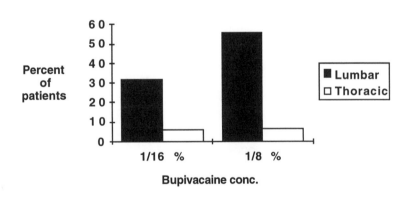

Figure 1. Motor block impairing ambulation using epidural bupivacaine infusions.

Washington Medical Center. In the future, it is possible that ropivacaine will provide analgesia similar to bupivacaine with even less impact on motor function.

A variety of opioids are commonly combined with bupivacaine. The commonest in the United States are fentanyl and morphine. Concentrations vary widely in the hands of different users. Monitoring of patients receiving epidural mixtures of opioids and local anesthetics should include strategies to detect side effects or problems associated with both components.

Epidural analgesic techniques are not all equal in efficacy. Table 2 shows the author's impression of the relative efficacy of a number of epidural drugs used alone or in combination. Among the factors which predict a need for greater efficacy are site and type of surgery, patient age, and prior opioid tolerance. In general, the more effective a drug or combination, the more frequent and severe the side effects and problems they may cause.

Table 2. Relative efficacy of epidural agents.

Effective	More Effective	Most Effective
Fentanyl $\leq 75\ \mu g/h$	Fentanyl $\geq 100\ \mu g/h$	Morphine
Meperidine ≤ 10 mg/h	Meperidine ≤ 20 mg/h	Bupiv 0.125% + fentanyl 4 μg/ml
Bupiv 0.0625% + fentanyl 2 μg/ml	Bupiv 0.0625% + fentanyl 4 μg/ml	Bupiv 0.25%
	Bupiv 0.125%	

PSYCHOLOGICAL AND OTHER METHODS

Following surgery, patients may suffer "discomfort" from causes unrelated to their incisions. Some of these may be physical, such as headaches or sensations arising from nasogastric tubes, surgical drains, and intravenous catheters. Others will be the result of non-organic causes such as anxiety, fear, or insomnia. Therapy for these latter problems can enhance patients' overall sense of well-being and, in some cases result in less "pain" being reported.

A number of studies have shown that psychological support in the form of discussion, reassurance, and the provision of information preoperatively result in less anxiety, less opioid use after surgery, and a shorter hospital stay compared with control groups (23-25). Hospitals are designed usually for the convenience of the staff, and sometimes leave patients feeling "depersonalized" and helpless. Measures which restore freedom, control, and participation in care, even involving simple self-care tasks, are likely to be beneficial.

No currently available approach to postoperative pain control achieves these goals in all patients after all kinds of surgery. Regardless of how analgesia is provided, compromises are frequently necessary.

MAKING THE CHOICE

Needless to say, the optimal use of any technique requires knowledge, skill, experience, and attentiveness to individual patient responses. With these elements, a variety of approaches to the treatment of postoperative pain can produce satisfactory results. By contrast, even with the most modern and sophisticated techniques, ordering the same analgesic doses and administration intervals for all patients while failing to regularly assess their efficacy will yield sub-optimal results. It is beyond the scope of this section to consider all available forms of therapy for postoperative pain. Major emphasis will be given to factors which should influence the choice between two of the newer methods of pain control—patient-controlled analgesia (PCA) and epidural opioid analgesia (EOA). In choosing the best technique, a number of factors must be considered. These can be categorized as: 1) clinical, 2) patient-related, and, 3) institutional factors.

CLINICAL FACTORS

It is well know that certain surgical procedures result in more pain than others. Incisions involving the upper abdomen or thorax are expected to cause more pain than operations on the hand or foot. The postoperative pain therapist should be aware of the growing evidence that although PCA produces analgesia that is frequently superior to intramuscular narcotics given on an "as needed" basis, it may not produce as much pain relief as EOA. Two studies report this finding in women following cesarean section (26,27), while the same observation has been made after open knee surgery (28) and after cholecystectomy (29) For some patients, the additional analgesia available with EOA may be of critical importance. This is particularly true when severe pain may compromise pulmonary function leading to atelectasis and pneumonia. Examples include patients with rib fractures or pain resulting from abdominal and thoracic incisions. Those with underlying medical conditions such as respiratory insufficiency or obesity may also derive particular benefit from the best available analgesia. In these situations, the need for profound analgesia is of major importance and may make EOA the preferred choice.

Other factors may favor the selection of PCA for analgesia. It does not require the extra time and skill that is necessary for the anesthesiologist to place epidural catheters. The question of who will reinject epidural catheters day and night does not apply. The time required to educate ward nurses is less for PCA than for EOA. In some patient populations side effects such as nausea, pruritus, and urinary retention are more common and more severe with EOA than with PCA.

Certain clinical issues in patient selection remain controversial. What approach for postoperative pain control should be recommended in patients with narcotic tolerance and/or drug-seeking behavior? This subject will be discussed in another presentation.

Another area of controversy involves the management of postoperative pain in patients with coagulopathies or who are scheduled to receive anticoagulants to facilitate vascular or cardiac surgery. EOA may be of great benefit to some of these patients, but is it safe? There is no clear scientific answer. Each patient should be considered individually with careful weighing of possible risks and expected benefits.

Although EOA and PCA can result in improved analgesia, both techniques are associated with a number of side effects. With EOA, pruritus, nausea and vomiting, and urinary retention are common. Sedation occurs infrequently. With PCA, the same side effects occur but in many situations they tend to be less frequent and less severe. Both techniques can result in respiratory depression which, if not recognized early, can be life-threatening. It is beyond the scope of this article to discuss these side effects in detail. Frequently they can be prevented or controlled, but when they occur they can be a major determinant of patient comfort and satisfaction with the management of their postoperative pain.

Effective methods for controlling pain are associated with risks. Traditional fears of addiction to opioids in hospitalized patients with acute pain are unfounded and are not a justifiable reason to withhold adequate analgesia (20). Lack of understanding of the nature of opioid-induced respiratory depression has also lead to inadequate analgesia in countless patients. With well organized clinical services established to provide modern analgesia, the risks associated with EOA and PCA may be no higher than with intramuscular narcotic injections. Careful patient selection, appropriate choice of drugs and dosage, nurse education, and adequate medical supervision can result in the safe application of both these methods throughout a modern hospital.

PATIENT-RELATED FACTORS

Each patient facing surgery is a unique human being. Many will harbor concerns, fears, expectations, recollections of previous experience with pain, preferences, and possibly, limitations. These factors alone or in combination may be of paramount importance when choosing a method of pain control. For example, although epidural morphine might produce superior analgesia after a major abdominal operation, a patient with a morbid fear of "a needle in the back" may be better treated in some other way. Or, a patient scheduled for a procedure ordinarily well suited to PCA will not obtain satisfactory analgesia if he or she is unwilling, or does not have the mental capacity to self-administer medication for pain.

Most people admitted to hospital for surgery are accustomed to an independent life style. On arrival in hospital, basic human rights involving eating, mobility, privacy, and even control over bodily functions may be taken over by hospital staff. Uncertainty about what to expect, fear about the surgery, and isolation from a familiar and controllable environment are compounded by the sudden experience of a new source of stress - postoperative pain. PCA allows patients to self-administer an analgesic, giving back, at least in one area, a sense of control over their care. Without having to negotiate with others for pain medication, more immediate pain relief is obtained. For people who are distressed by loss of "control" in the hospital setting, PCA will be greatly appreciated and viewed as superior to other methods that involve less control.

By contrast, some patients enter hospital with the belief and expectation that their needs should be evaluated and met by their doctors and nurses. Such patients are likely to be threatened by PCA and the responsibility they must assume to treat their own pain. Their fears and concerns are likely to lead to inadequate pain control. Such patients are likely to be more comfortable receiving EOA or other forms of therapy that require the doctors and nurses to regularly assess pain and administer doses of drugs as they judge them to be necessary.

INSTITUTIONAL FACTORS

New services developed to improve the treatment of acute pain in hospitalized patients have been described and are of current interest to anesthesiologists. Establishing such a service involves a considerable administrative commitment. It includes a close liaison with nurses to develop appropriate educational and procedural standards, as well as interactions with surgeons, hospital pharmacists, and those providing the surgical anesthetics. A well-planned and organized service is essential to optimal comfort and safety using EOA, PCA, and other methods of therapy. Until such organized care is possible, it may be best to delay introduction of sophisticated methods of pain control.

REFERENCES

1. Caplan RA, Ready LB, Oden RV, Matsen FA, Nessly ML, Olsson GL: Safety and efficacy of transdermal fentanyl for postoperative pain management: a double-blind study. JAMA 261:1036-1039, 1989
2. Sevarino FB, Naulty JS, Sinatra R, Chin ML, Paige D, Conry K, Silverman DG: Transdermal fentanyl for postoperative pain management in patients recovering from abdominal gynecological surgery. Anesthesiology 77:463-466, 1992
3. Rung G, Graf G, Riemondy S, Failner B, Kauffman G, Mostrom J: Transdermal fentanyl for analgesia after upper abdominal surgery. Anesth Analg 76:S362, 1993
4. Sandler AN, Baxter AD, Katz J, Samson B, Friedlander M, Norman P, Koren G, Roger S, Hull K, Klein J: A double-blind, placebo-controlled trial of transdermal fentanyl after abdominal hysterectomy. Analgesia, respiratory, and pharmacokinetic effects. Anesthesiology 81:1169-1180, 1994
5. Ready LB: How many acute pain services are there in the United States and who is managing patient-controlled analgesia? (letter). Anesthesiology 82:322, 1995
6. Fleming BM, Coombs DW: A survey of complications documented in a quality-control analysis of patient-controlled analgesia in the postoperative patient. J Pain Symptom Manage 7:463-469, 1992
7. Schug SA, Torrie JJ: Safety assessment of postoperative pain management by an acute pain service. Pain 55:387-391, 1993
8. Ashburn MA, Love G, Pace NL: Respiratory-related critical events with intravenous patient-controlled analgesia. Clinical Journal of Pain 10:52-56, 1994
9. Etches RC: Respiratory depression associated with patient-controlled analgesia: a review of eight cases. Can J Anaesth 41:125-132, 1994
10. Jebeles JA, Reilly JS, Gutierrez JF, Bradley EL, Kissin I: The effect of pre-incisional infiltration of tonsils with bupivacaine on the pain following tonsillectomy under general anesthesia. Pain 47:305-308, 1991
11. Ejlersen E, Andersen HB, Eliasen K, Mogensen T: A comparison between preincisional and postincisional lidocaine infiltration and postoperative pain. Anesth Analg 74:495-498, 1992
12. Ding Y, White PF: Post-herniorrhaphy pain in outpatients after pre-incision ilioinguinal-hypogastric nerve block during monitored anaesthesia care. Can J Anaesth 42:12-15, 1995
13. Selander D: Catheter technique in axillary plexus block. Acta Anaesthesiol Scand 21:324, 1977
14. Rosenblatt RM: Continuous femoral anesthesia for extremity surgery. Anesth Analg 59:631, 1980

15. Cousins MJ, Mather LE: Intrathecal and epidural administration of opiates. Anesthesiology 61:276-310, 1984
16. Rawal N, Sjöstrand U, Christoffersson E, Dahlström B, Arvill A, Rydman H: Comparison of intramuscular and epidural morphine for postoperative analgesia in the grossly obese: influence on postoperative ambulation and pulmonary function. Anesth Analg 63:583-592, 1984
17. Chein BB, Burke RG, Hunter DL: An extensive experience with post-operative pain relief using postoperative fentanyl infusion. Arch Surg 126:692-695, 1991
18. Harukuni I, Yamaguchi H, Sata S, Naito H: The comparison of epidural fentanyl, epidural lidocaine, and intravenous fentanyl in patients undergoing gastrectomy. Anesth Analg 81:1169-1174, 1995
19. Rawal N, Arnér S, Gustafsson LL, Allvin R: Present state of extradural and intrathecal opioid analgesia in Sweden: a nationwide follow-up survey. Br J Anaesth 59:791-799, 1987
20. Miller RR, Greenblatt DJ: Drug Effects in Hospitalized Patients. New York: John Wiley and Sons, 1976, pp 151-152
21. Ready LB, Loper KA, Nessly M, Wild L: Postoperative epidural morphine is safe on surgical wards. Anesthesiology 75:452-456, 1991
22. Kehlet H: Pain relief and modification of the stress response. Acute Pain Management. Edited by Cousins, MJ, Phillips, GD. New York: Churchill Livingstone, 1986, pp 49-75
23. Egbert LD, Battit GE, Turndorf H, Beecher HK: The value of the preoperative visit by an anesthesiologist. JAMA 185:553-555, 1963
24. Egbert LD, Battit GE, Welch CE, Bartlett MK: Reduction of postoperative pain by encouragement and instruction of patients. N Engl J Med 270:825-825, 1964
25. Schmitt FE: Psychological preparation in surgical patients. Nurs Res 22:108-116, 1973
26. Eisenach JC, Grice SC, Dewan DM: Patient-controlled analgesia following cesarean section: a comparison with epidural and intramuscular narcotics. Anesthesiology 68:444-448, 1988
27. Harrison DM, Sinatra R, Morgese L, Chung JH: Epidural narcotic and patient-controlled analgesia for post-cesarean section pain relief. Anesthesiology 68:454-457, 1988
28. Loper KA, Ready LB: Epidural morphine after anterior cruciate ligament repair: a comparison with patient-controlled intravenous morphine. Anesth Analg 68:350-352, 1989
29. Loper KA, Ready LB, Nessly M, Rapp SE: Epidural morphine provides greater pain relief than patient-controlled intravenous morphine following cholecystectomy. Anesth Analg 69:826-828, 1989

APPENDIX

TECHNIQUES FOR GRADING PAIN INTENSITY BEFORE AND AFTER TREATMENT*

TECHNIQUE	HOW PAIN IS GRADED	APPLICATION
Five point global scale	0 = none 1 = a little 2 = some 3 = a lot 4 = worst possible	Routine bedside evaluation.
Verbal quantitative scale	0 . . . . 5 . . . . 10 None Worst Possible What number describes your pain?	Routine bedside evaluation.
Visual analog scale (10 cm line, slide rule devices)	No Worst Possible Pain Pain Place a mark on the line to show how much pain you are having.	Routine bedside evaluation When "hard copy" desirable. Can be used with children age 6 years and older.
Behavioral and Physiologic Parameters	Restlessness, grimacing, vocalization, sweating, lacrimation, pupil dilatation, tachycardia, hypertension, dyscoordinate mechanical ventilation may all signs of pain. (These signs have not been validated so should be used with caution.)	Unconscious, unresponsive, confused, critically ill patients.
Observer-generated assessment of function	Can patient perform important functions associated with recovery (deep breathing, cough, spirometry, range of motion in joints, ambulation)? Yes/No.	Adjunct to patient-generated subjective pain reports. Should be used in all patients.

(Continued)

APPENDIX (CONT.)

Global satisfaction question	Are you satisfied with your pain relief? Yes/No.	Clarification of confusing responses; for unsophisticated patients.
Observer-generated pediatric pain scales	Observe facial expression, crying, cardio- respiratory responses. Compare with children who are not in pain.	Neonate to age 3 years and some age 3-6 years.
Patient-generated pediatric pain scales		Over age 6 years and some age 3-6 years.
a. <u>Pictorial</u>:		
Faces	Point at (or circle, or color) the face that shows how you feel.	
Draw a Picture of Your Pain	Estimate location, character, intensity from drawing.	
b. <u>Numeric</u>		
"Pieces of Hurt" (poker chips)	Poker chips represent pain that child can "give" to therapist.	
Hurt Thermometer	Similar to visual analogue scale for adults.	

* Many problems can be mislabelled as "pain". The reports of pain obtained using these techniques must be interpreted carefully. Pain should be assessed both at rest and during stimulation (deep breathing, coughing, ambulation).

PATIENT-CONTROLLED ANALGESIA (PART I): HISTORICAL PERSPECTIVE*

P. F. White

Despite advances in our understanding of the pathophysiology of acute postoperative pain and the pharmacology of analgesic drugs, postoperative pain is not always effectively treated. Since the early report on the under treatment of pain by Marks and Sachar (1), there are numerous publications describing inadequate management of postoperative pain (2,3). It is now recognized that under treatment of postoperative pain may be due to a number of factors related to knowledge, skills and attitudes of health care personnel, including concerns for side effects of analgesic drugs. In addition, the inherent pharmacokinetic and pharmacodynamic variability among patients contributes to differences in their analgesic requirements. Furthermore, variability in the patients' perception of pain contributes to difficulty in determining the appropriate dose of analgesic drugs.

It has been known for many years that intramuscular (IM) opioids administered either as needed or as scheduled injections are not optimally effective in relieving pain. It is difficult to accurately predict individual needs for analgesics because they are governed by a complex interplay of pharmacokinetic, pharmacodynamic, anthropometric, and personality factors. In addition, there is a progressive decline in the need for analgesics during the postoperative course. Individualization of analgesic therapy is crucial in treatment of postoperative pain. Patient-controlled analgesia (PCA) allows titration of analgesic drugs to the individual patients' requirements and is designed to accommodate the wide range of analgesic requirements that can be anticipated when managing postoperative pain (4). The use of PCA systems in the postoperative period has become increasingly popular for hospitalized patients over the past 15 years. The development of sophisticated microcircuitry for electronic PCA devices, and simplified non-electronic PCA devices, as well as a better understanding of the pharmacologic and patient characteristics influencing the

*Adapted from Joshi GP, White PF. Patient-Controlled Analgesia (Chapter 35). In Management of Acute Pain (M Ashburn and LJ Rice, Editors), New York: Churchill Livingston, 1997; pp 1-35.

T. H. Stanley et al. (eds.), Pain Management and Anesthesiology, 95–101.

efficacy of PCA has lead to an explosion of interest in the use of PCA as an analgesic modality for both hospitalized and ambulatory patients.

HISTORICAL BASIS FOR PCA THERAPY

The concept of "demand analgesia" was first described by Sechzer in 1968 when he described the administration of intravenous (IV) opioids for postoperative analgesia in small incremental doses on patient demand by a nurse observer. Sechzer observed that this "demand analgesia" system provided improved pain relief with smaller total drug dosages than conventional IM therapy. It was also noted that the postoperative analgesic requirement was cyclical and varied considerably among patients. Another early clinical application of PCA was described by Scott who allowed obstetrical patients to control their own IV infusion rate of meperidine to achieve pain relief. In 1970, Forrest and colleagues described an experimental device (Demand Dropmaster, Stanford, CA) that automatically administered IV analgesic drugs when activated by pressing a button on a handgrip. Shortly thereafter, instruments allowing patients to self-administer small IV doses of opioids were introduced and tested for clinical use. These early PCA devices consisted of electronically controlled infusion pumps connected to timing devices that could be activated by the patient using a thumb button. When triggered, the PCA device delivered a preset amount of opioid analgesic medication. Despite the primitive nature of the initial PCA devices, most patients were able to safely and effectively control the administration IV opioid analgesics and achieve effective pain relief. The use of demand analgesia (versus conventional IM therapy) decreased the incidence of substantial postoperative pain from 20-40% to less than 5%. When the demand analgesia group returned to IM therapy, the incidence of inadequate analgesia increased to 30% even though many of these patients received larger amount of analgesic medication.

The essential features of a PCA device should include: 1) a secure drug reservoir of sufficient capacity that allows repeated doses of analgesic drugs without the intervention of a nurse or physician, 2) an accurate infusion pump that is able to deliver a prescribed dose of analgesic drugs, 3) a remote activation push button with which the patient can trigger the device, 4) a microprocessor that allows programming of a variable demand (bolus) dose that is delivered in response to the patient demand, 5) a delay or lockout interval between successive doses to prevent the patient from administering a second dose until they perceived the effect of the pervious dose, and 6) a connecting tubing system which prevents drug siphoning (e.g., back-check valve).

The Cardiff Palliator (Graseby Dynamics Ltd.) was the first commercially available PCA device that was developed by investigators at the Welsh National School of Medicine. It utilized digital electronics to control the dose and lockout interval and had a interfacing microprocessor-based annotating chart recorder. In the mid-1970s more sophisticated microprocessor-controlled PCA devices, the On-Demand Analgesia Computer (ODAC, Janssen Scientific Instruments, Belgium) and the Prominject (Pharmacia AB, Sweden), with additional programmable features and integral printers were introduced for clinical use. The ODAC had a pneumograph that was used to suspend the drug administration if the patient's respiratory rate decreased below a critical value. In addition, administration of a concurrent (background) infusion that was either a fixed-rate infusion or an infusion that varied automatically according to patient's demand rate was possible with the ODAC. Subsequently several other microprocessor-based devices were developed, including the Abbott LifeCare PCA, Bard Harvard PCA, Leicester Micropalliator, and the Programmable On-Demand Analgesia Computer (PROPAC). More recently, simplified, non-electronic, disposable PCA systems have been introduced into clinical practice. These PCA devices appear to be more cost-effective for use during the postoperative period. They are well-accepted by patients and nurses in both the hospital and outpatient setting.

The first International Workshop on patient-controlled analgesia was held at Leeds Castle, England, in 1984, during which experience with these early devices was presented. Following the introduction of PCA as a new approach to postoperative pain management, there has been a widespread utilization of PCA for treatment of cancer pain, obstetric pain, and as an investigative tool (e.g., evaluation of equianalgesic dosage in drug trials and comparison of analgesic techniques). Although analgesic therapy using PCA was initially administered only via the IV route, different routes of administration (e.g., oral, intranasal, subcutaneous, or epidural) have been used to provide adequate analgesia.

EFFICACY OF PCA THERAPY

It has been proposed that for PCA to provide adequate analgesia the serum opioid concentrations should remain within a "therapeutic" window. The lower level of this so-called window represents the minimal serum concentration that provides satisfactory analgesia [minimal effective analgesic concentration (MEAC)] and the upper level represents the serum concentration at which adverse effects occur. These two concentrations vary between patients and also in the same patient over time. Age, sex, location of surgery, length of time after surgery and cardiovascular status have been implicated in altering these parameters. Importantly, the MEAC may be increased by movement or during physical therapy or decreased by distraction (e.g., electrical stimulation techniques). The administration of IM opioids intermittently yields widely fluctuating blood concentrations in phase with the dosing interval. Although continuous infusion of analgesic drugs decrease the fluctuations in the plasma concentrations and may improve the management of postoperative pain, frequent adjustments in the infusion rate would be required because of variability in the severity of pain with time.

The effectiveness of PCA therapy is based on use as a part of a feedback control system. PCA minimizes the variability in plasma concentrations because of the availability of on-demand and repetitive administration of small doses of the analgesic drugs. The patients will use the PCA when the plasma concentration falls below the MEAC and they can titrate their plasma concentrations around the MEAC to maintain consistent analgesia. Tamsen and colleagues performed several important pharmacokinetic and pharmacodynamic studies. Both the analgesic requirement and resultant therapeutic concentrations were highly variable. Neither age, sex, body weight nor the rate of drug elimination appeared to be related to the therapeutic concentrations. Relatively constant plasma concentrations were maintained by the patients when they were allowed to self-administer meperidine and morphine in the postoperative period.

IV- PCA VERSUS IM INJECTIONS

The widespread acceptance of PCA analgesia is due to the many positive reports describing its safety and efficacy. The early studies comparing IV-PCA with IM injections were flawed as these investigations were based on small samples or had included historic control groups. In addition, several studies used different analgesics in the comparator groups. Bennett and colleagues reported adequate analgesia with minimal sedation with the use of PCA. Although there was a ten-fold variation in the analgesic requirements in the obese, the use of PCA in this patient population improved postoperative pulmonary function. More importantly, these investigators found that significantly less medication was required in the postoperative period by patients receiving PCA when compared to a matched group of patients receiving IM analgesia. The same group reported significantly less pain, less sedation and greater activity in patients using PCA therapy in subjective testing after surgical procedures involving a flank incision. In one study, these investigators found evidence for a circadian variation in analgesic requirement in the postoperative period with maximal medication usage occurring in the morning and minimal usage during sleep.

Overall, PCA appears to provide superior pain relief than IM therapy. It may also have a beneficial effect on surgical outcome. For instance, Keeri-Santzo reported that PCA improved early mobilization, cooperation with physical therapy and significantly shortened hospital stay after thoracotomy in patients receiving PCA. A more recent study collaborated these findings following abdominal procedures. Compared to intermittent IM morphine, IV PCA morphine resulted in better postoperative pain control, early ambulation and rapid recovery of respiratory function, reduced the incidence of complications and early discharge from hospital with subsequent smoother convalescence at home.

Wasylak et al. proposed several explanations to account for improved recovery in PCA-treated patients. Early self-titrated pain control may alter the course of the metabolic response, reduce the deleterious side effects of opioids by avoiding high serum concentrations, and provide a more consistent matching of opioid availability to changing needs after surgery. Ready further suggested that PCA may affect the process by providing the patient with a greater sense of control. Although some studies have demonstrated that PCA improved recovery (i.e., fewer postoperative pulmonary or thromboembolic complications, shorter hospital stay), others suggest that any effective pain management strategy is equivalent in this respect. However, investigators could not demonstrate an earlier discharge with PCA following other types of surgery. Interestingly, IV-PCA was found to provide better analgesia than IM injections, but its use resulted in more fatigue and less vigor.

In a study involving elderly men, Egbert reported less confusion and lower incidence of pulmonary infections in patients receiving PCA therapy compared to IM therapy. However, the use of PCA did not significantly alter the measured psychological parameters compared with IM injections. These authors concluded that the improved analgesia was the result of pharmacologic effects, independent of psychological factors. Early studies also suggested that superior postoperative pain control with PCA therapy modifies the metabolic response to surgery. However, Moller et al. found that despite superior pain relief with PCA fentanyl compared with continuous infusion, there was no difference in the catabolic response to abdominal surgery.

Boulanger et al. observed that both IV-PCA and IM injections provided adequate pain relief when equianalgesic doses of meperidine were administered. However, a greater number of patients receiving IM injections required dosage adjustments compared to the IV-PCA group. Although there were no differences in the side effects profile, the duration

100

of hospital stay was lower in the PCA group. In addition, both the patients and nursing staff preferred IV-PCA therapy.

Compared to IM administration, PCA therapy provided effective analgesia after colon surgery with less morphine requirements and less sedation with patients feeling more comfortable and satisfied. However, there were no differences in the side effects or duration of hospitalization between PCA and conventional IM analgesia. Similarly, in a recent study involving patients undergoing cholecystectomy, Kenady et. al. found no significant differences in length of hospital stay or dose of morphine between patients receiving IV-PCA or IM injections. However, patients using PCA reported significantly improved subjective pain relief and spent a smaller percentage of time "in pain" during each of the first two postoperative days.

SUMMARY

The clinical management of acute pain has been impeded by traditions and misconceptions which have resulted in suboptimal application to the patient of the currently available methods of pain control. Standard regimens fail because of the wide, unpredictable variability in pain intensity, patient characteristics, and pharmacological responses. Treatment needs to be individualized for each patient. Patients have to be made aware that they should expect adequate pain relief and should communicate their analgesic needs to their care givers. PCA allows a patient to balance analgesic levels with the degree of pain relief required. PCA changes the role of the postoperative patient from passive to active, permitting patients in pain to cope actively for themselves. Moreover, it demonstrates that an integration of technological advances with psychological principles can improve patient satisfaction with care delivery.

Originally the scope of PCA was limited to IV therapy for postoperative analgesia in adults, but its proven efficacy, its range of applications have expanded to include oral, sublingual, SC, IM and epidural routes. PCA is now used in pediatric surgery, obstetrics, trauma, burns patients, cancer patients and variety of medical conditions. PCA has also been found valuable for scientific pain studies (e.g., to determine predictors of postoperative pain, drug interactions and pharmacokinetic experiments). Although the benefits of PCA may be associated with the technique itself, in part they may also be dependent on Health care professionals who are knowledgeable and skilled in its use. There is widespread misconception that pain relief with PCA is completely automatic and thus there is no need for specialized acute pain service management. In fact, PCA can only be used optimally when it is accompanied by regular, expert nursing and medical supervision.

REFERENCES

1. Marks RM, Sachar EJ: Undertreatment of medical inpatients with narcotic analgesics. Ann Intern Med 78:173, 1973
2. Owen H, McMillan V, Rogowski D: Postoperative pan therapy: a survey of patients' expectation and their experiences. Pain 41:303, 1990
3. Donovan M, Dillon P, McGuire L: Incidence and characteristics of pain in a sample of medical-surgical inpatients. Pain 30:69, 1987
4. White PF: Use of patient-controlled analgesia for management of acute pain. JAMA 259:243, 1988

PERIPHERAL TREATMENT OF ACUTE PAIN

H. Kehlet and J.L. Pedersen

Acute pain is mediated by physical stimuli and trauma-induced release of algesic substances such as protons, bradykinin, serotonin, arachidonic cascade metabolites, nerve growth factor (NGF), purines, and others. Several of these nociceptive mediators contribute to the inflammatory response and the sensitization of nociceptors (1,2). Subsequently, the nociceptive input induces central neuron changes such as increased receptive field sizes, increased responsiveness to nociceptive stimuli, decreased nociceptive thresholds, and recruitment of novel input. These central mechanisms may amplify the intensity and duration of acute pain (3). Although both the peripheral nervous system and the CNS may be targets for acute pain control, a logical step in the initial treatment of acute pain states would be at the site of injury. This paper is a short review on clinical experiences with peripheral treatment of acute pain, i.e., at the surgical wound site. The review will not include studies of peripheral nerve blocks.

The most important method for peripheral control of acute postoperative pain is incisional (wound-site) or intra-wound admin-istration of *local anesthetics*. This approach is safe, and analgesic effects have been documented in more than 15 controlled trials (4,5). The analgesic effect is best documented in small to moderate size surgical procedures, but the technique is less or not effective in major surgery. The explanation of the smaller effect in major surgery has not been established, but is probably due to pain arising from other sites than the wound and/or that relatively large wounds cannot be infiltrated sufficiently because of the risk of toxic side effects when large amounts of local anesthetic are necessary. The local anesthetic is more effective when given in the deeper layers (fascia, muscle) compared with subcutaneously, suggesting that postoperative pain may originate from these deeper layers (6). Unfor-tunately, the effects are relatively short-lived (about 3-16 hours) and there is a crucial need for a local anesthetic with a more prolonged effect. Presently, slow release preparations, where the local anesthetic is incor-porated into liposomes or micropheres seem most promising (7,8).

T. H. Stanley et al. (eds.), Pain Management and Anesthesiology, 103–108.
© *1998 Kluwer Academic Publishers. Printed in the Netherlands.*

The use of local anesthetics intra-articularly is also well established, but again the analgesic effect is brief. The use of intra-peritoneal local anesthetics in laparoscopic cholecystectomy or gynecological procedures has been evaluated in more than 14 randomized studies, but most, except a few have been negative (9,10). Probably, additional infiltration of the parietal peritoneum may improve analgesia in such laparoscopic procedures (11). It is controversial whether preemptive incisional or intraperitoneal local anesthetic administration is more effective than administration at the end of surgery.

The demonstration of increased opioid receptor expression on the peripheral nerve terminals in post-inflammatory states has led to evaluation of peripheral administration of *opioids* in more than 30 controlled studies, mainly in arthroscopic procedures (12,13). The analgesic effect is not consistent, and suggest that a possible effect is only moderate (13). Also, the trials comparing identical doses of morphine given intra-articularly vs. systemically have not demonstrated consistent improvement of analgesia with peripheral administration (12). On the other hand a prolonged effect of peripheral opioid administration, lasting up to 24 hours, has been demonstrated in several studies. Although more randomized data are required to reach definite conclusions, the treatment may be recommended for routine use in arthroscopic procedures, since it is inexpensive and without side effects. The use of "peripheral" opioid treatment with intraperitoneal or intrapleural administration or in surgical incisions has not been demonstrated to provide superior analgesic effects compared with systemic use (11,12).

The additional analgesic effect of intraarticular opioids combined with other analgesic agents, i.e., local anesthetics is not consistent, although most studies suggest an improvement of analgesia since local anesthetics are effective in the early and opioids in the later postoperative phase (13).

Since primary hyperalgesia may be partly mediated by arachidonic cascade metabolites, a rational approach may be peripheral (wound) administration of inhibitors. *NSAID's* provide peripheral and central mediated analgesic effects and are effective in postoperative pain treatment following systemic administration. Recently, several studies have been published investigating the analgesic effect of peripheral administration of NSAID's (incisional, intravenous anesthesia and intra-articularly). However, the results are not consistent, and therefore suggest either a small or no additional analgesic effect compared with systemic use (16-28). Since the additional analgesic effect of peripheral administration apparently is limited and because the potential side effects with incisional administration (bleeding, impaired wound healing) have not been evaluated, it is too early to give recommendations for clinical use of incisional/intraarticular administration of NSAID's.

Glucocorticoids inhibit the trauma-induced release of several algesic substances such as arachidonic cascade metabolites, cytokines, etc. In major abdominal surgery systemic administration of high-dose of prednisolone may reduce pain and various parameters of the systemic inflammatory response such as IL-6, hyperthermia and PGE2-responses as well as pulmonary function may be improved (29,30). Furthermore, local corticosteroid injection may have powerful analgesic and anti-inflammatory effects in rheumatic disorders (31). Peripheral (wound site) administration of glucocorticoids have also been demonstrated to reduce pain and swelling after dental procedures (32,33). Recently, we have performed a double-blind controlled trial to demonstrate that intra-articular administration of methylprednisolone 40 mg together with 150 mg bupivacaine and 4 mg morphine significantly reduced pain, leg muscle strength, use of crutches and convalescence (sick leave) compared with intra-articular saline or the same dose of bupivacaine and morphine alone (34). Local administration of glucocorticoids may therefore be an interesting approach to reduce inflammation and pain in certain procedures. However, more data are needed on safety aspects, as regards wound healing and risk of infection, since such safety data so far only are available from dental procedures and the common use of a single dose glucocorticoid intra-articularly in rheumatic disorders (31).

The sympathetic nervous system may be involved in the changes in nociceptive function at the site of injury in certain chronic pain states following nerve injury. In preliminary studies, *clonidine*, which may inhibit norepinephrine release at the nerve endings, has been shown to have analgesic effects when administered intra-articularly in arthroscopic procedures (35) or topically in patients with hyperalgesia with chronic sympathetically maintained pain (36).

Ketamine has slight analgesic effects after systemic administration, probably because of its NMDA antagonistic effects. Local administration of ketamine may enhance the analgesic effects of bupivacaine in patients undergoing herniorrhaphy (37) and hyperalgesia in superficial burn injury in human volunteers (38,39). The effect may be mediated by antagonism with peripheral NMDA receptors, and/or local anesthetic effects but obviously more data are needed from different surgical procedures to establish the analgesic efficacy as well as the safety.

No clinical studies are available on the local, wound site use of *bradykinin* or *substance-P antagonists, leukotriene synthetase inhibitors,* etc.

In summary, the peripheral use of analgesics may be of value in the treatment of acute postoperative pain. However, so far the experience is limited and has mostly been focused on analgesia, whereas no conclusive data are available on safety aspects except for the incisional use of local anesthetics and opioids. Further studies are needed with multimodal peripheral treatment in individual surgical procedures (40). In addition, the development and assessment of slow release preparations of different analgesics administered at the site of injury should receive attention in the future.

REFERENCES

1. Dray A. Inflammatory mediators of pain. Br J Anaesth 1995;75:125-131.
2. Steen KH, Steen AE, Kieysel HW, et al. Inflammatory mediators potentiate pain induced by experimental tissue acidosis. Pain 1996;66:163-170.
3. Woolf CJ. Somatic pain—pathogenesis and prevention. Br J Anaesth 1995;75:169-176.
4. Dahl JB, Møiniche S, Kehlet, H. Wound infiltration with local anaesthetics for postoperative pain relief—a review. Acta Anaesthesiol Scand 1994;38:7-14.
5. Callesen T, Kehlet H. Post-herniorrhaphy pain—a review. Anesthesiology (in press).
6. Yndgaard S, Holst B, Bjerre-Jepsen K, et al. Subcutaneously versus subfascially administered lidocaine in pain treatment after inguinal herniotomy. Anesth Analg 1994;79:324-327.
7. Grant GJ, Vermeulen K, Zakowski M, et al. Prolonged analgesia and decreased toxicity with liposomal morphine in a mouse model. Anesth Analg 1994;79:706-709.
8. Curley J, Castillo J, Hoz J, et al. Prolonged nerve blockade—injectable biodegradable bupivacaine/polyester micropheres. Anesthesiology 1996;84:1401-1410.
9. Pasqualucci A, De Angilis V, Contardo R, et al. Preemptive analgesia: intraperitoneal local anesthetic in laparoscopic cholecystectomy. Anesthesiology 1996;85:11-20
10. Mraovic B, Jurisic T, Kogler-Majeric V, et al. Intraperitoneal bupivacaine for analgesia after laparoscopic cholecystectomy. Acta Anaesthesiol Scand 1997;41:193-196.
11 Alexander DJ, Ngoi SS, Lee L, et al. Randomised trial of periportal peritoneal bupivacaine for pain relief after laparoscopic cholecystectomy. Br J Surg 1996;83:1223-1225.

12. Stein C, Yassouridis A. Peripheral morphine analgesia. Pain 1997;71:119-121.
13. Kalso E, Tramér MR, Carroll D, et al. Pain relief from intraarticular morphine after knee surgery: a qualitative systematic review. Pain 1997;71:127-134.
14. Schulte-Steinberg H, Wenenger E, Jokisch D, et al. Intraperitoneal versus intrapleural morphine or bupivacaine for pain after laparoscopic cholecystectomy. Anesthesiology 1995;82:634-640.
15. Rosenstock C, Andersen G, Antonsen K, et al. Analgesic effect of incisional morphine following inguinal herniotomy on the spinal anesthesia. Reg Anesth 1996;21:93-98.
16. Reuben SS, Connelly NR. Postoperative analgesia for outpatient arthroscopic knee surgery with intraarticular bupivacaine and ketorolac. Anesth Analg 1995;80:1154-1157.
17. Reuben SS, Steinberg RB, Kreitzer JM, et al. Intravenous regional anaesthesia using lidocaine and ketorolac. Anesth Analg 1995;81:11-113.
18. Knudsen KE, Bronfeldt S, Mikkelsen S, et al. Peritonsillar infiltration with low-dose tenoxicam after tonsillectomy. Br J Anaesth 1995; 75:286-288.
19. Reuben SS, Connelly NR. Postarthroscopic meniscus repair analgesia with intraarticular ketorolac or morphine. Anesth Analg 1996; 82:1036-1039.
20. Jones NC, Pugh SC. The addition of tenoxicam to prilocaine for intravenous regional anaesthesia. Anaesthesia 1996;51:446-448.
21. Ben-David B, Baune-Goldstein U, Goldik Z, et al. Is preoperative ketorolac a useful adjunct to regional anesthesia for inguinal herniorrhaphy? Acta Anaesthesiol Scand 1996;40:358-363.
22. Elhakim M, Fathy A, Elkott M, et al. Intraarticular tenoxicam relieves postarthroscopy pain. Acta Anaesthesiol Scand 1996;40:1223-1226.
23. Lundell JC, Silverman DG, Brull SJ, et al. Reduction of post-burn hyperalgesia after local injection of ketorolac in healthy volunteers. Anesthesiology 1996;84:502-509.
24. Reuben SS, Duprat KM. Comparison of wound infiltration with ketorolac versus intravenous regional anesthesia with ketorolac for postoperative analgesia following ambulatory hand surgery. Reg Anesth 1996;21:565-568.
25. Cook TM, Tuckey JP, Nolan JP. Analgesia after day-case knee arthroscopy. Double-blind study of intraarticular tenoxicam, intraarticular bupivacaine and placebo. Br J Anaesth 1997;78:163-168.
26. Connelly NR, Reuben SS, Albert M, et al. Use of preincisional ketorolac in hernia patients, intravenous versus surgical site. Reg Anesth 1997;22:229-232

27. Corpataux J-B, Gessel EF, Donald FA, et al. Effect of postoperative analgesia of small dose lysine-acetylsalicylate added to prilocaine during intravenous regional anesthesia. Anesth Analg 1997;84:1081-1085.

28. Mikkelsen SS, Knudsen KE, Kristensen BB, et al. Comparison of tenoxicam by intramuscular injection or wound infiltration for analgesia after inguinal herniorrhaphy. Anesth Analg 1996;83:1239-1243.

29. Schulze S, Sommer P, Bigler D, et al. Effect of combined prednisolone, epidural analgesia and indomethacin on systemic response after colonic surgery. Arch Surg 1992;127:325-331.

30. Schulze S, Andersen J, Overgård H, et al. Effect of prednisolone on the systemic response and wound healing after colonic surgery. Arch Surg 1997;132:129-135.

31. Gray RG, Tennenbaum J, Gottlieb NL. Local corticosteroid injection treatment in rheumatic disorders. Sem Arthr Rheum 1981;10:231-254.

32. Skelbred P, Løkken P. Reduction of pain and swelling by a corticosteroid injected 3 hours after surgery. Eur J Clin Pharmacol 1982;23:141-146.

33. Baxendale BR, Vater M, Lavery KM. Dexamethasone reduces pain and swelling following extraction of third molar tooth. Anaesthesia 1993;48:961-964.

34. Rasmussen S, Larsen AT, Thomsen, ST, et al. Intraarticular glucocorticoid reduces pain, inflammatory response and convalescence after arthroscopic menisectomy (submitted).

35. Gentili M, Juhel A, Bonnet F, et al. Peripheral analgesic effect of intraarticular clonidine. Pain 1996;64:593-596.

36. Davis KD, Treede RD, Raja, SN, et al. Topical application of clonidine relieves hyperalgesia in patients with sympathetically maintained pain. Pain 1991;47:309-317.

37. Tverskoy M, Oren M, Vaskuvich M, et al. Ketamine enhances local anesthetic and analgesic effects of bupivacaine by peripheral mechanism: a study in postoperative patients. Neurosci Lett 1996;215:5-8.

38. Warncke T, Jørum E, Stubhaug A, et al. Local treatment with the N-methyl-D-aspartate receptor antagonist ketamine, inhibit development of secondary hyperalgesia in man by a peripheral action. Neurosci Lett 1997;227:1-4

39. Pedersen JL, Galle T, Kehlet H. Effect of local vs systemic ketamine on hyperalgesia after burn injury (submitted).

40. Kehlet H, Dahl JB. The value of multi-modal or balanced analgesia on postoperative pain relief. Anesth Analg 1993;77:1048-1056.

PATIENT-CONTROLLED ANALGESIA (PART II): UPDATE ON ITS CLINICAL USAGE*

P. F. White

With the rapid growth in acute and chronic pain management services, anesthesiologists find themselves dealing with an intriguing variety of analgesia techniques. IV-PCA can be used with a variety of opioid analgesics and different modes of administration, giving it enhanced flexibility in the management of individual patient's analgesic needs. On-demand analgesia has gained popularity as a result of its effectiveness when utilized via the oral, sublingual, intranasal, IM, IV, subcutaneous (SC) and epidural routes (1-14).

The use of on-demand epidural analgesia (PCEA) has received significant attention with numerous reports concerning its efficacy in the treatment of postoperative pain. This technique has been most commonly used in pregnant women to provide analgesia both during labor and delivery and after cesarean section. In contrast to obstetric patients, PCEA in nonobstetric patients had a dose-sparing effect. Boudreault et al. reported that epidural administration of bupivacaine combined with fentanyl provided effective analgesia following laparotomy. However, the dose of fentanyl necessary to achieve adequate analgesia was reduced when it was administered by intermittent bolus PCA than by continuous infusion. Owen et al. compared the effects of fentanyl administered by PCEA with or without a background infusion of the drug and also a fixed-rate continuous epidural infusion in patients undergoing abdominal surgery. Although the pain scores and sedation scores did not differ between the three treatment groups, epidural PCA fentanyl caused less oxygen desaturation than the continuous infusion techniques. In a recent study, PCEA was compared to IV-PCA with fentanyl for post-thoracotomy pain. There was no difference between the two groups in respiratory rates, $PaCO_2$ values, pain scores or changes in bedside pulmonary function tests (i.e., FVC and FEV1). However, fentanyl requirements were significantly

---

*Adapted from Joshi GP, White PF. Patient-Controlled Analgesia (Chapter 35). In Management of Acute Pain (M Ashburn and LJ Rice, Editors), New York: Churchill Livingston, 1997; pp 1-35.

T. H. Stanley et al. (eds.), Pain Management and Anesthesiology, 109–123.
© 1998 *Kluwer Academic Publishers. Printed in the Netherlands.*

less when given via the epidural route, supporting the concept of a direct spinal cord site of action for epidural fentanyl. A subsequent study comparing IV-PCA morphine with PCEA fentanyl for the treatment of post-thoracotomy pain reported that patients receiving IV-PCA morphine experienced more sedation on postoperative day one, whereas pruritus was more frequent in the epidural fentanyl group. Controversy surrounds the question as to whether post-thoracotomy pain should be managed via epidural catheter placed in the lumbar versus the thoracic region. A recent study found no difference in post-thoracotomy analgesia when sufentanil was administered at the thoracic or lumbar level.

While IM-PCA has been evaluated by placing a small-gauge cannula in the deltoid muscle of the non-dominant arm, the SC route of PCA administration appears to have advantages and is effective with morphine, hydromorphone and oxymorphone. SC-PCA represents a clinically acceptable alternative to IV-PCA in the treatment of postoperative pain in both inpatients and outpatients. A recent study comparing the IV and SC routes of administration for PCA in children, reported that subcutaneous route was as effective and safe as IV-PCA. However, the SC route was associated with decreased requirements of morphine and a lower incidence of hypoxemia. The authors concluded that the SC route may offer advantages over the IV route by providing feedback on successful demands for analgesia and enhancing the appropriate and effective use of PCA. The use of SC route of administration provides many advantages of IV-PCA without the need for maintaining a continuous IV access. However, SC route required higher analgesic dosages compared to IV-PCA. Potential side effects associated with the SC route include pain secondary to a large volume of fluid, slow onset of analgesia, delayed respiratory depression resulting from a "depot" effect, and infection at the site of injection.

Oral PCA was initially described in patients with chronic cancer pain. Recently, Litman et. al., reported the successful use of oral PCA in adolescents by placing a limited number of analgesia tablets by the patient's bedside, giving them some degree of independence and self-control over their postoperative treatment while in the hospital. On demand administration of sublingual buprenorphine and intranasal fentanyl has also been reported. Patient-controlled spinal analgesia is a new area of on-demand pain management. In addition to opioids, other drugs (e.g., clonidine and metoclopramide) have also been used for patient-controlled administration.

CLINICAL USE OF PCA THERAPY

The American Society of Anesthesiologists Task Force on Pain Management recently published a list of important elements of IV-PCA orders. There are several standard parameters that are usually programmed into the modern PCA device [e.g., demand (bolus) dose, lockout (delay) interval, background (basal) infusion rate, and 1- and 4-hr limits]. In addition, there is often a loading dose prescribed prior to initiating PCA therapy. The quantity of analgesic medication available to the patient will primarily depend on the demand dose and lockout interval. The settings for the demand dose and lockout interval are influenced by the choice of the analgesic drug and choice of appropriate settings based on clinical experience.

SELECTION OF PCA MEDICATION

The desirable pharmacologic properties of an opioid analgesic for PCA therapy include: 1) a rapid onset of analgesic action such that the patient can maintain control of their pain and not have to wait for pain relief, or have to continually press the on-demand button, 2) high efficacy in providing pain relief (the potency of the drug is of less concern since the medication can be administered in varying size bolus doses as needed), 3) an intermediate duration of action to improve controllability, and 4) absence of tolerance or significant side effects. Although the ideal PCA analgesic is not available, a wide variety of parenteral analgesics including both opioid agonists and agonist-antagonists have been used with the available PCA delivery systems.

Of the many opioids used in PCA therapy, morphine and meperidine have been most extensively investigated. Morphine is still most commonly used opioid. Although the reduced incidence of side effects and high patient satisfaction reported with the use of meperidine has increased its usage, it may be ineffective in controlling severe postoperative pain. The duration of methadone and buprenorphine may be too long, whereas fentanyl and its newer analogs are short-acting when administered in incremental doses. Fentanyl (15-75 µg), sufentanil (2-10 µg) and alfentanil (100-300 µg) can also be effectively used as on-demand analgesics when combined with a background (or basal) infusion. Nevertheless, the number of demands will be higher than morphine, meperidine or hydromorphone due to their shorter duration of action. The demand frequency was unacceptably high in one study of PCA alfentanil. Owen et al. reported inadequate analgesia with PCA and basal infusion of alfentanil. In another study, the same authors reported effective analgesia with alfentanil PCA. However, the concurrent administration of fixed-rate infusion with PCA did not proportionately reduce the number of demands made by the patients which resulted in higher doses being received by patients with higher infusion rate.

The margin of safety or the therapeutic index are important determinants in prescribing opioids. The side effect profile of opioids at equipotent doses would be another rational basis for drug choice. Some authors favor alfentanil because its use is associated with less sedation than with other opioids. On the other hand, in a study comparing PCA sufentanil, alfentanil and morphine, sufentanil provided a rapid onset of analgesia, less sedation and less depression of oxygen saturation. However, Hill and colleagues recently reported no difference between morphine, fentanyl and alfentanil with respect to ventilatory drive and sedation. Sinatra et al. evaluated the analgesic effectiveness and safety of morphine, meperidine and oxymorphone in patients undergoing cesarean section. Oxymorphone had a rapid onset with a uniform level of analgesia, but patients receiving morphine achieved the highest level of analgesia. In another study, the same authors demonstrated that both morphine and oxymorphone provided similar pain relief, however, there was more nausea with oxymorphone and more sedation and pruritus with morphine. Oxymorphone is limited by its high incidence of nausea and high costs. Hydromorphone is an opioid intermediate in lipid solubility between morphine (less lipid-soluble than hydromorphone) and fentanyl (more lipid-soluble than hydromorphone). It has a rapid analgesic onset, low incidence of side effects, and a low risk of delayed respiratory depression. Therefore, hydromorphone can be used as an alternative to morphine.

Agonist-antagonist opioids, such as butorphanol and nalbuphine, produce "ceiling" or plateau effects with respect to both respiratory depression and analgesia. In clinical circumstances where agonist-antagonist opioids could provide acceptable analgesia (i.e., mild-to-moderate pain), these drugs may be less likely to produce clinically-significant respiratory depression than pure μ-receptor agonists. However, nalbuphine used as PCA was unable to provide adequate pain relief and was associated with excessive sedation. Compared to morphine and meperidine, nalbuphine PCA provided similar analgesia at rest, with no difference in the frequency of side effects. However, morphine was significantly better in controlling pain during movement and deep breathing. Until we gain better insights into PCA medication profiles, selection of the "right drug" for PCA therapy will be made on theoretical, pharmacokinetic, economic or prejudicial grounds.

LOADING DOSE

PCA is essentially a maintenance therapy which should begin with a loading dose. Before initiating the PCA, the analgesic medication is titrated to achieve adequate pain control and make the patient comfortable. The loading dose is typically administered in the Post Anesthesia Care Unit (PACU) once the patient has recovered from anesthesia and has been given appropriate instructions in the use of PCA therapy (in addition to preoperative instructions). An adequate loading dose titrated to pain relief can result in decreased postoperative morbidity. It should not be necessary to administer a loading dose if adequate pain relief has been achieved intraoperatively and the patient is comfortable in the PACU.

DEMAND (BOLUS) DOSE

The demand dose is the amount of drug the patient receives every time the PCA device is activated. The incremental bolus dose depends on the kinetics of the analgesic drug used. The size of the demand dose influences the patient's perception of effectiveness of PCA therapy. If the demand dose is too small, patients will be unable to achieve adequate pain relief. Because there is evidence of operant conditioning with PCA, if the demand dose is inadequate the patients do not make the connection between effective pain relief and the PCA device. On the other hand, if the demand dose is too high, patients may experience undesirable side effects and thus may be discouraged from using the PCA device. The size of the incremental bolus should be large enough to provide adequate analgesia but not so large as to prevent feedback. Thus, the optimal dose for use with PCA is the "minimum" dose that produces adequate analgesia consistently without causing subjective or objective side effects.

The most appropriate size of the demand dose has been the source of considerable debate. An initial demand dose of morphine 1 mg, has been recommended by several investigators. In one study, patients were started on PCA with an initial demand dose of morphine 0.6 mg/square meter of body surface area with the dosage adjusted up or down by a factor of 50% until satisfactory analgesia was achieved with minimal side effects. At the termination of the study, a median demand dose of morphine 1 mg was determined to be appropriate. In a prospective study, Owens et al. compared the demand doses of morphine 0.5 mg, 1 mg and 2 mg and confirmed that a demand dose of morphine 1 mg was most appropriate. The demand dose for other opioids should be equianalgesic to morphine 1 mg .

Ideally, patients should not be required to make too frequent demands in order to attain adequate analgesia. It is estimated that a

114

patient receiving PCA therapy will need at least one adjustment in the size of the bolus dose. Most modern PCA devices monitor the total number of attempts (premature as well as the actual [successful] delivered doses). This information is helpful in determining the appropriateness of the analgesic regimen. If the patient reports significant pain and has made numerous attempts, it suggests that an increase in the size of the demand dose may be required or that the patient simply does not understand how to effectively utilize the PCA device.

LOCKOUT (DELAY) INTERVAL

The lockout interval is the minimum time between two demand doses. In order to prevent the patient from receiving a second dose of analgesic medication before the effects of the previous dose had been experienced, a mandatory lockout or delay interval is programmed into all PCA devices. The duration of the lockout interval is based upon the time of onset of the analgesic effect. Ideally, the patients will demand repeated doses until their pain is relieved. Furthermore, it is assumed that the patient will not push the demand button once an adequate analgesic level is achieved. If the lockout time too long adequate analgesia can not be obtained as the serum opioid concentrations fall below the MEAC before the next demand dose can be administered. In one study, patients did not request more than 9 demands per hour. This may be related to patient concerns of overdosage or decreased confidence in the PCA therapy.

Importantly, the lockout interval depends on the size of the demand dose. Although lockout intervals for morphine in various studies range from 2 to 20 min, there are few well-conducted studies investigating this aspect of PCA therapy. The initial lockout interval for demand dose of morphine 1 mg should be 6 min. The lockout interval of other opioids will depend on their lipophilicity and pharmacokinetics. The ratio of incremental boluses delivered versus patient demands may provide a measure of adequacy of pain relief. To achieve maximum efficacy, this ratio should approach one. If the number of patients demands are significantly greater than the number of boluses delivered, the lockout interval is too long or the patient fails to understand how to use the PCA device.

BACKGROUND (BASAL) INFUSION

Most modern PCA devices are able to deliver a fixed-rate continuous infusion to supplement conventional PCA therapy. Ideally, a concurrent basal opioid infusion with PCA should be helpful in maintaining a consistent therapeutic "analgesic" level of the drug and improve the quality of analgesia. Patients who are excessively sedated as a result of residual anesthetic effects or fatigued after surgery may underdose themselves with opioid medication when using PCA therapy and thus, often awaken with pain. Furthermore, patients who are comfortable at rest may experience distressing pain with sudden increase in physical activity. Another perceived advantage of using a background infusion is that it improves continuity of analgesia and provides analgesia during sleep. The use of a continuous infusion at night-time was thought to facilitate sleep and improve sleep patterns by reducing the number of occasions when patients are awakened by pain that requires subsequent use of the PCA device. However, carefully controlled studies have failed to validate these theoretical advantages.

Early PCA investigators advocated concurrent basal opioid infusion with PCA as a way of improving sleep and the quality of pain relief during physical activity. However, using continuous infusion PCA to enhance sleep may be ill-advised since sleep may enhance respiratory depression and sedation given at bedtime may further potentiate the opioid's central nervous system depressant effects. In addition, continuous infusion may reduce the inherent safety of PCA that is, with increasing sedation there is decrease in demands (negative feedback). The use of basal infusion may also result in larger amounts of opioid being administered and an increase in the incidence of opioid-related side effects. Recent studies suggest that there is no advantage to a continuous infusion of opioids combined with PCA. Furthermore, there may be potential harmful effects of bolus plus infusion techniques. Owen et al. compared morphine PCA with or without continuous infusion at 1.5 mg/hr over a period of 24 hr postoperatively. They concluded that a use of continuous infusion did not decrease the number of bolus demands nor the pain scores. In addition, patients receiving continuous infusion had a higher incidence of respiratory depression. In another study, basal infusion of morphine 2 mg/hr increased the incidence of nausea without improving the degree of pain relief.

Parker et. al. studied 230 adult women randomized to receive IV-PCA morphine alone or IV-PCA morphine with a continuous infusion of morphine 0.5, 1.0 or 2.0 mg/hr. Patients receiving the 2.0 mg/hr infusion used significantly more morphine from 9 to 72 hours after their operation than the control group. The presence of a constant infusion did not significantly decrease the number of patient demands or supplemental bolus doses. These investigators concluded that the use of a continuous opioid infusion in combination with a conventional PCA regimen did not improve pain management compared with PCA alone after abdominal hysterectomy. In more recent studies comparing PCEA with and without a background continuous infusion, investigators have also concluded that although both groups had high quality analgesia, the addition of a continuous infusion conferred no additional benefit to the patient. In patients receiving a basal infusion, if PCA bolus doses are not utilized, the basal infusion rate is too high. On the other hand, if the number of bolus demands are too frequent, there may be an advantage in adding (or increasing) the basal infusion.

PCA THERAPY WITH ADJUVANT DRUGS

There have been numerous clinical reports describing the use of nonopioid analgesic medication as an adjuvant to conventional opioid-based PCA. A combination of opioid and nonopioid analgesics as a part of multimodal or balanced analgesia may be effective in decreasing the opioid-related side effects. With the availability of parenteral preparations of non-steroidal anti-inflammatory drugs (NSAIDs) and reports of their opioid-sparing action, the use of these drugs has become more widespread. The other adjunct medications which have been administered with opioid analgesics include local anesthetics and alpha-2 agonists.

The use of IV ketorolac has prompted a number of investigations into its opioid-sparing effects on the PCA opioid requirement. It may be possible to reduce the opioid doses by supplementing analgesia by ketorolac. Grass et al. reported the use of ketorolac as an adjunct to PCEA fentanyl after radical retropubic prostatectomy. In addition to PCEA patients received either IM ketorolac or placebo every 6 hr. Pain scores at rest were lower in the combination group during the first 4 hr but were similar thereafter. Pain scores with activity were lower in the ketorolac group on both the first and second postoperative day. Bladder spasm pain occurred less frequently and recovery of gastrointestinal function occurred sooner in the ketorolac group. Finally, PCEA fentanyl usage was less in the ketorolac group throughout the study. Combination of IV ketorolac with PCA morphine for the management of surgical pain after lower abdominal pain decreased resting pain scores and there was a trend toward decreased morphine self-administration.

Combination of IM ketorolac with IV-PCA provided better pain relief with reduced morphine requirements than placebo. Furthermore, continuous IM infusion of ketorolac was better than intermittent IM ketorolac. Intravenous diclofenac reduced fentanyl requirements but the degree of analgesia and the incidence of side effects was unaltered compared with PCA fentanyl alone for the management of pain after total hip replacement. Propacetamol, an injectable prodrug of acetaminophen, demonstrated a morphine-sparing effect in orthopedic patients receiving PCA morphine. In pediatric patients, a single intraoperative dose of IV ketorolac appeared to decrease opioid use, provided superior analgesia and decreased the frequency of urinary retention during the first 12 hr of PCA therapy with morphine. A recent study compared analgesic efficacy of PCA ketorolac with that of PCA morphine after abdominal surgery. The authors concluded that although IV-PCA ketorolac was well-tolerated, it had limited effectiveness as the sole postoperative analgesic. Thus, NSAIDs should be used as adjuvants and not sole analgesics for the management of moderate-to-severe postoperative pain.

Clonidine, a centrally acting alpha-2 agonist, has been shown to have analgesic-like properties and thus may be an effective adjunct to opioid PCA therapy. De Kock and colleagues evaluated the analgesic efficacy of clonidine administered during surgery (loading dose of 4 µg/kg followed by 2 µg/kg/hr until the end of the surgery) in patients undergoing abdominal surgery. The authors concluded that clonidine improved the quality of PCA morphine without increasing the frequency of side effects. In contrast, oral clonidine 300 µg administered 1 hr before and 12 hr after surgery tended to reduce PCA morphine requirements but did not improve the pain scores. Moreover, its use was associated with significant sedation and reduced heart rate. Clonidine 3 µg/ml added to PCEA sufentanil 2 µg/ml following cesarean section did not reduce the pain scores but resulted in significant reduction in the 24 hr consumption of sufentanil. Oral-transcutaneous clonidine reduced the postoperative PCA morphine requirements by 50%, in elderly men undergoing radical prostatectomy procedures. Local anesthetics can also be used with PCA as a part of a multimodal (or balanced) analgesic technique. Continuous local anesthetic infusions reduce PCA morphine requirements by 40-50%. Recently, metoclopramide has been used an analgesic adjunct to PCA morphine. Single dose of metoclopramide 10 mg IV reduced pain and morphine requirements.

In summary, opioid requirements necessary to achieve adequate pain relief are related to patient characteristics, the drug and the PCA settings. Once the patients pain is adequately treated with a loading dose of morphine, PCA should be initiated with a demand dose of 1 mg and lockout interval of 6 min is initiated. If the analgesia is inadequate, encouragement of further usage of PCA and/or increase the demand dose to 1.5 mg should be considered. Alternatively, the lockout interval can be decreased to 5 min. If a demand dose of 1.5 mg with a lockout interval of 5 min is not adequate, addition of an adjuvant such as NSAIDs or clonidine may be beneficial. A multimodal approach to providing analgesia should be advantageous in providing superior analgesia with fewer drug-induced side effects. Occasionally it may be necessary to add basal infusion (0.5-1 mg/hr) or change the opioid medication. Furthermore, it is important to look for other treatable causes of increase in severity of pain. It is necessary to establish protocols to allow for effective and safe use of PCA therapy. This should include patient monitoring and occurrence of side effects (4 hr assessments of pain level using pain scores, degree of sedation, and respiratory rate). The total usage of opioid and the frequency of PCA demands (successful and unsuccessful) should also be noted.

SIDE EFFECT AND SAFETY ISSUES WITH PCA THERAPY

Since its introduction in clinical practice, PCA has become the one of the most commonly used technique for postoperative pain management. Reports of large series of patients using on-demand analgesia have confirmed the safety of PCA devices. In a study evaluating the use of PCA in 1122 patients, Fleming and Coombs observed a complication rate of only 0.7%. The complications observed by the authors were related to drug overdose or interaction including respiratory depression, seizure, hypotension, hallucination and somnolence, allergic reaction, nausea and vomiting, decreased intestinal motility, and urinary retention.

It is unlikely that any postoperative pain therapy, including PCA, based on the use of opioids will be totally free from opioid-related side effects such as nausea, vomiting, pruritus, and sedation. A major factor limiting the use of PCA is the concern of respiratory depression. All routes of administration and techniques based on opioid analgesia result in some degree of oxygen desaturation. However, patients receiving PCA therapy were reported to have fewer episodes of severe oxygen desaturation (SaO_2 < 90%) than with either IM or epidural analgesia. Fentanyl administered by PCEA caused less oxygen desaturation than fentanyl administered as a continuous infusion or PCA plus basal infusion. The reduced incidence of severe hypoxemia with the use of PCA may be the result of improved analgesia. Mild carbon dioxide retention has been observed with both epidural and IV-PCA morphine. Although rare, severe respiratory depression have occurred with PCA usage. Etches reported 8 cases of serious respiratory depression in among 1800 patients who has received PCA therapy. The occurrence of these side effects was related to the dose, rate, and method of opioid administration and age and preoperative patient status. Hypovolemia may result in erratic absorption and potential for adverse effects. Patients with morbid obesity and/or labile hemodynamic status are unsuitable for PCA therapy because of a high possibility of respiratory depression. Severe bradypnea during the use of PCA buprenorphine has been reported. Since buprenorphine has a slow onset and long duration of action, the patient pressed the demand button an excessive number of times before obtaining adequate pain relief. Opioid-related side effects including urinary retention and gastrointestinal dysfunction (e.g., colonic pseudo-obstruction) may occur during PCA therapy. There is recent evidence suggesting the development of tolerance to PCA administered opioids, although it may not be as rapid as continuous infusion. Thus, increasing doses of opioids may be required to achieve same degree of analgesia with prolonged use. Recently, case reports of pulmonary embolus and myocardial infarction, presumably masked by the use of PCA have been described. A sudden increase in the use of PCA warrants a careful investigation of whether the pain is due to any cause other than surgical pain.

Problems that occur with PCA can be classified into operator errors, patient errors, and mechanical errors. The most common cause of overdosage with PCA is operator error such as misprogramming or improper loading of drug reservoir. Equipment failure with resultant respiratory depression has also been reported. A random computer error leading to runaway infusion of meperidine resulted in overdose. Accidental activation of a PCA device has been reported to occur by electronic noise interference when a power cord was reinserted. In one report, disengagement of a glass syringe from the PCA device lead to massive opioid overdose. The weight and ease of movement of plungers of syringes make siphoning possible and thus it is necessary to incorporate antisyphon and unidirectional valves in PCA devices. Similarly, incorporation of a two-way pressure-driven valve in the tubing which obstructs the gravitational flow of medication but does not impede the pump-driven flow is also necessary.

Patient error was demonstrated in a patient who overdosed herself by pressing the PCA demand button thinking that it was the nurse call button. Activation of the PCA device by any person other than the patient may have disastrous consequences as the basic safety of the PCA is bypassed. There are instances when spouse-controlled or parent-controlled activation have resulted in significant adverse effects. In a recent survey of patient visitors, half of the visitors stated that they would push the demand button if they felt their loved-one was in pain. Tampering of the PCA device has also been reported.

Patients with renal failure are at a risk of developing opioid-related side effects because of accumulation of active metabolites (e.g., morphine-6-glucuronide or normeperidine). Thus, patients whose renal function is deteriorating should be monitored very closely for opioid-related side effects. Normeperidine-induced seizures have also been reported in patients with normal renal function. A recent study suggests that doses of meperidine exceeding 25 $\mu g/kg/24$ hr may be associated with toxicity, especially in the presence of renal impairment. Therefore, patients should not receive more than 100 mg of meperidine every 2 hr for more than 24 hr. In addition, the continuous infusion of meperidine should be discouraged.

Recently, Ashburn and colleagues described the results of a study involving a large group of patients (3785) receiving PCA therapy for a total of 11,521 patient-care days. There were 14 critical events, of which 4 led to increased patient care. There were 8 programming errors (all involving misprogramming of the continuous infusion), 3 involved family members activating the device, 3 were results of an error in clinical judgment, and 1 involved a patient tampering with the device (with 1 event involving more than one error). Of the 4 events that led to increased patient care, 2 involved a family member activating the device, 1 was the result of a programming error, and 1 was the result of an error in clinical judgment. All patients who experienced a critical event had an uneventful recovery. The authors concluded that PCA therapy has the risk of potentially serious complications and requires constant physician and nursing care with an active quality assurance program. Others have described computerized methods of monitoring adverse events associated with PCA therapy to allow quality assurance and critical appraisal of the efficacy and potential adverse effects of PCA therapy. Appropriate patient selection, monitoring and follow-up is important to optimize PCA therapy and minimize the incidence of adverse effects.

NAUSEA ASSOCIATED WITH PCA

Since opioids are most commonly administered using PCA systems, the incidence of postoperative nausea and vomiting (PONV) is predictably high, with incidences as high as 80% reported. A wide variety of antiemetic drugs have been used to prevent or treat this problem. Several studies have evaluated the antiemetic efficacy of droperidol added to PCA morphine. However, these drugs may be associated with side effects such as increased sedation, hypotension and extrapyramidal symptoms. Addition of droperidol in morphine PCA after a prophylactic dose at induction reduced the degree of nausea and the incidence of request for rescue antiemetic, but resulted in a greater degree of sedation. Similarly, addition of droperidol (5 mg) in PCA morphine (30 mg) following a single dose of droperidol (1.25 mg) at the end of surgery resulted in a greater degree of sedation without improving the antiemetic effect.

Gan et al. did not find any difference in the incidence of PONV and sedation between droperidol 1.25 mg administered as a single dose at the end of the surgery or a small dose (0.16 mg) given concurrently with each dose of PCA morphine from placebo. Other investigators used even smaller doses of droperidol (0.1 mg) with each dose of PCA morphine and observed significant reduction in the incidence of PONV. A placebo-controlled, randomized trial, the efficacy of three prophylactic antiemetic regimens (droperidol, metoclopramide and tropisetron) evaluated the prevention of PONV during PCA therapy with morphine. The frequency and severity of PONV, as well as the need for rescue antiemetics, incidence of side effects and overall patient satisfaction were assessed. Droperidol was most efficacious in reducing the incidence of PONV for entire 36 hr of the study period. Tropisetron reduced the incidence and severity of PONV but the effect of single bolus dose lasted only 18 hr, while metoclopramide was only marginally effective. Because butyrophenones are structurally similar to opioids they may have a weak opioid agonist effect which may result in opioid-sparing activity. However, other authors have not been able to demonstrate any opioid-sparing effect of droperidol.

A recent study demonstrated that simultaneous titration of promethazine (0.625 mg/PCA dose, an average of 17.6 mg/24 hr) and morphine decreased nausea associated with PCA therapy. Doyle et al. studied the efficacy of transdermal hyoscine in reducing the incidence of PONV in children 6-14 yr receiving epidural PCA morphine following abdominal surgery. They concluded that the hyoscine-treated children had a significantly lower incidence of PONV compared to the placebo group, however, the treatment group had a significantly increased incidence of sedation and dry mouth. However, in another study in adults, the use of transdermal hyoscine with PCA morphine reduced the incidence of PONV only minimally (88% to 78%). Addition of metoclopramide (0.5 mg/ml) to morphine reduced the incidence of severe PONV during the first 6 hr, but the overall incidence of PONV was not affected.

SUMMARY

It is essential that Health care personnel using PCA devices have a full appreciation of the drug pharmacology and basic pharmacological principles before designing and implementing PCA therapy. Proper use of PCA requires a coordinated system of management, clearly delineated protocols, and ongoing education of physicians, nurses, patients and parents. The rare mishaps that have occurred with PCA have been due almost entirely to human error, not machine malfunction. Opioid-related side effects can occur, so it is important to implement standardized algorithms for management of side effects. The use of PCA does not obviate the need for ongoing assessment of patients by nurses and physicians. Careful monitoring should prevent the advent of most mishaps with PCA. Patients should be monitored for side effects and efficacy of treatment and the equipment used. There will likely be continued utilization of PCA as long as it continues to enjoy a good safety record and its applications will continue to expand in the future.

REFERENCES

1. White PF: Use of a patient-controlled analgesia infuser for the management of postoperative pain. Chapter 10.   In: Patient-Controlled Analgesia (Harmer, Rosen and Vickers, Eds.), Blackwell Scientific Publications Ltd., London, 1985, pp 140-148.
2. White, PF: Patient-controlled analgesia. In: Problems in Anesthesia (D.L. Brown, Ed.), J.B. Lippincott Co., Philadelphia, 1988, pp 339-350.
3. White PF: Patient-controlled analgesia: An update on its use in the treatment of postoperative pain. Chapter 5. In: Clinics of North America (R.V. Oden, Ed.). W.B. Saunders Co., Philadelphia, 1989, pp 63-78.
4. White PF: Patient-controlled analgesia delivery systems. Chapter 7. In: Patient-controlled analgesia (Ferrante, Ostheimer, Covino, Eds.). Blackwell Scientific Publications, Boston, 1990, pp 70-81.
5. White PF: Alternative routes for PCA in the management of acute pain. Chapter 22.   In: Patient-controlled analgesia (Ferrante, Ostheimer, Covino, Eds.), Blackwell Scientific Publications, Boston, 1990, pp 223-227.
6. Owen H, White PF: Overview of patient-controlled analgesia. Chapter 13.   In: Acute pain—mechanisms and management (Sinatra R, Hord A, Eds.), Mosby Yearbook Co, St. Louis, 1992, pp 151-164.
7. White PF: Patient-controlled analgesia—A new approach to the management of postoperative pain. Sem Anesth 4:255-266, 1985.
8. White PF: Postoperative pain management with patient-controlled analgesia. Sem Anesth 5:116-122, 1986.
9. White PF: Mishaps with patient-controlled analgesia (PCA). Anesthesiology 66:81-83, 1987.
10. White PF: Use of patient-controlled analgesia for management of acute pain. JAMA 259:243-247, 1988.
11. Parker RK, Holtmann B, White PF: Patient-controlled analgesia: Does a concurrent opioid infusion improve pain management after surgery? JAMA 266:1947-52, 1991.
12. Parker RD, Sawaki Y, White PF: Epidural patient-controlled analgesia: Influence of bupivacaine and hydromorphone basal infusion on pain control after cesarean delivery.   Anesth Analg 75:740-746, 1992.
13. Ghouri AF, Taylor E, White PF: Patient-controlled sedation—a comparison of midazolam, propofol and alfentanil during local anesthesia. J Clin Anesth 4:476-479, 1992.

14. Perry F, Parker RK, White PF, Clifford PA: Role of psychological factors in postoperative pain control and recovery with patient-controlled analgesia. Clin J Pain 10:57-63, 1994.

ORGANIZATION AND OPERATION OF AN ACUTE PAIN SERVICE

L. B. Ready

INTRODUCTION

The optimal care of surgical patients includes effective control of incisional pain. Despite advances in knowledge of pathophysiology, pharmacology of analgesics, and the development of more effective techniques for postoperative pain control, many patients do not receive adequate analgesia. The reasons for inadequate treatment are many. These include deficiencies in knowledge and skills on the parts of health care providers, patients, and those responsible for the management of health care systems, including governmental agencies. It has only recently been recognized that there are wide variations from patient to patient in the amount of pain that is experienced in response to a particular insult. There are also great differences in responsiveness to particular therapeutic approaches. We and others have described the development and experience of postoperative pain management services (1-56). The purpose of this presentation is to provide additional detail regarding the original organizational and operational aspects of this type of service as well current trends.

ORGANIZATION

HOSPITAL LOCATIONS WHERE CARE IS PROVIDED

Our initial experience with postoperative pain control was using epidural opioid analgesia (EOA) in patients following extensive thoracic surgery. These were typically patients who, because of their age and a variety of underlying medical problems, were scheduled for postoperative admission to our intensive care unit. It soon became apparent that the benefits of superior analgesia to these patients extended beyond the time that ICU care was needed. It was also clear that there were many additional patients undergoing painful surgical procedures who could benefit from postoperative EOA, but who did not require ICU admission. We therefore

T. H. Stanley et al. (eds.), Pain Management and Anesthesiology, 125–135.
© 1998 *Kluwer Academic Publishers. Printed in the Netherlands.*

126

gradually expanded availability of EOA to all post-surgical wards in the hospital, preceded in all cases by the development of nursing protocols and procedures, and by careful and detailed nurse training. Patient-controlled analgesia (PCA) was similarly introduced gradually to all post-surgical wards, preceded by the development of nursing protocols and appropriate nurse training. Standard orders have been developed for use throughout our institution both for EOA and PCA. Their purpose is to provide a consistent and familiar approach to care in all areas while minimizing the risk of errors of omission or duplication in the orders.

SAFETY ISSUES

1. Monitoring: Although early reports mentioned the occurrence of sudden respiratory arrest in patients receiving EOA, all recent reports of which we are aware describe slowly increasing ventilatory insufficiency. Our experience now exceeds 12,000 surgical patients treated with a variety of epidural opioids (some with local anesthetics added) and an additional 3,000 patients who received a single injection of epidural or subarachnoid morphine following cesarean section. In the few cases of respiratory depression we have observed, gradually increasing somnolence was a prominent feature. Our current monitoring practice relies primarily on well trained nurses who check both respiratory rate and a simple bedside sedation scale hourly for the first 24 hours in all patients receiving an epidural or intrathecal narcotic (57).

2. Order-writing: To avoid potentially dangerous duplication, it is necessary to establish that all pain-related orders, including orders for sedatives, hypnotics, and other CNS depressants, come from one source. In our case it is the Acute Pain Service. Responsibility for analgesic therapy reverts to the surgeon when patients can obtain satisfactory pain relief with oral analgesics.

3. Medical Support: Clinical rounds on all patients on the Acute Pain Service are made each morning and thereafter throughout the day as necessary. For each patient, quality of analgesia and side effects are assessed, effective narcotic dose is noted, the epidural catheter site is inspected, and chart documentation of care is completed. Acute Pain Service physicians are available at all times to answer questions from ward nurses, consult with surgeons, or see patients who are experiencing problems with any aspect of their pain relief.

Nursing Policies and Procedures

Developing hospital-wide nursing policies and procedures helps standardize clinical practice using techniques such as EOA and PCA. Standardization promotes safety and creates a framework from which individualized patient care follows. Policies, the foundation or "ground rules" for practice, accompanied by step-wise procedures which outline the "how to" are located in manuals on each nursing unit. The polices and procedures (alternately called nursing protocols) also serve as ongoing educational and informational references.

MANPOWER AND TRAINING

Pain Management Physicians

A postoperative pain management service makes considerable demands, both administrative and clinical, on those responsible for its operation. Initial administrative duties include liaison with nursing services in the development of policies and protocols, standard orders, monitoring practice, and medical responsibility. Hospital administration must be consulted to initiate the purchase or leasing of equipment (e.g., PCA pumps). Teaching programs for ward nurses must be developed, updated as needed, and frequently offered. Mechanisms for disseminating information to surgeons and surgical patients are necessary. An educational program is also needed for the operating room anesthesiologists. In an academic department, the education of medical students, anesthesiology residents, and fellows must be planned. Appropriate research should be encouraged and supported early in the evolution of a new service. Once a program has been established, physicians must be available to provide daily patient care and a call response capability. In a busy hospital this can easily become a full time activity.

Operating Room Anesthesiologists

Close cooperation and communication are essential between the operating room anesthesiologist and the postoperative pain management team which assumes responsibility for analgesia when surgery is completed. Recommendations for postoperative analgesia including benefits, risks, and alternatives are best made to patients at the time of the preanesthetic visit.

NURSES

1. EOA: Ongoing education is integral to patient safety. Nursing education must precede implementation of EOA or PCA in the clinical setting. Our education program for nursing management of patients receiving EOA consists of a video program accompanied by written material and practical experience under supervision. The nurse education video is entitled Epidural Analgesia: the Basics and Beyond. Those interested in more information should call the Health Sciences Center for Educational Resources, University of Washington, Seattle, WA (206) 685-1186.

2. PCA: The educational thrust for nurses when introducing PCA is the set-up and operation of PCA pumps. Most companies marketing PCA devices provide educational resources and inservice training for nursing staff. We use a video tape to assist in educating new nursing staff.

SURGEONS

For reasons of patient safety, the standard orders for EOA and PCA specify that all orders for pain control and sedatives are to be given by the pain service. Responsibility for analgesic therapy reverts to the surgeon when patients can obtain satisfactory pain relief with an oral analgesic. To facilitate a smooth transition, the surgeon is asked to write oral analgesic orders immediately after surgery to become effective when EOA or PCA are discontinued.

PHARMACISTS

To facilitate prompt, safe care, the hospital pharmacy must become familiar with special preparations of narcotics for epidural injection or infusion, and the loading and operating procedures for a number of pumps sometimes used for administering them. They can assure drug compatibility when local anesthetics and narcotics are mixed and can alert physicians if they identify the possibility of adverse drug interactions. They must develop reliable stocking and dispensing procedures for narcotics administered by PCA pumps. Controlled substance regulations must be followed while using these new methods of narcotic administration.

FUTURE DIRECTIONS OF ACUTE PAIN SERVICES

There is no doubt that changes in acute pain management practices will be needed to keep pace with changing times. An example of such a change might be that experts in acute pain management provide leadership within their institutions in developing programs to meet the needs of all patients. In the past, when such programs were established, all the therapy provided tended to be the sole clinical responsibility of the experts that developed the programs. An alternative approach could be programs that are developed and administered by the "experts" but which make provision for acute pain management in uncomplicated patients by primary physicians. In such a program the experts direct more of their clinical attention more toward treatment of more complex patients. The Acute Pain Service at the University of Washington Medical Center has developed such a program to guide PCA use throughout the institution (tables 1-2, figures 1-3). The importance of collaboration with others in developing such programs, in particular collaboration with nurses, deserves repeated emphasis.

Table 1. UWMC PCA Program.

Program Goals

- To facilitate use of PCA in a way that best meets the needs of patients at UWMC
- To define and maintain standards of practice with regard to effective and safe use of PCA
- To permit management of PCA in "routine" patients by primary services wishing to do so
- To ensure management of PCA in "complex" patients by the pain service
- To ensure adequate education for all physicians prescribing PCA, and for all nurses caring for patients using PCA
- To ensure bedside nurses have access to medical expertise
- To minimize pharmacy-related problems
- To provide ongoing assessment of the success of the program

---

Table 2 .

Role of the Pain Service
(Physicians and CNS)

- Develop and supervise the program
- Develop and distribute educational
  resources with revisions as needed:
    - physicians
    - nurses
- Develop preprinted orders with revisions as needed
- Liaison with primary care services
- Liaison with pharmacy
- Liaison with unit nurses
- Liaison with hospital administration
- Manage equipment-related issues
- Develop CQI program and collaborate
  in its application
- Manage "routine" PCA patients when requested
- Manage all "complex" PCA patients
- Provide consultation when difficulty is
  experienced with "routine" PCA patients
- Manage epidural analgesia, nitrous oxide, local
  anesthetic techniques, etc.

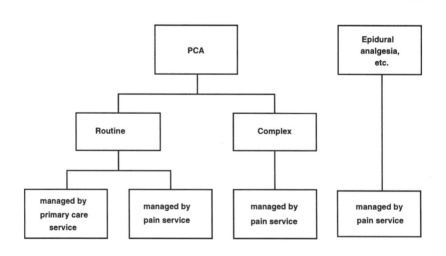

Figure 1. Patients in Acute Pain

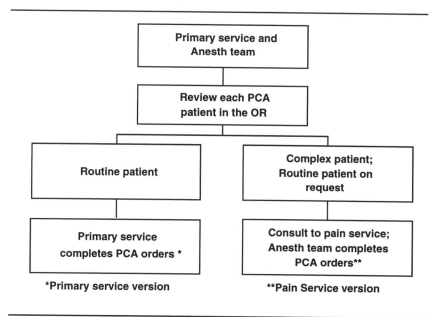

Figure 2.

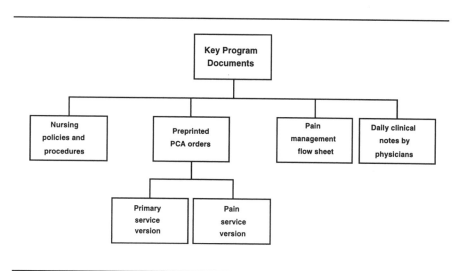

Figure 3.

REFERENCES

1. Bejarano P, Duque C, Griego J, Alvarez OL: "Naughty goblins" during the establishment of a PCA program. Abstracts - 7th World Congress on Pain 392, 1993

2. Berde C, Sethna NF, Masek B, Fosburg M, Rocklin S: Pediatric pain clinics: recommendations for their development. Pediatrician 16:94-102, 1989

3. Breivik H, Högström H, Curatoto M, Weiss S, Zbinden A, Thomson D: Developing a hospital-wide postoperative pain service. Acta Anaesth Scand 37(S100):223, 1993

4. Brenn BR, Rose JB: Pediatric pain services: monitoring for epidural analgesia in the non-intensive care unit setting (letter). Anesthesiology 83:432-433, 1995

5. Cartwright PD, Helfinger RG, Howell JJ, Siepmann KK: Introducing an acute pain service. Department of Anaesthesia, Princess Royal Hospital, Telford. Anaesthesia 46:188-191, 1991

6. Chein BB, Burke RG, Hunter DL: An extensive experience with postoperative pain relief using postoperative fentanyl infusion. Arch Surg 126:692-695, 1991

7. Cross DA, Hunt JB: Feasibility of epidural morphine for postoperative analgesia in a small community hospital. Anesth Analg 72:765-768, 1991

8. Dear G, Sullivan F, Muir M, Ginsberg B: National survey of epidural analgesia in hospital based pain services (abstract). Anesth Analg 82:S87, 1996

9. Delilkan AE, Vijayan R: Experience with an acute pain service in a developing country. Abstracts - 7th World Congress on Pain 395, 1993

10. Domsky M, Kwartowitz J: Efficacy of subarachnoid morphine in a community hospital. Reg Anesth 17:279-282, 1992

11. Ginsberg B, Sullivan F, Muir M, Dear G: Monitoring practices following epidural opioids for acute pain management (abstract). Anesth Analg 82:S131, 1996

12. Gould TH, Harmer M, Lloyd SM, Lunn JN, Rees GAD, Roberts DE, Webster JA: Policy for controlling pain after surgery: effects of sequential changes in management. Br Med J 305:1187-1193, 1992

13. Hart L, Macintyre PE, Winefield H, Rousefell BF, Runciman WB: Re-evaluation of patient, medical and nursing staff attitudes to postoperative opioid analgesia after the establishment of an acute pain service: stage 2 of a longitudinal study. Abstracts - 7th World Congress on Pain 397, 1993

14. Hoopman P: Nursing considerations for acute pain management. Postoperative Pain Management. Edited by Ferrante, FM, Vade Boncouer, TR. New York: Churchill Livingstone, 1993, pp 605-612

15. Hughes JH: Comments on low cost acute pain services (letter). Pain 59:154, 1994

16. Judge M, Merry AF: The assessment of the impact of the introduction of an acute pain management service. Abstracts - 7th World Congress on Pain 398, 1993

17. Kinnear SB, Macintyre PE, Hart L, Webb RK: Pain relief for cholecystectomy patients before and after the start of an acute pain service - stage 2 of a longitudinal study. Abstracts - 7th World Congress on Pain 397, 1993

18. Lauder GR, Sutton D: The acute pain service and GP referral practices [letter]. Anaesthesia 48:454, 1993

19. Le Sage EM: Financial Aspects of Acute Pain Management. Postoperative Pain Management. Edited by Ferrante, FM, VadeBoncouer, TR. New York: Churchill Livingstone, 1993, pp 599-604

20. Macintyre PE, Ready L: Acute Pain Management: a Practical Guide. London: W B Saunders, 1996

21. Macintyre PE, Runciman WB, Webb RK: An acute pain service in an Australian teaching hospital: the first year. Med J Aust 153:417-421, 1990

22. Mackey DC, Ebener MK, Howe BL: Patient-controlled analgesia and the acute pain service in the United States: health-care financing administration policy is impeding optimal patient-controlled analgesia management (letter). Anesthesiology 83:433-434, 1995

23. McKenna M, Murphy DF: The role of the nurse in the acute pain service. Abstracts - 7th World Congress on Pain 398, 1993

24. O'Connor M, Warwick P, Culpeper VEA: Evaluation of the effectiveness of an acute pain team. Abstracts - 7th World Congress on Pain 394, 1993

25. Pasero CL, Hubbard L: Development of an acute pain service monitoring and evaluation system. QRB Qual Rev Bull 17:396-401, 1991

26. Ramsey DH: Perioperative pain: establishing an analgesia service. Problems in Anesthesia - Perioperative Analgesia. Edited by Brown, DL. Philadelphia: Lippincott, 1988, pp 321-326

27. Rawal N: Postoperative pain treatment on wards - Swedish experience. Acta Anaesth Scand 37(S100):6-8, 1993

28. Rawal N: Acute pain services in Europe - a 17-country survey. Reg Anesth 20-2S:85, 1995

29. Rawal N: Organization of an acute pain service - a low-cost alternative. Abstracts - 7th World Congress on Pain 398, 1993

30. Rawal N: Postoperativ Smärta Och Dess Behandling. Örebro: Kabi Pharmacia, 1991

31. Rawal N: Epidural and intrathecal opioids for postoperative pain management in Europe—a 17-nation survey. Reg Anesth 20-2S:45, 1995

32. Rawal N, Berggren L: Organization of acute pain services: a low-cost model. Pain 57:117-123, 1994

33. Ready LB: Acute pain service unit. Acta Anaesth Scand 37(S100):137-140, 1993

34. Ready LB: How well is patient-controlled analgesia managed? - in reply (letter). Anesthesiology 83:640, 1995

35. Ready LB: The acute pain service. Acta Anaesth Belg 43:21-27, 1992

36. Ready LB: How many acute pain services are there in the United States and who is managing patient-controlled analgesia? (letter). Anesthesiology 82:322, 1995

37. Ready LB, Edwards WT: Management of Acute Pain: a Practical Guide. Seattle: IASP Publications, 1992

38. Ready LB, Oden R, Chadwick HS, Benedetti C, Caplan RA, Wild LM: Development of an anesthesiology-based postoperative pain management service. Anesthesiology 68:100-106, 1988

39. Ready LB, Rawal N: Anesthesiology-based acute pain services: a contemporary view. Textbook of Regional Anesthesia and Analgesia. Edited by Brown, DL. Philadelphia: W. B. Saunders Company, 1996

40. Ready LB, Wild LM: Organization of an acute pain service: training and manpower. Anesthesiology Clinics of North America - Postoperative Pain. Edited by Oden, RV. Philadelphia: Saunders, 1989, pp 229-239

41. Saidman LJ: The anesthesiologist outside the operating room: a new and exciting opportunity (editorial). Anesthesiology 68:1-2, 1988

42. Salomäki TE, Laitinen JO, Nuutinen LS: Postoperative pain management on wards. Finnish experience. Acta Anaesth Scand 37(S100):9-11, 1993

43. Sandler AN: Acute pain -guidelines for care. Can J Anaesth 44:R137-R141, 1997

44. Schug SA, Haridas RP: Development and organizational structure of an acute pain service in a major teaching hospital. Aust N Z J Surg 63:8-13, 1993

45. Schug SA, Torrie JJ: Safety assessment of postoperative pain management by an acute pain service. Pain 55:387-391, 1993

46. Scott DA, Beilby DSN, McClymont C: Postoperative analgesia using epidural infusions of fentanyl with bupivacaine: a prospective analysis of 1,014 patients. Anesthesiology 83:727-737, 1995

47. Shapiro BS, Cohen DE, Covelman KW, Howe CJ, Scott SM: Experience of an interdisciplinary pediatric pain service. Pediatrics 88:1226-1232, 1991

48. Shipton E, A, Beeton AG, S MH: Introducing a patient-controlled analgesia-based acute pain service. S Afr Med J 83:501-505, 1993

49. Smith G: Pain after surgery. Br J Anaesth 67:233-234, 1991

50. Steude GM, Hasselbach N, Urbanski B: Complications associated with bupivacaine-fentanyl epidural infusions with PCEA for pain control in postoperative patients. Anesth Analg 80-S1:S473, 1995

51. VadeBoncouer TR, Ferrante FM: Management of a postoperative pain service in a teaching hospital. Postoperative Pain Management. Edited by Ferrante, FM, VadeBoncouer, TR. New York: Churchill Livingstone, 1993, pp 625-639

52. Warfield CA, Kahn CH: Acute pain management: programs in U.S. hospitals and experiences and attitudes among U.S. adults. Anesthesiology 83:1090-1094, 1995

53. Watt JW, Wiles JR: Does an acute pain service require a high dependency unit? [letter]. Anaesthesia 46:789-790, 1991

54. Wenrich J: Acute pain service in a community hospital. J Post Anesth Nurs 6:324-330, 1991

55. Wheatley RG, Madej TH, Jackson IJB, Hunter D: The first year's experience of an acute pain service. Br J Anaesth 67:353-359, 1991

56. Zimmermann DL, Stewart J: Postoperative pain management and acute pain service activity in Canada. Can J Anaesth 40:568-575, 1993

57. Ready LB, Loper KA, Nessly M, Wild L: Postoperative epidural morphine is safe on surgical wards. Anesthesiology 75:452-456, 1991

USE OF NON-OPIOID ANALGESIC TECHNIQUES *

P. F. White

"Slapping the patient on the face and telling him or her that 'it's all over' is a complete inversion of the truth. As far as the patient is concerned, it is often just the beginning" (1). Although the currently available armamentarium of analgesic drugs and techniques is impressive (2,3), management of acute postoperative pain poses some unique problems following ambulatory surgery (4). The increasing number and complexity of operations being performed on an outpatient basis are presenting the practitioner with new challenges with respect to acute pain management. Outpatients undergoing day-care procedures require an analgesic technique that is effective, has minimal side effects, is intrinsically safe, and can be easily managed away from the hospital or surgery center (5).

The adequacy of postoperative pain control is one of the most important factors in determining when a patient can be safely discharged from the outpatient facility. Since inadequately treated pain is a major cause of unanticipated hospital admissions after ambulatory surgery, the ability to provide adequate pain relief by simple methods that are readily available to the day-care patient in his or her home environment is one of the major challenges for providers of outpatient surgery and anesthesia. Unfortunately, there are very few well-controlled studies that have examined the incidence and severity of pain after outpatient surgery, or the adequacy of its treatment. Even in the majority of postsurgical inpatients, parenteral opiate analgesics administered for moderate or severe pain fail to achieve adequate pain relief. Not surprisingly, inadequate analgesia is the most common surgically-related cause of unanticipated hospital admission after ambulatory surgery.

Perioperative analgesia has traditionally been provided by opioid analgesics. However, aggressive use of opioids can be associated with an increased incidence of postoperative nausea and vomiting, which may in

*Adapted from Joshi GP, Fredman B, White PF: In Anesthesiology and Pain Management (Stanley TH and Ashburn MA, Eds.), Klumer Academic Publishers, Netherlands, 1994, pp. 151-169.

T. H. Stanley et al. (eds.), Pain Management and Anesthesiology, 137–152.
© 1998 *Kluwer Academic Publishers. Printed in the Netherlands.*

turn contribute to a delayed discharge from the day-care facility. In order to minimize these opioid-related adverse effects, "balanced" analgesia (6) involving the use of opioid and non-opioid analgesic drugs [local anesthetics and non-steroidal anti-inflammatory drugs (NSAIDs)] is becoming increasingly popular.

In this lecture, the rationale for the perioperative use of local anesthetics, NSAIDs and non-pharmacologic techniques will be discussed.

LOCAL ANESTHETIC TECHNIQUES

Peripheral nerve blocks and wound infiltration with local anesthetics are becoming increasingly popular adjuvants to general anesthesia because they can provide significant intraoperative and postoperative analgesia. These techniques can decrease the incidence of pain and reduce the requirements for narcotic analgesics in the perioperative period. Pain relief in the early postoperative period from the residual block of the local anesthetic techniques provides for a rapid and smooth recovery, enabling earlier ambulation and discharge. Local anesthesia and effective postoperative pain control can decrease the incidence of nausea and vomiting, and thereby, potentially lowering the incidence of unanticipated hospital admissions after ambulatory surgery. Struggling, crying, and restlessness can result in hematoma formation and thereby delay wound healing. Adequate pain control leads to decreased manipulation of the surgical site and thereby reduces swelling, hematoma formation, and infection (4).

Carefully controlled clinical studies are needed to identify the most efficient techniques and the most suitable local anesthetic and/or local anesthetic mixtures for peripheral blocks. Blockade of the ilioinguinal and iliohypogastric nerves with bupivacaine significantly decreases the anesthetic and analgesic requirements in children and adults undergoing inguinal herniorrhaphy (7-9). Infiltration of the ilioinguinal, iliohypogastric and genitofemoral nerves with 0.25% bupivacaine provided 6-8 h of effective analgesia after inguinal herniorrhaphy (10). In addition, pain from a Pfannenstiel's incision can be treated with bilateral blockade of the ilioinguinal and iliohypogastric nerves (11). Although, this technique can be useful in providing analgesia from the skin and layers of the anterior abdominal wall, it does not block visceral pain.

Subcutaneous ring block of the penis with 0.25% bupivacaine effectively provides analgesia after circumcision (12). For postcircumcision pain, penile block with a mixture of 1% lidocaine and 0.25% bupivacaine is as effective as 0.25% bupivacaine alone, however, with significantly lower serum levels of bupivacaine (13). Similarly, infiltration of the mesosalpinx in the area of the Yoon ring placement, with 0.5% bupivacaine or 1% etidocaine, significantly decreases the postoperative pain and cramping after laparoscopic tubal ligation (14,15). Pain after knee surgery has been successfully treated with femoral nerve blocks (16). However, complete anesthesia of the knee would require anesthetizing not only the femoral nerve but also the obturator, lateral femoral cutaneous, and sciatic nerves.

While subcutaneous infiltration of the operative site with local anesthetics remains a popular technique for decreasing the postoperative opioid analgesic requirement (17,18), other simplified local anesthetic delivery systems have been described in the anesthesia literature. Topical analgesia with lidocaine aerosol was found to be highly effective in decreasing pain, as well as the opioid analgesic requirement, after inguinal herniorrhaphy (19) (Figure 1). Instillation of 0.25% bupivacaine into the hernia wound provided similar postoperative pain relief as ilioinguinal/iliohypogastric nerve block in children (20). The simple application of topical lidocaine jelly, lidocaine ointment, or lidocaine spray

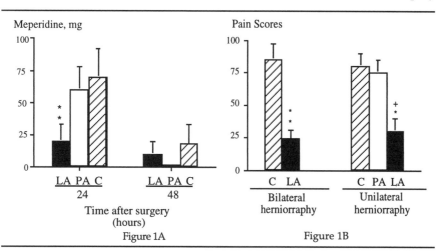

Figure 1A: Meperidine requirements in the first 24 hr after inguinal hernia repair were significantly reduced for patients treated with lidocaine aerosol (LA) in the wound, compared with patients treated with placebo aerosol (PA) or untreated control patients (C). Bars show mean requirement, whiskers demarcate SEM (**P < 0.01).

Figure 1B: 24 hr after surgery, pain scores on palpation of the herniorrhaphy wound were significantly less when treated with LA in the wound (left portion of panel). There was a significant reduction of pain scores with LA (**P<0.01). Seven patients having bilateral hernia repair (right portion of panel) were randomly assigned to treatment on one wide with LA or PA, while the other side was left untreated as a paired control. There was a significant response compared with control for LA (*P<0.05), and for LA versus PA (+P<0.05).

[Data from Sinclair et al. (19).]

has been shown to be as effective as nerve blocks and parenteral opioids in providing pain relief after outpatient circumcision (21,22) (Table 1). Although, pain relief was comparable with all topical techniques, children preferred lidocaine spray if repeated application was necessary. Intracavity and wound instillation of local anesthetics is another simple and effective

Table 1. Comparative effects of parenteral morphine, bupivacaine nerve block, and topical lidocaine for postoperative pain relief after outpatient circumcision[a].

	Control	Morphine Sulfate (.2 mg/kg)	Nerve Block (1.0-1.5 ml)	Lidocaine Jelly (0.5-1.0 ml)
Age (yr)	5 ± 2	5±2	4±2	4 ± 2
Pain in postanesthesia care unit (%)	92	27	7[b]	5[b]
Pain-free period (h)	1.1 ± 1.0	4.8 ± 1.7[b]	5.2 ± 1.7[b]	5.3 ± 1.9[b]
Analgesic doses (n)				
0-24 h	1.9 ± 1.0	2.0±0.9	1.5 ± 1.1	1.7 ± 1.1
24-48 h	1.5 ± 1.3	0.7 ± 1.1	1.0 ± 1.1[b]	0.7 ± 1.2[b]

[a] Mean values ± SD
[b] Significant difference from the control group, $p<0.05$
[Data from Tree-Trakarn and Pirayavaraporn (21).]

technique for providing pain relief during the early postoperative period. Intraperitoneal administration of local anesthetics (80 ml, 0.5% lidocaine and 0.125% bupivacaine with epinephrine) during laparoscopy was found to be an efficient method of reducing the intensity of postoperative scapular pain (23). Continuous (24,25) or intermittent perfusion (25-28) of the surgical wound with local anesthetic solutions is also an effective technique for pain control after superficial (non-cavitary) procedures. In contrast, several authors using various techniques of local anesthetic wound infiltration have failed to find significant differences in pain relief or narcotic usage (29, 30). The variable results may be due to differences in local anesthetic dose, timing, and concentration.

Local anesthetics are frequently injected into the knee joint to provide analgesia during arthroscopic surgery and to facilitate early recovery. Administration of bupivacaine, lidocaine, mepivacaine, or prilocaine either by single instillation or by controlled pressure-irrigation systems have been described (31-34). Although intraarticular bupivacaine, 25-40 ml, 0.25%, has been demonstrated to be a safe (35,36) and effective analgesic, the mean duration of analgesia is only two hours (37,38). In another study, intraarticular instillation of 30 ml of 0.5% bupivacaine reduced the opioid requirements and facilitated early mobilization after knee arthroscopy but did not significantly decrease the patients' perception of pain (39). However, the results in the postarthroscopy model are inconsistent (40-42).

In recent years, increasing evidence has been obtained to suggest that intraarticular morphine, either alone or in combination with bupivacaine, can produce effective and long-lasting analgesia following knee arthroscopy (43-46). Combining intraarticular bupivacaine 0.5% and ketorolac 60 mg, decreased pain on arrival in the PACU after arthroscopy compared to either the local anesthetic or NSAIDs alone. The combination, however, did not result in earlier discharge. There are few well-controlled studies and the results are controversial (47-49).

Although local anesthetic supplementation usually decrease the severity of pain in the immediate (50) period, patients may still complain of significant pain after discharge due to difficulty in anticipating the degree of pain at the time the patient is allowed to go home (51). Thus, a limitation to a single dose of local anesthetic is duration. These situations may arise when a long-lasting local anesthetic like bupivacaine is used. Combination of local anesthetic techniques with NSAIDs may be used as a part of multimodal therapy to achieve a better pain control throughout the perioperative period. The concept of "balanced analgesia" consists of administration of agents affecting the various physiological processes involved in nociception in order to produce more effective analgesia with fewer side effects (52).

Another factor which has encouraged the increased use of local anesthetic techniques is the concept of preemptive analgesia (53,54). Prophylactic neural blockade prior to surgical incision (and other noxious perioperative stimuli) may prevent the nociceptive input from altering the excitability of the central nervous system. The application of preemptive analgesic techniques is alleged to reduce postoperative pain and skeletal muscle spasm. Preincisional infiltration of bupivacaine in combination with general anesthesia was reported to be superior to spinal anesthesia in relieving postoperative pain (55). These findings suggest that inhibition of peripheral sensitization may be important in prevention of postoperative pain. Similarly, infiltration of the tonsillar bed with bupivacaine prior to tonsillectomy is reported to decrease both constant pain and pain on swallowing for up to 5 days after surgery (56). However, only a few controlled studies have compared neural block administered before and after the surgical stimulus (57).

In summary, wound infiltration and peripheral nerve blocks are found to be simple, safe and effective. Availability of new local anesthetic drugs, with less toxicity and long duration, which selectively block sensory neural fibers may further increase advantages of these techniques. Increasing use of local anesthetic techniques in combination with NSAIDs and opioid analgesics can markedly enhance the safety and efficacy of analgesic drugs in the perioperative period. A multimodal approach can decrease morbidity and permit earlier ambulation and discharge after elective operations. More importantly, improved analgesic techniques will increase patient satisfaction and enhance their perception of ambulatory anesthesia and surgery.

NON-STERIODAL ANTI-INFLAMMATORY DRUGS

Oral non-steriodal anti-inflammatory drugs (NSAIDs) have long been used in medicine for their anti-inflammatory, antipyretic and analgesic properties. With the introduction of parenteral preparations of NSAIDs, more widespread use of these drugs has been reported in the management of postoperative pain. NSAIDs block the synthesis of prostaglandins by inhibition of the enzyme cyclooxygenase (58). Prostaglandins mediate several components of the inflammatory response including fever, pain and vasodilation (59,60). In addition, NSAIDs also have prostaglandin-independent effects such as inhibition of neutrophil migration and lymphocyte responsiveness which contribute to their anti-inflammatory and analgesic properties (61).

Traditionally, the analgesic properties of NSAIDs have been attributed to their inhibitory effects on the synthesis of prostaglandins in the peripheral nerves. Inhibition of prostaglandin synthesis by NSAIDs decreases the tissue inflammatory response to surgical trauma and hence, reduces peripheral nociception and pain perception (62). However, recent *in vivo* animal studies suggest that the central response to painful stimuli may also be modulated by NSAIDs inhibition of prostaglandin synthesis (63). Several recent observations support this central antinociceptor effect of the NSAIDs. Firstly, NSAIDs produce a dose-dependent depression of the rat thalamic response to peripheral nociceptor input. Secondly, they interfere with transmitters or modulators other than prostaglandins in the nociceptive system and the spinal cord (64).

Since the NSAIDs have analgesic properties comparable to opioid compounds (65-67) without opioid-related side effects (68,69), anesthesiologists often administer these drugs as adjuvants during and after surgery.

When ketorolac and dezocine, a μ-receptor agonist-antagonist, were administered as adjuvants to propofol-N_2O anesthesia, both analgesic drugs were associated with improved postoperative analgesia and patient comfort when compared to fentanyl (70). However, ketorolac was associated with a lower incidence of nausea and vomiting, and patients tolerated oral fluids and were judged "fit for discharge" significantly earlier than those in the dezocine treatment group. Similarly, while ketorolac provided postoperative pain relief similar to that of fentanyl (71) it was associated with less nausea, somnolence, and an earlier return of bowel function when compared to fentanyl. Furthermore, the administration of ketorolac as an alternative to fentanyl for augmentation of local anesthesia during monitored anesthesia care resulted in significantly less postoperative pruritus, nausea or vomiting (72). However, when ketorolac was substituted for, or combined with fentanyl for minor gynecological procedures (73-75), it failed to significantly decrease intraoperative opioid requirements, shorten recovery times or decrease postoperative side effects. When ketorolac or saline were administered prior to induction, post-intubation, and in the Postanesthesia Care Unit (PACU) in patients undergoing laparoscopic cholecystectomy, ketorolac decreased immediate postoperative opioid requirements, but failed to influence either emetic sequelae or ventilatory function (76). These seemingly conflicting results can be explained by the timing and dose of ketorolac administered, as well as differences in surgical procedures.

Using shock wave lithotripsy to evaluate the effect of NSAIDs on visceral pain, diclofenac was administered as an adjuvant to a fentanyl-midazolam sedative technique. While diclofenac was associated with improved hemodynamic stability, only a marginal opioid-sparing effect could be demonstrated (77). Furthermore, when this drug was administered intravenously prior to outpatient arthroscopic surgery and compared to either fentanyl 1 mg/kg, IV, or placebo, diclofenac was associated with similar visual analog pain scores to fentanyl (78). However, following laparoscopic surgery, diclofenac had no effect on the recovery profile in the immediate postoperative period, but resulted in decreased pain and analgesic requirements 24 hours postoperatively (79).

Preoperative oral or rectal administration of NSAIDs is also effective in the management of postoperative pain. When oral naproxen was administered prior to laparoscopic surgery, postoperative pain scores, opioid requirements, and time to discharge were significantly shorter when compared to placebo (80). Furthermore, in the late recovery period and after discharge from the outpatient facility, oral ibuprofen (800 mg) or naproxen suppositories (500 mg), were associated with superior analgesia and less nausea compared to fentanyl, 75 mg, IV or placebo (81,82). Intra-articular injection of ketorolac produced no reduction in postoperative pain when compared to intraarticular bupivacaine (83). Similarly, there was no advantage in combining acetylsalicylic acid with local anesthetic during intravenous regional anesthesia (46).

At the extremes of age, opioid-related adverse effects may be of particular concern to the anesthesiologist. When diclofenac and acetaminophen were administered preoperatively to pediatric patients, both the preoperative incidence of restlessness and crying, as well as the postoperative meperidine requirements were lower in the diclofenac-treated patients (84). When oral ketorolac (0.9 mg/kg in juice) was com-pared to both acetaminophen and placebo for bilateral myringotomy pro-cedures in children, the ketorolac-treated patients recorded lower pain scores and required less analgesia in the early postoperative period (85). Similarly, in pediatric patients, the intraoperative administration of ketorolac as an adjuvant to general anesthesia provided postoperative analgesia comparable to morphine (86). The ketorolac-treated patients experienced less postoperative nausea and vomiting. As expected, when either morphine or ketorolac were administered to pediatric patients for postoperative pain relief, ketorolac-induced analgesia developed more slowly but was more sustained than morphine (87).

In a study designed to assess postoperative pain in elderly patients following orthopedic procedures, no significant difference could be demonstrated between patients receiving intramuscular ketorolac or papaveretum followed by the oral administration of either ketorolac or a paracetamol-dextropropoxiphene combination (88). Due to the weak anal-gesic properties of the NSAIDs they have limited use in the management of acute intraoperative pain. However, despite the seemingly conflicting reports in the literature, the NSAIDs are useful adjuvants in the man-agement of postoperative pain in the ambulatory setting. Importantly, it appears that the clinical efficacy of this group of analgesic drugs depends upon the time, route of administration, as well as the surgical procedure. Finally, since the NSAIDs may be associated with less postoperative nausea, vomiting and respiratory depression when compared to the opioid analgesic drugs, their use in outpatient anesthesia will contribute not only a shorter postoperative recovery period, but may also lead to improved patient comfort and safety.

NON-PHARMACOLOGIC TECHNIQUES

The use of transcutaneous electric nerve stimulation (TENS) or acupuncture-like transcutaneous electrical nerve stimulation (ALTENS) and percutaneous electrical nerve stimulation (PENS) have been described in the treatment of chronic pain. Given the inherent side effects produced by both opioid and non-opioid analgesics, as well as the local anesthetics, it is not surprising that the nonpharmacologic approaches to managing acute postoperative pain have been evaluated in the outpatient setting. The mechanisms by which TENS, ALTENS, and PENS may exert their analgesic action have not been completely elucidated. Possible mechanisms include: (i) an influence on descending pain inhibitory pathways, (ii) an inhibition of substance-P release in central nervous structures, (iii) and the release of endogenous opiate substances (89-92).

Transcutaneous electrical nerve stimulation has been reported to produce a 15-30% decrease in the postoperative opioid requirement (93). Pulmonary function was reportedly less depressed in TENS-treated patients than in a sham-treated group (94). In addition, Jensen et al. reported a more rapid recovery of joint mobility after outpatient arthroscopic surgery (95). Nevertheless, other investigative groups have reported no significant decrease in the requirement for opioid analgesic medication or improvement in the quality of postoperative pain control (96,97). When used after superficial surgical procedures, proper application of the stimulating electrodes and proper patient instruction appear to be important factors in achieving success with TENS (98). A double-blind prospective study involving PENS and ALTENS combined with a standardized intubation general anesthesia technique for retroperitoneal lymph node resection showed a reduction of the need for opiates intraoperatively and in the early postoperative period (99). TENS has been used as an adjuvant during and after minor outpatient surgical procedures. However, no well-controlled studies have documented the effectiveness of concomitant use of PENS and/or ALTENS with a conventional anesthetic or analgesic technique for pain relief during and after surgery. Clinical efficacy of this technique remains controversial because potential sources of bias and/or absence of a control (or sham) group precludes conclusive findings. Other nonpharmacologic approaches (e.g., cryoanalgesia, ultrasound, and hypnosis) have also been evaluated as potentially useful adjuvants to opioid analgesics in the early postoperative period (100-102). For most of these modalities, clinical studies have yielded conflicting or inconclusive data (103).

SUMMARY

As more extensive and painful surgery procedures (e.g., laparoscopic cholecystectomy, laminectomy, knee reconstructions, hysterectomies) are being undertaken on an outpatient basis, availability of sophisticated postoperative analgesic regimens are necessary to optimize the benefits of day-care surgery for both the patient and the health care provider. However, outcome studies are needed to evaluate the effect of these newer therapeutic approaches with respect to postoperative side effects, and other important recovery parameters. Recent studies suggest that factors other than pain *per se* must be controlled in order to reduce postoperative morbidity and facilitate the recovery process. Not surprisingly, the anesthetic technique can influence the analgesic requirement in the early postoperative period. Although opioid analgesics will continue to play an important role, the adjunctive use of both local anesthetic agents and non-steroidal anti-inflammatory analgesics will likely assume a greater role in the future. Use of drug combinations (e.g., opiates and local anesthetics, opiates and NSAIDs) may provide for improved analgesia with fewer narcotic-induced side effects than opioid analgesics alone. Finally, safer and simpler analgesic delivery systems are needed to improve our future ability to provide cost-effective pain relief after daycare surgery.

In conclusion, as a result of our enhanced understanding of the mechanisms of acute pain and the physiologic basis of nociception, the provision of "stress free" anesthesia with minimal postoperative discomfort is now possible for most patients undergoing elective surgical procedures. The aim of an analgesic technique should not only be to lower the pain scores but also to facilitate earlier mobilization and to reduce perioperative complications. If future clinical studies clarify the issues which have been raised by experimental work in animals, clinicians may be able to effectively treat postoperative pain using combination of "balanced," "preemptive," and "peripheral" analgesia.

REFERENCES

1. Armitage E. Postoperative pain-prevention or relief (Editorial). Br J Anaesth 1989;63:136-8.
2. White PF. Current and future trends in acute pain management. Clin J Pain 1989;5:51-58.
3. Wildsmith JAW. Symposium on aspects of pain. Br J Anaesth 1989;63:135.

4. White PF. Pain management after day-case surgery. Curr Opinion in Anesthesiol 1988;1:70-75.

5. Poler SM, Zelcer J, White PF. Postoperative pain management. In: White P, ed. Outpatient Anesthesia. New York: Churchill-Livingstone, 1990: 417-451.

6. Code W. NSAIDs and balanced analgesia. Can J Anaesth 1993;40(5):401-5.

7. Cross GD, Barrett RF. Comparison of two regional techniques for postoperative analgesia in children following herniotomy and orchiopexy. Anaesthesia 1987;42:845-49.

8. Langer JC, Shandling B, Rosenberg M. Intraoperative bupivacaine during outpatient hernia repair in children: A randomized double-blind trial. J Ped Surg 1987;22:267-70.

9. Ding Y, White PF. Outpatient herniorrhaphy: use of ilioinguinal-hypogastric nerve block (IHNB) with 0.25% bupivacaine during MAC (Abstract. Anesth Analg 1993;76:S80.

10. Hinkle HA. Percutaneous inguinal blocks for the outpatient management of post-herniorrhaphy pain in children. Anesthesiology 1987;67:411-12.

11. Blunting P, McConachie I. Ilioinguinal nerve blockade for analgesia after caesarean section. Br J Anaesth 1988;61:773-5.

12. Elder PT, Belman AB, Hannallagh RS, et al. Postcircumcision pain: A prospective evaluation of subcutaneous ring block of the penis. Reg Anesth 1984;9:48-9.

13. Sfez M, Le Mapihan Y, Mazoit X, et al. Local anesthetic serum concentration after penile block in children. Anesth Analg 1990;71:423-426.

14. Alexander CD, Wetchler BV, Thompson RE. Bupivacaine infiltration of the mesosalpinx in ambulatory surgical laparoscopic tubal sterilization. Can J Anaesth 1987;34:362.

15. Baram D, Smith C, Stinson S. Intraoperative etidocaine for reducing pain after laparoscopic tubal ligation. J Rep Med 1990;35:407-10.

16. Tierney E, Lewis G, Hurtig JB, et al. Femoral nerve block with bupivacine 0.25% for postoperative analgesia after open knee surgery. Can J Anaesth 1987;34:455-8.

17. Owens H, Galloway DJ, Mitchell KG. Analgesia by wound infiltration after surgical excision of benign breast lumps. Ann R Coll Surg Engl 1985;67:114-5.

18. Moss G, Regal ME, Lichtig L. Reducing postoperative pain, narcotics, and length of hospitalization. Surgery 1986;99:206-10.

19. Sinclair R, Cassuto J, Hogstrom S, et al. Topical anesthesia with lidocaine aerosol in the control of postoperative pain. Anesthesiology 1988;68:895-901.

20. Casey WF, Rice LJ, Hannallah RS, Broadman L, Norden JM, Guzetta P. A comparison between bupivacaine instillation versus ilioinguinal/iliohypogastric nerve block for postoperative analgesia following inguinal herniorrhaphy in children. Anesthesiology. 1990;72:637-639.

21. Tree-Trakarn T, Pirayavaraporn S. Postoperative pain relief for circumcision in children: Comparison among morphine, nerve block, and topical analgesia. Anesthesiology 1985;62:519-22.

22. Tree-Trakarn T, Pirayavaraporn S, Lertakyamee J. Topical analgesia for relief of post-circumcision pain. Anesthesiology 1987;67:395-9.

23. Narchi P, Benhamou D, Fernandez H. Intraperitoneal local anaesthetic for shoulder pain after day-case laparoscopy. Lancet 1991;338:1569-70.

24. Thomas DFM, Lambert WG, Lloyd WK. The direct perfusion of surgical wounds with local anaesthetic solution: An approach to postoperative pain? Ann R Coll Surg Engl 1983;65:226-29.

25. Gibbs P, Purushotam A, Auld C, Cuschieri RJ. Continuous wound perfusion with bupivacaine for postoperative wound pain. Br J Surg 1988;75:923.

26. Hashemi K, Middleton MD. Subcutaneous bupivacaine for postoperative analgesia after herniorrhaphy. Ann R Coll Surg Engl 1983;65:38-9.

27. Levack ID, Robertson GS. The direct perfusion of surgical wounds with local anaesthetic solution. Ann R Coll Surg Engl 1984;66:146.

28. Levack ID, Holmes JD, Robertson GS. Abdominal wound perfusion for the relief of postoperative pain. Br J Anaesth 1986;58:615.

29. Cameron AEP, Cross FW. Pain and morbidity after inguinal herniorrhaphy: Ineffectiveness of subcutaneous bupivacaine. Br J Surg 1985;72:68-9.

30. Aull L, Woodward ER, Rout RW, et al. Analgesia and postoperative hypoxemia after gastric partion with and without bupivacaine. Can J Anaesth 1990;37:S53.

31. Butterworth JF, Carnes RS, Samuel MP, Janeway D, Poehling GG. Effect of adrenaline on plasma concentrations of bupivacaine following intra-articular injection of bupivacaine for knee arthroscopy. Br J Anaesth 1990;65:537-9.

32. Dahl MR, Dasta JF, Zuelzer W, McSweeney TD. Lidocaine local anesthesia for arthroscopic knee surgery. Anesth Analg 1990;71:670-4.

33. Hultin J, Hamberg P, Stenstrom A. Knee arthroscopy using local anesthesia. Arthroscopy 1992;8:239-41.

34. Wredmark T, Rolf L. Arthroscopy under local anaesthesia using controlled pressure-irrigation with prilocaine. J Bone Joint Surg. 1982;64-B:583-5.

35. Katz JA, Keading CS, Hill JR, Henthorn TK. The pharmacokinetics of bupivacaine when injected intra-articularly after knee arthroscopy. Anesth Analg 1988;67:871-5.

36. Solanki DR, Enneking FK, Ivey FM, Scarborough M, Johnston RV. Serum bupivacaine concentrations after intraarticular injection for pain relief after knee arthroscopy. Arthroscopy 1992;8:44-7.

37. Chirwa SS, MacLeod BA, Day B. Intraarticular bupivacaine (Marcaine) after arthroscopic meniscectomy: a randomized double-blind controlled study. Arthroscopy 1989;5:33-5.

38. Kaeding CC, Hill JA, Katz J, Benson L. Bupivacaine use after knee arthroscopy: pharmacokinetics and pain control study. Arthroscopy 1990;6:33-9.

39. Smith I, Van Hemelrijck J, White PF, Shively R. Effects of local anesthesia on recovery after outpatient arthroscopy. Anesth Analg 1991;73:536-9.

40. Milligan KA, Mowbray MJ, Mulrooney L, Standen PJ. Intra-articular bupivacaine for pain relief after arthroscopic surgery of the knee joint in daycase patients. Anaesthesia 1988;43:563-4.

41. Hughes DJ. Intra-articular bupivacaine for pain relief in arthroscopic surgery. Anaesthesia 1985;40:821.

42. Henderson RC, Campion ER, DeMasi RA, Taft TN. Postarthroscopy analgesia with bupivacaine. Am J Sports Med 1990;18:614-7.

43. Joshi GP, McCarroll SM, Cooney CM, Blunnie WP, O'Brien TM, Lawrence AJ. Intra-articular morphine for pain relief after knee arthroscopy. J Bone Joint Surg 1992;74-B:749-51.

44. Stein C, Comisel K, Haimeri E, et al. Analgesic effect of intraarticular morphine after arthroscopic knee surgery. N Engl J Med 1991;325:1123-6.

45. Khoury GF, Chen ACN, Garland DE, Stein C. Intraarticular morphine, bupivacaine, and morphine/bupivacaine for pain control after knee videoarthroscopy. Anesthesiology 1992;77:263-6.

46. Corpataux J, Van Gessel E, Forster A, Gamulin Z. Does the addition of acetylsalicylic acid to local anesthetic during the Beir block improve postoperative analgesia? Anesthesiology 1992;77:A811.

47. Stein C. Peripheral mechanisms of opioid analgesia. Anesth Analg 1993;76:182-91.

48. Raja SN, Dickstein RE, Johnson CA. Comparison of postoperative analgesic effects of intraarticular bupivacaine and morphine following arthroscopic knee surgery. Anesthesiology 1992;77:1143-47.

49. Heard SO, Edwards WT, Ferrari D, et al. Analgesic effect of intraarticular bupivacaine or morphine after arthroscopic knee surgery: A randomized, prospective, double-blind study. Anesth Analg 1992;74:822-6.

50. Smith I, Shively RA, White PF. Effects of ketorolac and bupivacaine on recovery after outpatient arthroscopy. Anesth Analg 1992;75:208-12.

51. Meridy HW. Criteria for selection of ambulatory surgery patients and guidelines for anesthetic management: A retrospective study of 1553 cases. Anesth Analg 1982;61:921-26.

52. Dahl JB, Rosenberg J, Dirkes WE, Mogensen T, Kehlet H. Prevention of postoperative pain by balanced analgesia. Br J Anaesth 1990;64:518-20.

53. Wall PD. The prevention of postoperative pain. Pain 1988;33:289-90.

54. Woolf CJ. Recent advances in the pathophysiology of acute pain. Br J Anaesth 1989;63:139-46.

55. Tverskoy M, Cozacov C, Ayache M, Bradley EL, Kissin I. Postoperative pain after inguinal herniorrhaphy with different types of anesthesia. Anesth Analg 1990;70:29-35.

56. Jebeles J, Reilly J, Gutierrez J, Bradley E, Kissin I. The effect of preincisional infiltration of tonsils with bupivacaine on the pain following tonsillectomy under general anesthesia. Pain 1991;47:305-8.

57. Dahl JB, Kehlet H. The value of pre-emptive analgesia in the treatment of postoperative pain. Br J Anaesth 1993;70:434-439.

58. Vane JR. Inhibition of prostaglandin synthesis as a mechanism of action for the aspirin-like drugs. Nature New Biol 1971;231:232.

59. Moncada S, Vane JR. Arachidonic acid metabolites and the interactions between platelets and blood-vessel walls. N Engl J Med 1979;300:1142.

60. Trang LE. Prostaglandins and inflammation. Semin Arthr Rheum 1980;9:153.

61. Abramson SB, Weissman G. The mechanisms of action of nonsteriodal anti-inflammatory drugs. Arthr Rheum 1989;32:1-9.

62. Dahl J, Kehlet H. Non-steroidal anti-inflammatory drugs: Rationale for use in severe postoperative pain. Br J Anaesth 1991;66:703-12.

63. Malmberg AB, Yaksh TL. Hyperalgesia mediated by spinal glutamate or substance P receptor blocked by spinal cyclooxygenase inhibition. Science 1992;257:1276-8.

64. Jurna I, Brune K. Central effect of the non-steroid anti-inflammatory agents, indomethacin, ibuprofen, and diclofenac, determined in C fibre-evoked activity in single neurons of the rat thalamus. Pain 1990;41:71-80.

65. Yee JP, Koshiver JE, Albon C, et al. Comparison of intramuscular ketorolac tromethamine and morphine sulphate for analgesia of pain after major surgery. Pharmacotherapy 1986;6(5):253-61.

66. O'Hara DA, Fragen RJ, Kinzer M, et al. Ketorolac tromethamine as compared with morphine sulphate for the treatment of postoperative pain. Clin Pharm Ther 1987;41:556-61.

67. Powell H, Smallman JMB, Morgan M. Comparison of intramuscular ketorolac and morphine in pain control after laparotomy. Anaesthesia 1990;45:538-42.

68. Murray AW, Borckway MS, Kenny GNC. Comparison of the cardiorespiratory effects of ketorolac and alfentanil during propofol anesthesia. Br J Anaesth 1989;63:601-3.

69. Kenny GNC, Mcardle CS, Aitkin HH. Parenteral Ketorolac: Opiatesparing effect and the lack of cardiorespiratory depression in the perioperative patient. Pharmacotherapy 1990;10:127S-31S.

70. Ding Y, White PF. Comparative effects of ketorolac, dezocine and fentanyl as adjuvants during outpatient anesthesia. Anesth Analg 1992;75:566-71.

71. Wong H, Carpenter R, Kopacz, et al. A randomized double-blind evaluation of ketorolac tromethamine for postoperative analgesia in ambulatory surgery patients. Anesthesiology 1993;78:6-14.

72. Bosek B, Smith D, Cox C. Ketorolac or fentanyl to supplement local anesthesia. J Clin Anesth 1992;4:480-3.

73. Ding Y, White PF. Use of ketorolac and fentanyl during ambulatory surgery. Anesthesiology 1992;77:A5.

74. Ding Y, Fredman B, White PF. Use of ketorolac and fentanyl during outpatient gynecological surgery. Anesth Analg 1993;in press.

75. Green CR, Pandit SK, Kothary SP, et al. No fentanyl sparing effect of intraoperative iv ketorolac after laparoscopic tubal ligation. Anesthesiology 1992;77:A7.

76. Liu J, Ding Y, White PF, et al. Effects of ketorolac on postoperative analgesia and ventilatory function after laparoscopic cholecystectomy. Anesth Analg 1993;76:1061-6.

77. Fredman B, Jedeikin R, Olsfanger D, et al. The opioid-sparing effect of diclofenac sodium in outpatient extracorporeal shock wave lithotripsy (ESWL). J Clin Anesth 1992;5:141-4.

78. McLoughlin C, McKinney MS, Fee JPH, et al. Diclofenac for day-care arthroscopy surgery: comparison with standard opioid therapy. Br J Anaesth 1990;65:620-3.

79. Gillberg LE, Harsten AS, Stahl LB. Preoperative diclofenac sodium reduces post-laparoscopy pain. Can J Anaesth 1993;40(5):406-8.

80. Comfort VK, Code WE, Rooney ME, Yip RW. Naproxen premedication reduces postoperative tubal ligation pain. Can J Anaesth 1992;4:349-52.

81. Rosenblum M, Weller RS, Conrad PL, et al. Ibuprofen provides longer lasting analgesia than fentanyl after laparoscopic surgery. Anesth Analg 1991;73:255-9.

82. Dueholm S, Forrest M, Hjortso E, et al. Pain relief following herniotomy: a double-blind randomized comparison between naproxen and placebo. Acta Anaesthesiol Scand 1989;33:391-4.

83. Monahan SJ, Johnson CJ, Downing JE, Fontenot KJ, Buhrman WC. Post arthroscopy analgesia with intra-articular ketorolac. Anesthesiology 1992;77:A854.

84. Baer GA, Rorarius MGF, Kolehmainen S, et al. The effect of paracetamol or diclofenac administered before operation on postoperative pain and behavior in small children. Anaesthesia 1992;47:1078-80.

85. Watcha MF, Ramirez-Ruiz M, White PF, et al. Perioperative effects of oral ketorolac and acetaminophen in children undergoing bilateral myringotomy. Can J Anaesth 1993;39:649-54.

86. Watcha MF, Jones MB, Lagueruela RG, et al. Comparison of ketorolac and morphine as adjuvants during pediatric surgery. Anesthesiology 1992;76:368-72.

87. Maunaksela E, Kokki H, Bullingham RES. Comparison of intravenous ketorolac with morphine for postoperative pain in children. Clin Pharmacol Ther 1992;52:436-43.

88. Smallman JMB, Powell H, Ewart MC, et al. Ketorolac for postoperative analgesia in elderly patients. Anaesthesia 1992;47:149-52.

89. Takeshige C, Sato T, Mera T, Hisamitsu T, Fang J. Descending pai inhibitory system involved in acupuncture analgesia. Brain Research Bulletin 1992;29:617-34.

90. Yonehara N, Sawada T, Matsura H, Inoki R. Influence of electro-acupuncture on the release of substance P and the potential evoked by tooth pulp stimulation in the trigeminal nucleus caudalis of the rat. Neuroscience Letters 1992;142:53-56.

91. Cheng SS, Pomeranz BH. Electro-acupuncture analgesia is mediated by stereospecific opiate receptors and is reversed antagonists of type I receptors. Life Science 1980;26:631-8.

92. Mayer DJ, Price DD, Rafii A. Antagonism of acupuncture analgesia in man by narcotic antagonist naloxone. Brain Research 1979;121:368-72.

93. Tyler E, Caldwell C, Ghia JN. Transcutaneous electrical nerve stimulation: an alternative approach to the management of postoperative pain. Anesth Analg 1982;61:449.

94. Ali J, Yaffe C, Serrette C. The effect of transcutaneous nerve stimulation on postoperative pain and pulmonary function. Surgery 1981;89:507.

95. Jensen JE, Conn RR, Hazelrigg G, Hewett JE. The use of transcutaneous neural stimulation and isokinetic testing in arthroscopic knee surgery. Am J Sports Med 1985;13:27.

96. McCallum MI, Glynn CJ, Moore RA, et al. Transcutaneous electrical nerve stimulation in the management of acute postoperative pain. Br J Anaesth 1988;61:308.

97. Smedley F, Taube M, Wastell C. Transcutaneous electrical nerve stimulation for pain relief following inguinal hernia repair: a controlled trial. Eur Surg Res 1988;20:233.

98. Cooperman AM, Hall B, Mikalacki K, et al. Use of transcutaneous electrical stimulation in the control of postoperative pain. Am J Surg 1977;133:185.

99. Kho HG, van Egmond J, Zuang CF, Lin GF, Zhang GL. Acupuncture anaesthesia: Observations on its use for removal of thyroid adenomata and influence on recovery and morbidity in a Chinese hospital. Anaesthesia 1990;45:480-5.

100. Khiroya RC, Davenport HT, Jones JG. Cryoanalgesia for pain after herniorrhaphy. Anaesthesia 1986;41:73.

101. Hashish I, Hai HK, Harvey W, et al. Reduction of postoperative pain and swelling by ultrasound treatment: a placebo effect. Pain 1988;33:303.

102. Houle M, McGrath PA, Moran G, Garrett OJ. The efficacy of hypnosis- and relaxation-induced analgesia on two dimensions of pain for cold pressor and electrical toothe pulp stimulation. Pain 1988;33:241.

103. Wood GJ, Lloyd JW, Bullingham RES, et al. Postoperative analgesia for day-case herniorrhaphy patients: a comparison of cryoanalgesia, paravertebral blockade and oral analgesia. Anaesthesia 1981;36:603.

PAIN MANAGEMENT IN CHILDREN

L. J. Rice

> *Pain is an unpleasant sensory and emotional experience associated with tissue damage (actual or potential) or described in terms of such damage*
>
> International Association for the Study of Pain

DO CHILDREN EXPERIENCE PAIN DIFFERENTLY?

Children experience pain differently than do adults. Adults experience a needle as a brief, uncomfortable, inconvenience; while children regard it as the epitome of all the evil of their disease (1). The emotional component of pain is very strong—a child may "feel" the absence of visitors or the missed class activity to be much more painful than the traction and broken leg in the hospital. Children with cancer have stated that they would rather die than receive another needle.

Cognitive and emotional development, prior painful experiences, ability to communicate, family interactions and psychological defense mechanisms are a few of the important variables to be considered with pediatric pain. Children may cope with pain by withdrawing, rather than crying or asking for medication, whereas most adults seek pain relief (2,3).

DO CHILDREN EXPRESS PAIN DIFFERENTLY?

The problems of pediatric pain assessment are complicated by children's changing but relatively limited cognitive ability to understand measurement instructions or to articulate descriptions of their pain. Discrimination between pain and distress may be very challenging, particularly in the younger pediatric patient.

Children also express pain differently. Both of these differences are magnified at younger ages. Part of the challenge of caring for children is that things change as they develop. The problems of pediatric pain assessment are complicated by children's changing but relatively limited cognitive ability to understand measurement instructions or to articulate

T. H. Stanley et al. (eds.), Pain Management and Anesthesiology, 153–166.

descriptions of their pain.   Discrimination between pain and distress may be very challenging, particularly in the younger pediatric patient.

In addition, it is recognized that the emotional component of pain is very strong in children.   Nonpharmacologic methods of pain management are therefore very important.   While the most important of these is minimal separation from parents, other methods such as reassurance, cuddling, stroking , and distraction should also be employed.   Security objects should be kept with the children.   Early education of children expected to undergo multiple painful procedures should be an important part of an overall care plan.   Avoidance of procedure and needle pain is also very important in this patient population.

Pain assessment tools exist, but need to be applied in a systematic fashion.   Older children can employ visual analogue pain scales in the same way as adults do.   Other clinically useful tools exist for pain assessment for children 3-7 years of age.   Several faces scales that have pictures of real children or simple drawings can be employed.   These faces are arranged from smiling or happy views to crying or sad views.   After instructions, children are asked to select the face that most closely resembles the way they feel at the time of questioning.

Children less than 4 years of age cannot reliably assess pain; physiologic/behavioral scales are employed for those children.   Nuances of validation of pain assessment tools are less important than selecting tools for use in your clinical setting, educating all practitioners as to their use, and employing them routinely.   Many institutions now have a pain assessment column on the vital signs sheet, and assess children in pain at regular intervals.   Recognizing that assessment, intervention, and reassessment are the keys to good pain management is an important step.   Quality assurance evaluation of pain management of pediatric outpatients and inpatients is the only way to ensure that your institution is providing optimal pain management for these patients.   Cognitive and emotional development, prior painful experiences, ability to communicate, family interactions and psychological defense mechanisms are a few of the important variables to be considered with pediatric pain.   Children may cope with pain by withdrawing, rather than crying or asking for medication, whereas most adults seek pain relief.

WHAT ARE MY PHARMACOLOGIC OPTIONS?

NON-OPIOID ANALGESICS

Nonopioid analgesics; usually acetaminophen or a nonsteroidal antiinflammatory agent (NSAID) are useful for the treatment of mild-to-moderate discomfort (such as in many ambulatory procedures) as well as reducing the need for opioids in more severe pain (4-6).

Acetaminophen has traditionally been employed in the same doses for oral or rectal administration. These doses have been based on a model of fever treatment rather than pain treatment. It will take at least an hour to achieve peak plasma levels with the oral route, and up to 3 hours with a bolus rectal dose. As with many medications, rectal absorption is very inefficient and doses of 10-15 mg/kg are highly ineffective.

Acetaminophen in doses of 15-20 mg/kg orally or 20-25 mg/kg rectally (after a first dose of 45 mg/kg) every 4 hours, with a maximum dose of 2.5 g/24 hours produces relatively low plasma levels with good analgesia (7). Oral acetaminophen may be given as a premedication and rectal acetaminophen may be administered after induction of general anesthesia in order to achieve effective blood levels in the immediate postoperative period.

Nonsteroidal antiinflammatory drugs can cause gastritis and interfere with platelet function, which may contribute to clinically important adverse events in children suffering severe tonsillitis or pharyngitis. Ketorolac has been administered by both the intravenous and intramuscular routes (8,9). Since a child will often deny pain rather than submit to an IM injection, intravenous administration of ketorolac has become very popular, in spite of the fact that it is an off-label use of the drug. Intramuscular doses of 0.75 mg/kg provide highly effective postoperative analgesia, as do IV doses of 1 mg kg as a loading dose, with 0.5 mg/kg administered every 6 hours thereafter. This medication is rarely employed in children in its oral formulation.

There have been few reported problems with gastritis or renal failure in pediatric patients receiving ketorolac. Although the bleeding time is not increased following administration of this drug, there is an increasing tendency to avoid its administration in surgical procedures that place a large stress on platelets and clotting mechanisms, such as tonsillectomy and adenoidectomy.

Indomethacin is available for IV administration, and because of its use in premature infants to promote closure of the patent ductus arteriosus, there has been considerable clinical pediatric experience with this agent. Use of a continuous infusion of indomethacin has been shown to provide excellent adjunctive pain relief in postoperative patients, and provide greater patient satisfaction than PRN narcotics alone (10).

Ibuprofen, at a dose of 10 mg/kg was reported to be superior to acetaminophen in reducing pain scores and severity of other symptoms in children suffering severe tonsillitis or pharyngitis. Aspirin is usually avoided in pediatric patients because of the association with the use of this agent to treat febrile illness and the development of Reye's syndrome. In addition, there is a higher incidence of platelet dysfunction and gastrointestinal side effects than with other NSAIDs.

OPIOID PAIN MEDICATIONS

Conventional pain management has involved on-demand administration of oral or parenteral analgesics. Narcotics are usually given to treat rather than to prevent pain. The most common postoperative modality of narcotic administration is still the PRN intramuscular injection. However, under-utilization of analgesics under these circumstance has been well documented, particularly in pediatric patients. Other disadvantages of this approach to analgesia include wide fluctuations in blood concentrations of analgesic medication during each dosing interval, as well as the discomfort caused by intramuscular injections, which are painful and disliked by both children and adults.

ORAL OPIOIDS

Codeine can be administered orally or parenterally, and provides effective control of mild-to-moderate postoperative pain. The bioavailability of codeine following oral administration is around 60%. Orally administered codeine (0.5-1.0 mg/kg) is often combined with acetaminophen (10-15 mg/kg). This combination reduces the overall codeine requirement, thus limiting dose-dependent side effects. Although available, this medication is rarely used in its intravenous form as it has no advantage over morphine, and may be associated with a higher incidence of nausea and vomiting. Oxycodone (0.2 mg/kg) is available only as a tablet, and is also often combined with acetaminophen or an NSAID. This agent appears to cause less nausea than codeine at equipotent doses.

Methadone, in a dose of 0.1 mg/kg has also been successfully employed as an oral analgesic postoperatively, although it is more frequently employed for the treatment of chronic pain (11). This narcotic is known for its slow elimination, prolonged duration of analgesia, and high oral bioavailability. Because a single dose of intravenous or oral methadone can provide analgesia for 12-36 hours, it is a convenient way to provide prolonged analgesic without requiring an intramuscular injection.

INTERMITTENT INTRAVENOUS OPIOIDS

Fentanyl, with its short action and quick onset, is the most frequently employed opioid analgesic for pediatric ambulatory surgery patients. It is most often titrated in doses of 0.5-1 µg/kg. The rapid onset of analgesia and short duration of actions rarely delay discharge in an ambulatory surgery setting. It is frequently employed in combination with rectal acetaminophen, or regional analgesic techniques in this setting.

Morphine continues to be the most popular opioid analgesic for treatment of postoperative pain in pediatric inpatients. As with any respiratory depressant agent, preterm infants and very young infants are more susceptible to the respiratory effects of this opioid, and titration of small doses should be employed (12). Intravenous doses of 0.05-0.2 mg/kg are employed in older children, usually administered by low infusion over 20 minutes, at 4-6 hour intervals. As with any intermittently administered agent, fluctuating blood levels with concomitant fluctuating analgesia will occur.

Preliminary work by Berde and colleagues indicates that intermittent intravenous administration of long-acting narcotic analgesics such as methadone may provide prolonged pain relief in postoperative pediatric patients (11). Berde recommends an intravenous loading dose of 0.1-0.2 mg/kg, followed by titration of 0.05 mg/kg increments every 10-15 minutes until analgesia is achieved. Supplemental methadone can be administered by intravenous infusion over 20 minutes every 12 hours as needed. An •alternative "reverse prn" schedule has been employed as well; the nurse asks the child if he has pain, and administers methadone on a "sliding scale" as needed. In theory, the choice of this opioid should provide more stable blood levels of medication as well as more consistent analgesia, without requiring as many doses as intermittent morphine would need to achieve the same effect.

CONTINUOUS INTRAVENOUS INFUSIONS OF OPIOIDS

Continuous morphine infusions following major surgery have been evaluated in children from 3 months to 12 years of age (12,13). After loading with intravenous fentanyl 1-2 µg/kg, an infusion of morphine 14 µg/kg/hr was begun, to be adjusted by the nursing staff for optimum pain control. Pain scores and plasma morphine levels were recorded. A mean serum level of 6.54 ng/ml provided effective pain relief in all children, but the steady-state blood concentration of morphine showed a large interpatient variation (4.67-9.58 ng/ml). A satisfactory and constant analgesic state was noted within six hours. No clinical signs of respiratory depression or other side effects were noted, even in the youngest child. Lynn and colleagues evaluated the use of continuous morphine infusion doses of 10-30 µg/kg/hr following cardiac surgery and concluded that serum morphine levels less than 30 ng/ml did not interfere with weaning from mechanical ventilation (14). No study has compared continuous infusions with other modalities of narcotic administration.

Hendrickson and colleagues compared the safety and quality of postoperative analgesia provided by intermittent IM injection with continuous intravenous infusion of morphine in children 1-16 years of age (15). As might be expected, the children in the intravenous group received greater amounts of drug, but were more comfortable than those in the group who got "shots." There was no difference in complications (nausea, urinary retention, ileus, respiratory depression) between the groups. Subcutaneous administration of concentrated opioids has also proven successful.

PATIENT-CONTROLLED ANALGESIA

Patient controlled analgesia (PCA) has received enthusiastic acceptance in both adult and pediatric populations, even though pain scores are not necessarily improved when compared to prn intravenous narcotic administration, timed intramuscular administration or epidural local anesthetics or narcotics (16). In spite of this lack of improved pain scores, patients have uniformly preferred PCA to other pain management programs. This is particularly true in the adolescent population, where control is an important part of personality development. Patients, nurses, and parents uniformly preferred PCA to prn intravenous narcotic administration, and no adverse side effects were noted (17).

With the advent of more sophisticated pumps, allowing a background continuous infusion of narcotic with the patient adding small boluses as needed, the major complaint of pain upon awakening from sleep, impossible to avoid with on-demand analgesic delivery systems, should be alleviated. In this video game era, even five year olds appear to understand and appreciate the chance to take care of their own pain medication. "Parent controlled analgesia," where a parent who is rooming-in with a young child is allowed to control the PCA administration, is also under investigation.

CAN I USE REGIONAL ANESTHETIC TECHNIQUES IN CHILDREN?

Although more research is required of all forms of pain treatment for pediatric patients, there exist numerous studies addressing the use of regional analgesia for acute pain in the postoperative period. This may reflect the increasing attention paid to outpatients, as regional analgesia methods are particularly applicable to this population. All regional anesthetic techniques have been successfully employed for pain relief in pediatric patients. The most common techniques were discussed in the lecture on regional anesthesia; due to space limitations interested readers are referred to standard texts; however a few of the more common pediatric regional anesthetic techniques will be mentioned (18-20).

A. TOPICAL BLOCKS

Indications:	Anesthesia to intact skin, exposed mucous membranes.
Cautions:	Known sensitivity to prilocaine (EMLA), cooperation (iontophoresis)
Drugs/Doses:	Enough to have good contact with target tissue. Follow directions for EMLA.
Technique:	Merely removing sensation so that the child does not feel the needle will not decrease the fear of the needle. EMLA is a combination of lidocaine 2.5% and prilocaine 2.5% in an oil-in-water emulsion cream that will penetrate intact skin to a depth of 5 mm. This white cream should be placed on the skin 1 hour prior to the procedure, covered with an occlusive dressing, and left alone. Iontophoresis of lidocaine requires an apparatus for about 10 minutes and causes a "tingly" sensation that can be troublesome to the child as the apparatus must be used for 10 minutes.
	Topical analgesia has also been used for analgesia of mucous membranes, such as following tonsillectomy or circumcision, and for analgesia of exposed nerve and muscle tissue, such as inguinal herniorrhaphy. Intratracheal lidocaine is often employed for bronchoscopy. Finally, topical analgesia is being explored for other uses: lidocaine placed on the tympanic membrane prior to myringotomy, and for attenuation of the oculocardiac reflex in children undergoing strabismus surgery.

B. ILIOINGUINAL/ILIOHYPOGASTRIC NERVE BLOCK

Indications:	Inguinal herniorrhaphy, orchidopexy.

Cautions: Undesirable femoral nerve block, hematoma if wound edge infiltration.

Drugs/Doses: Bupivacaine 0.25-0.5%, with or without Epi. 2-10 ml, depending on size of patient.

Techniques: 1. Wound edge infiltration by surgeon at end of dissection prior to closure.

2. Instillation by surgeon at end of dissection prior to closure (enough to fill wound).

3. Identify anterior superior iliac spine (ASIS). Find spot 1-2 cm medial and 1-2 cm inferior. Place 23-gauge needle directed 45° lateral toward the ASIS and "pop" through the fascia (very superficial). Lay down a "fan-shaped" wall of local anesthetic from lateral to medial at this level. You should not see a "cainoma" on the skin.

C. PENILE NERVE BLOCK

Indications: Circumcision, hypospadias repair, retraction of foreskin.

Cautions: AVOID EPINEPHRINE!

Drugs/Doses: Bupivacaine 0.25% PLAIN. 2 ml for infant to 10 ml for adolescent.

Techniques: 1) Topical at end of case for circumcision using lidocaine jelly or bupivacaine, remembering that the local anesthetic agent must contact the suture edges/exposed mucous membrane to be effective.

2) Ring the base of the penis with a raised superficial wheal of local anesthetic.

3) Retract penis towards the feet and insert needle 90° to the skin, just below symphysis pubis into the shaft of the penis. You will feel the "pop" as the needle crosses Buck's fascia. Inject half the dose at 11 o'clock and half at 1 o'clock, and a final ml on the underside of the penis.

D. FASCIA ILIACUS COMPARTMENT BLOCK

Indications: Femoral shaft fracture or osteotomy, skin graft from front of thigh, quadriceps muscle biopsy.

Drugs/Doses: Bupivacaine 0.25% or Lido 1%/Tetra 0.1%. Volumes of 5 ml for infant up to 25 ml for adolescent. For rapid onset/long duration, 10 mg of tetracaine in each 10 ml of lidocaine will last 18-24 hours, but will have strong motor block.

Techniques: Mark inguinal ligament (ASIS to pubic tubercle). Insert a needle at the junction of the lateral 1/3 and the medial 2/3 of that line, 0.5-1 cm below the inguinal ligament. A 22/23-gauge block needle is best to feel the 2 "pops" as the needle is inserted at a right angle to the skin, although a 23-gauge needle will also work. The 2 "pops" are the needle piercing the fascia lata and iliacus to enter the compartment. There should be no resistance to injection, and no visible skin wheal.

E. FEMORAL BLOCK

Indications: Femoral shaft fracture or osteotomy, quadriceps muscle biopsy.

Cautions: Failed block if injection is made on a sartorius movement or if the current is too strong.

Drugs/Doses: Bupivacaine 0.25% or Lido 1%/Tetra 0.1%. Volumes of 5 ml for infant up to 20 ml for adolescent. For rapid onset/long duration, 10 mg of tetracaine in each 10 ml of lidocaine will last 18-24 hours, but will have strong motor block.

Techniques: Feel pulse of femoral artery. Remember NAVAL (Nerve, Artery, Vein And Lymphatics)means that the nerve is lateral to the artery. A nerve stimulator (in a patient who is NOT muscle-relaxed) should be attached to a 1-1/2 to 3 inch needle, depending on how much tissue is between the skin and the nerve. The nerve stimulator should be set to the lowest setting that you feel a twitch, on 1/sec repeat. The needle should be advanced just lateral to the artery, just below the inguinal ligament until a twitch is noted on the patella. Beware the sartorius twitch. If the twitch does not fade after 2 ml, the needle is incorrectly placed.

F. AXILLARY BLOCK

Indications: Surgery on arm and hand.

Cautions: Avoid on supracondylar fracture or other fracture associated with frequent nerve injuries because of the need for peripheral nerve block in the postoperative period.

Drugs/Doses: Bupivacaine 0.25 % or Lido 1%/Tetra 0.1%. O.5 ml/kg up to 40 ml will usually include the musculocutaneous nerve. For rapid onset/long duration, 10 mg of tetracaine in each 10 ml of lidocaine will last 18-24 hours, but will have strong motor block.

Techniques: The brachial plexus is very superficial in children. Twitch to the fingers can often be found when the nerve stimulator is applied to the skin over the axilla in a child who has not been administered a neuromuscular block. The technique that you employ should be the same that you employ in your successful adult blocks. If you employ a paresthesia in adults, use the nerve stimulator as mentioned above in the child. The brachial pulse can easily be palpated for a transarterial approach.

G. SINGLE-SHOT CAUDAL BLOCK

Indications: Surgery below the diaphragm, especially in the sacral and lower lumbar areas.

Cautions: Aberrant sacral anatomy. 15% failure rate for children >7 years of age. Sacral analgesia means a "numb stripe" down the back of the legs, sole of feet and in perineum. Would you want this additional decreased sensation if you were a 7-year-old boy and there was an alternate block?

Drugs/Doses: See references. Bupivacaine 0.25%, up to a dose of 20 ml, provides optimal analgesia with no delay in discharge if the block is performed prior to the onset of surgery. Epinephrine probably does not prolong the duration of the block.

Technique: Place the child lateral or supine. Lateral position same as for spinal in adults. Identify sacral cornua (one way is to identify posterior superior iliac spines and use them to make an equilateral triangle pointing south). Note that the sacral cornua are almost always above the gluteal fold—most common reason for failed block is local anesthetic place too low, with coccyx mistaken for sacral hiatus. Place 23-gauge needle (for volumes less than 10 ml) or 18-gauge needle (for 20 ml syringe) with syringe attached through the sacrococcygeal ligament at 45° angle to skin until a "pop" is felt. Bring needle angle down to parallel to the skin and advance 1 mm until the entire bevel of the needle is through the skin. Following careful (and negative) aspiration for blood and CSF, easy injection of a small aliquot of local anesthetic (2 ml) with no change in ECG monitoring should be followed by incremental injection of the remainder of the local anesthetic. Alternatives to the needle are a 23-gauge butterfly needle or a 22/20-gauge intravenous needle/catheter, with the catheter easily slipped off after needle placement. Injection of local anesthetic should be easy; and resistance indicated incorrect needle placement.

H. CONTINUOUS CAUDAL BLOCK

Indications: Surgery below the diaphragm for an inpatient who will benefit from prolonged pain relief.

Cautions: Aberrant sacral anatomy. Problems retrieving the catheter (?spica cast). Institutional ability to provide appropriate nurse and physician supervision. Need to maintain clean dressing area in young infants. Watch out for motor block, accumulation of local anesthetic, respiratory depression (opioids).

Drugs/Doses: See references.

Technique: Similar to single-shot. Use of a commercial kit and catheter provide appropriate drapes as this block must be carried out using sterile gloves, prep and drape. A Crawford needle of appropriate length (usually 2 inches) or an IV catheter through which the epidural catheter will pass (check first!) is placed as described above. The catheter is then advanced 2-3 cm. Some experts believe that the catheter can be reliably advanced even farther in infants. It is important to secure the catheter well, reinforce the hub/catheter connection, and dress the catheter to avoid soilage. Nursing care is even more critical here than with most analgesia techniques.

I. LUMBAR EPIDURAL BLOCK

Indications: Surgery below the diaphragm for an inpatient who will benefit from prolonged pain relief.

Cautions: Aberrant sacral anatomy. Problems retrieving the catheter (?spica cast). Institutional ability to provide appropriate nurse and physician supervision. Watch out for motor block, accumulation of local anesthetic, respiratory depression (opioids).

Drugs/Doses: See references.

Technique: Similar to adults, although the epidural space is closer to the skin. Use of a commercial kit and catheter provide the necessary equipment in one place. A clear drape (provided in most pediatric kits) is helpful. A Tuohy needle of appropriate length (usually 2 inches for children less than 30 kg, and adult 3-1/2 inches above that) is placed using saline loss of resistance. Because of reports of air emboli in pediatric patients, a technique of saline loss of resistance rather than air is prudent. The catheter is then advanced 2-3 cm. Some experts believe that the catheter can be reliably advanced even farther in infants. It is important to secure the catheter well, reinforce the hub/catheter connection, and dress the catheter so that the catheter-skin junction is visible. Nursing care is even more critical here than with most analgesia techniques.

CONCLUSION

Any method used for pain relief in the adult patient can be adapted for pain relief in the pediatric patient. Children have the same right to pain relief as do adults, even if their pain is more difficult to assess. More frequent use of NSAIDs, as well as many more studies of opioid administration, especially long acting narcotic analgesics, continuous infusions and patient or parent controlled analgesia are required. An increased response to the challenge of acute pain treatment with regional analgesic techniques in the pediatric outpatient will also be useful, with more continuous catheter techniques employed in hospitalized patients. Certainly, we have the responsibility to provide optimum pain relief for all patients, not just those who can complain in a way that is easy to understand.

REFERENCES

1. Lewis N: The needle is like an animal. Children Today (Jan-Feb):18-21, 1978.
2. Holder KA, Patt RB: Taming the pain monster: pediatric postoperative pain management. Pediatr Ann 24:163-16, 1995.
3. Siegel LJ, Smith KE: Children's strategies for coping with pain. Pediatrician 16:110-118, 1989.
4. Roberts NV, Goresky GV. The management of postoperative pain in children following outpatient surgery. In: White PW (Ed): Ambulatory Anesthesia and Surgery. London: Ballière Tindall Ltd, 1996.
5. Yaster M, Sola JE, Pegoli W, Paidas CN. The night after surgery: postoperative management of the pediatric outpatient—surgical and anesthetic aspects. Pediatr Clin North Am 41:199-220, 1994.
6. Maunuksela E-L: Nonsteroidal anti-inflammatory drugs in pediatric pain management. In: Pain in infants, children and adolescents. Edited by Schechter NL, Berde CB, Yaster M. Baltimore, William and Wilkins, pp135-143, 1993.
7. Birmingham PK, Tobin MJ, Henthorn TK, et al: Twenty-four hour pharmacokinetics of rectal acetaminophen in children: an old drug with new recommendations. Anesthesiology 87:244-252, 1997.
8. Houck CS, Berde CB, Anand KJS: Pediatric pain management. In: Pediatric anesthesia. Edited by Gregory GA. New York, Churchill Livingstone, pp743-772, 1994.
9. Maunuksela E-L, Kokki H, Bullingham RES: Comparison of intravenous ketorolac with morphine for postoperative pain in children. Clin Pharmacol Ther 52:436-443, 1992

10. Maunuksela E-L, Olkkola KT, Korpela R: Does prophylactic intravenous infusion of indomethacin improve the management of postoperative pain in children. Can J Anaesth 35:123-127, 1988

11. Berde CB, Beyer JE, Bournaki MC, et al: Comparison of morphine and methadone for prevention of postoperative pain in 3- to 7-year old children. J Pediatr 119:136-141, 1991

12. Millar AJW, Rode H, Cywes S: Continuous morphine infusion for postoperative pain in children. S Afr Med J 72:386-398, 1987

13. Beasley SW, Tibballs J: Efficacy and safety of continuous morphine infusion for postoperative analgesia in the paediatric surgical ward. Aust N Z J Surg 57:233-237, 1987

14. Lynn AM, Opheim KO, Tyler DC: Morphine infusion after pediatric cardiac surgery. Crit Care Med 12:863-866, 1984

15. Hendrickson M, Myre L, Johnson DG, et al: Postoperative analgesia in children: a prospective study of intermittent intramuscular injection versus continuous intravenous infusion of morphine. J Pediatr Surg 25:185-191, 1990

16. Gillespie JA, Morton NS: Patient-controlled analgesia for children: a review. Paediatr Anaesth 2:51-59, 1992

17. Sinatra RS, Savarese A: Parenteral analgesic therapy and patient-controlled analgesia for pediatric pain management. In: Acute pain: mechanisms and management. Edited by Sinatra RS, Hord AH, Ginsberg B, Preble LM., St. Louis, Mosby Year Book, pp453-469, 1994

18. Sethna NS, Berde CB: Pediatric regional anesthesia. In: Pediatric anesthesia. Edited by Gregory GA. New York, Churchill Livingstone, 1994, 281-318, 1994

19. Rice LJ: Regional anesthesia. In: Motoyama E, Davis P, editors: Smith's anesthesia for infants and children, ed 6, St. Louis, CV Mosby Co, 403-442, 1996

20. Dalens BJ. Pediatric Regional Anesthesia, 4th ed. In: Miller RD, ed. Anesthesia. New York: Churchill Livingstone, 1565-1591, 1994.

EFFECT OF POSTOPERATIVE PAIN RELIEF ON SURGICAL OUTCOME

H. Kehlet

Despite much progress within the anesthetic and surgical specialities, major surgical procedures may still be followed by undesirable sequelae such as cardiac, pulmonary, thromboembolic and infective complications. The most important pathogenic factors to determine surgical outcome are various perioperative risk factors and pathophysiological responses included in the general surgical stress response to injury (1). Since trauma-induced nociceptive impulses may initiate autonomic and somatic reflex responses and modify organ functions including those of the endocrine organs, various techniques of postoperative pain relief may therefore alter (inhibit) the surgical stress response, and thereby improve organ dysfunction and overall outcome (1,2). Of the available pain treatment techniques, regional anesthesia with local anesthetics, and especially continuous epidural techniques, are the most powerful analgesic and stress reducing techniques, followed by other epidural regimens (opioids, clonidine etc.), PCA opioids and NSAID's (2).

The effect of various pain relieving techniques on surgical outcome has been extensively reviewed in recent years (2,3) and results based upon randomized controlled trials will briefly be updated and summarized here. Pain treatment techniques will be divided into sections including NSAID treatment, PCA opioid treatment, and single dose and continuous regional anesthetic techniques.

NSAID treatment has relatively minor effects on surgical stress responses (2), and effects on outcome are therefore mostly expected to be related to the well documented opioid sparing effect (20-30%), thereby potentially reducing morbidity parameters such as nausea, vomiting, ileus, sedation, sleep disturbances, bladder dysfunction etc. Although NSAID's are effective and safe, if relevant precautions are taken in patients at risk for side effects (4), there is no definite proof for a reduction in postoperative morbidity following analgesic treatment with NSAID's (5). However, in about 20-30% of major controlled studies the data support a reduction in the above mentioned opioid related side effects (5). Ibuprofen treatment did not improve survival or morbidity in sepsis

167

T. H. Stanley et al. (eds.), Pain Management and Anesthesiology, 167-172.
© 1998 Kluwer Academic Publishers. Printed in the Netherlands.

patients, despite reduction of temperature, heart rate and oxygen consumption (6). Further studies are needed in well defined surgical populations, predominantly within the ambulatory or semi-ambulatory setting where the opioid sparing effect of NSAID's may be most relevant.

PCA opioid treatment provides a high degree of patient satisfaction, but pain relief during mobilization is inferior to that with epidural combination techniques. Also, the effect on stress responses and organ dysfunctions are limited. Correspondingly, plenty of controlled studies have not been able to demonstrate a clinically significant advantageous effect of PCA opioid techniques on surgical outcome compared with other analgesic treatments (1,2).

Central neural blockade techniques. Many controlled clinical studies in the lower body procedures have demonstrated single dose epidural and spinal anesthesia to reduce intraoperative blood loss by about 30% and to reduce thromboembolic complications by about 30-50%, including the risk of graft thrombosis after peripheral vascular surgery. Although mortality is reduced in acute surgery for hip fracture (2,3) no positive effect has been demonstrated in peripheral vascular surgery (7), or on postoperative mental dysfunction (2,3).

The analgesic effect of continuous epidural techniques is superior to that of other analgesic techniques, especially on mobilization induced pain when balanced techniques are used with combinations of local anesthetics and opioids (2,3,8). Also, such powerful analgesia is well documented to have the potential to improve postoperative pulmonary function, cardiac dysfunction and gastrointestinal ileus (2,3). It is therefore most surprising and disappointing that data from controlled clinical studies comparing outcome parameters in patients undergoing major procedures and receiving continuous epidural analgesia with local anesthetics, opioids or a combination versus systemic opioid treatment alone, have not convincingly been able to demonstrate clinical relevant advantages (1-3) (Figure 1). It may be argued that this is due to insufficient design of many of these studies by the lack of use of epidural local anesthetic-opioid combination techniques, by insufficient duration of analgesia, a limited number of patient studied, and by the inclusion of a variety of surgical procedures. Although this criticism is relevant, and most will agree that there is a need for more large size well-designed controlled studies, existing data so far suggest that such analgesic techniques will not per se lead to major improvement of surgical outcome, despite the otherwise well-documented potential beneficial effects of different organ functions. It is therefore necessary to reconsider the potential advantages of regional anesthetic/analgesic techniques into a more global context, together with

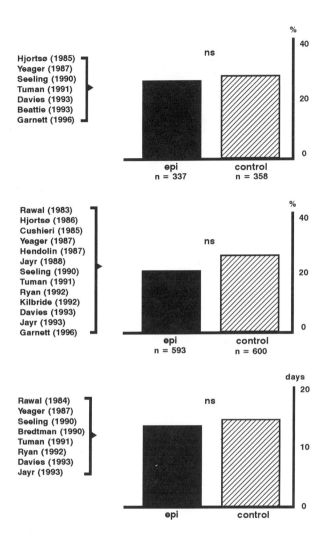

Figure 1. Effect of continuous epidural analgesic techniques on cardiac complications (upper part), pulmonary infection (middle part) and postoperative hospital stay (lower part) after major abdominal/thoracic surgery. Data from controlled studies including (30 patients (for references see ref. 2 and 3).

other factors that may contribute to perioperative morbidity (1). Furthermore, it may be asked whether future outcome studies should be designed differently than in the past.

THE MULTI-MODAL APPROACH TO CONTROL POSTOPERATIVE
PATHOPHYSIOLOGY AND REHABILITATION

As observed in many other medical conditions, it has become clear that unimodal treatment of such complex problems as perioperative morbidity and pain relief cannot be expected to have major efficacy, but instead should be replaced by a multi-modal effort to develop an accelerated and low morbidity stay program (1). This concept is based upon the fact that several postoperative factors may delay recovery, including pain (which can be effectively treated), nausea, vomiting and ileus, postoperative organ dysfunction (the surgical stress syndrome), hypoxemia and sleep disturbances, immobilization-induced side effects on pulmonary and skeletal muscle function, semistarvation-induced side effects on the gastrointestinal mucosal integrity and skeletal muscle function, fatigue etc. (1). All these factors may lead to a postoperative cascade to dependency, fatigue and prolonged convalescence and specific organ morbidity (Table 1). In the discussion of the effect of postoperative analgesia on surgical outcome, effective pain treatment should therefore be integrated into a multi-modal effort to enhance rehabilitation, including the use of enforced mobilization and early oral nutrition, facilitated by pain treatment techniques (1). In recent years, small pieces of information have been gathered from different institutions and types of operation (colonic surgery, cholecystectomy, inguinal herniotomy, vascular surgery, orthopedic procedures etc.) where the multi-modal approach to control postoperative pathophysiology and rehabilitation, and effective functional pain relief, has been evaluated (1). Despite that these data mostly come from uncontrolled, descriptive studies, they suggest an important clinical beneficial effect to be obtained by this strategy. However, obviously these findings need to be confirmed in future controlled clinical studies or in a multi-center collaborative design.

Summarizing, we have therefore entered the second round of the debate on the effect on pain relief on surgical outcome, and where a reconsideration of the many factors which may contribute to perioperative morbidity is required. It has become clear that a multi-modal effort will be needed to demonstrate positive outcome effects as well as the provided pain relief should be effective to allow early mobilization and oral nutrition. Such an approach will require an organization with increased collaboration between anesthesiologists and surgeons, and will also require a thorough revision of the perioperative care program, to be adjusted to the use of scientifically proved procedures and eliminating those which are not founded on valid data and which may retard rehabilitation (1). In muscle function, semistarvation-induced side effects on the gastrointestinal mucosal integrity and skeletal muscle function, fatigue etc. (1). All these factors may lead to a postoperative cascade to dependency, fatigue and prolonged convalescence and specific organ morbidity (Table 1). In the discussion of the effect of postoperative analgesia on surgical outcome, effective pain treatment should therefore be integrated into a multi-modal effort to enhance rehabilitation, including the use of enforced mobilization and early oral nutrition, facilitated by pain treatment techniques (1). In recent years, small pieces of information have been gathered from different institutions and types of operation (colonic surgery, cholecystectomy, inguinal herniotomy, vascular surgery, orthopedic procedures etc.) where the multi-modal approach to control postoperative pathophysiology and rehabilitation, and effective functional pain relief, has been evaluated (1). Despite that these data mostly come from uncontrolled, descriptive studies, they suggest an important clinical beneficial effect to be obtained by this strategy. However, obviously these findings need to be confirmed in future controlled clinical studies or in a multi-center collaborative design.

Summarizing, we have therefore entered the second round of the debate on the effect on pain relief on surgical outcome, and where a reconsideration of the many factors which may contribute to perioperative morbidity is required. It has become clear that a multi-modal effort will be needed to demonstrate positive outcome effects as well as the provided pain relief should be effective to allow early mobilization and oral nutri-

---

Table 1. Factors which may contribute to postoperative fatigue, convalescence and dependency ("the postoperative cascade to dependency").

• surgical stress	• traditions, restrictions
• pain	• tubes, drains, etc)
• immobilization	• nausea, ileus
• sleep disturbances	• impaired oral nutrition
↓	↓
• impaired pulmonary function	
• hypoxemia	
• myocardial ischemia	• infectious complications
• loss of muscle function	• loss of muscle function
↘	↙

- • fatigue
- • convalescence
- • dependency

tion. Such an approach will require an organization with increased collaboration between anesthesiologists and surgeons, and will also require a thorough revision of the perioperative care program, to be adjusted to the use of scientifically proved procedures and eliminating those which are not founded on valid data and which may retard rehabilitation (1). In addition, more data are needed on the potential advantages as well as deleterious effects and safety aspects of the various analgesic techniques on postoperative recovery of body organ functions (9).

REFERENCES

1. Kehlet H. Multi-modal approach to control postoperative pathophysiology and rehabilitation—a review. Br J Anaesth 1997;78:606-617.
2. Kehlet H. Modification of responses to surgery and anesthesia by neural blockade: clinical implications. In: Cousins MJ, Bridenbaugh PO (eds.). Neural Blockade in Clinical Anesthesia and Management of Pain. Third ed., Philadelphia, Lippincott 1998 (in press).
3. Liu S, Carpenter RL, Neal JM. Epidural anesthesia and analgesia—their role in postoperative outcome. Anesthesiology 1995;82:1474-1506.
4. Merry A, Power I. Perioperative NSAID; towards greater safety. Pain Reviews 1995;2:268-291.
5. Kehlet H, Rung GW, Callesen T. Postoperative opioid analgesia—time for a reconsideration? J Clin Anesth 1996;8:441-445.
6. Bernard GR, Wheeler AP, Russell JA, et al. The effects of ibuprofen on the physiology and survival of patients with sepsis. N Engl J Med 1997:226:912-918.
7. Bode RH, Lewis KP, Zarich SW, et al. Cardiac outcome after peripheral vascular surgery: comparison of general and regional anesthesia. Anesthesiology 1996;84:3-13.
8. Kehlet H, Dahl JB. The value of multi-modal or balanced analgesia on postoperative pain relief. Anesth Analg 1993;77:1048-1056.
9. Symposium on "Future directions of acute pain management." Reg. Anesth 1996;21(6 Suppl):1-157.

PAIN ASSESSMENT IN KIDS—THE FIFTH VITAL SIGN

L. J. Rice

> I often say that when you can measure what you are speak-
> ing about, and express it in numbers, you know something
> about it, but when you cannot measure it, when you
> cannot express it in numbers, your knowledge is of a
> meager and unsatisfactory kind; it may be the beginning of
> knowledge, but you have scarcely, in your thoughts,
> advanced to the stage of science, whatever the matter may
> be.
>
> Lord Kelvin, quoted in Thomas (1)

IS ASSESSMENT THE SAME AS MEASUREMENT?

The International Association for the Study of Pain defines pain as "an unpleasant sensory and emotional experience associated with tissue damage (actual or potential) or described in terms of such damage" (2). The inclusion of "emotional" in this definition means that there does not need to be an overt abnormality to have pain. It also implies that the severity of pain is what the one experiencing the unpleasant sensation says that it is. Since children have varying abilities to communicate, and these abilities change as they develop, self-report of pain is not possible in young pediatric patients. Measurement implies the use of a tool to precisely and objectively quantitate a parameter—the height of a bridge, the square footage of a house. Assessment, on the other hand, is less precise and more subjective. Pain is a subjective phenomenon, influenced by the individual's experience, social and cultural attitudes, personality, coping skills, developmental level, and the perceived consequence of the pain complaint, among other influences (3). Assessment is a broader concept than measurement (4).

WHAT PARAMETERS ARE USED FOR PAIN ASSESSMENT?

The most reliable pain assessment is the self-report of the patient (a cognitive tool). Children older than seven years can reliably self-report

T. H. Stanley et al. (eds.), Pain Management and Anesthesiology, 173–184.
© 1998 Kluwer Academic Publishers. Printed in the Netherlands.

pain using tools similar to those employed in adult patients. Children between 4 and 7 years can usually self-report pain (after appropriate education) with tools specifically designed and validated for that age group (5). Younger children require tools that assign pain scores based on physiologic or behavioral observations, or a combination of the two (6). While behavioral ratings can be used to assess overt pain behavior, self-report procedures are necessary to assess the covert aspects of the experience of pain (7). It is often difficult to differentiate between pain and anxiety with a behavioral pain assessment tool.

Seven dimensions of acute pain should be considered when assessing pain (8). Most pain assessment tools and scores try to assign a numerical value to just one of these dimensions. Cognitive, physiological, sensory, behavioral, affective, sociocultural and environmental factors all affect pain assessment. Familiarity with the child's age and level of development, family situation, cultural background and clinical condition assists the health care worker to make a judgment of that specific child at that specific time in that specific medical environment having undergone that specific painful experience (surgical, medical or trauma).

Use of prior experience and an understanding of the amount of pain that a similar surgical experience would cause the health care worker, allows that individual to avoid the classic scenario where pain assessment tools or even self-report may not be reliable. This scenario is that of a young child who not only does not complain of pain, but may deny it when asked. This child lies silently, still and rigid after an abdominal operation or with a perforated appendix, scoring zero for pain at rest on any pain assessment tool. This child may be afraid to move in case it hurts, and even more afraid that a complaint of pain would lead to an intramuscular injection—the dreaded "shot"!

HOW OFTEN DO WE NEED TO DO THIS PAIN ASSESSMENT?

Pain assessments should be performed and recorded at appropriate intervals, just like all other vital signs. Hourly pain assessments may be necessary for children who have just undergone a major surgical procedure and are receiving complex pain management (epidural, opioid infusion or patient-controlled analgesia PCA). This evaluation should include assessment of pain treatment efficacy, side effects such as sedation, respiratory depression and cardiovascular changes, emesis), as well as checks of the infusion delivery system (9). It would be appropriate for these observations to be increased in frequency if the assessed analgesia is poor or if there are excessive adverse effects; less frequent if pain assessment scores are low and there are no adverse effects noted.

Children receiving less sophisticated pain treatments or with less pain stimuli might have observations at 2 or 4 hourly intervals, with other vital signs or routine checks of the intravenous infusion. It should be remembered that there are other causes of pain and discomfort than surgical pain; headache, full bladder, or lack of parental or peer visits may be just as painful as the osteotomy site—but treatment is certainly different.

The modern approach to pain management includes proactive planning and multimodal therapy. This proactive approach, reinforced by good patient, family and staff education means putting pain control to the top of the priorities of both medical and nursing practice. If pain assessment finds that pain is at unacceptable levels, an intervention and reassessment after appropriate time must be planned. The assessment-intervention-reassessment cycle is the cornerstone of proper pain management. An important part of this intervention plan is preemptive pain treatment. If a planned medical or nursing intervention is recognized to be painful, treatment should be planned in a timely fashion in advance of the intervention. For example, a dorsal penile nerve block may be administered half an hour prior to the planned circumcision of a newborn infant, while acetaminophen would need to be administered orally 1 hour prior or rectally 3 hours prior to the procedure, and a sucrose pacifier could be started minutes before the procedure. Eutectic Mixture of Lidocaine (EMLA cream) might be placed on a planned intravenous catheter site an hour prior to placement, or iontophoresis of lidocaine utilized 10-20 minutes prior. A suggestion to an older patient to begin using her PCA button half an hour prior to removal of the nasogastric tube or physical therapy might also be an appropriate preemptive pain treatment scheme.

Ensuring that adequate loading and maintenance doses of acetaminophen, non-steroidal antiinflammatory agents (NSAIDS) and opioids have been prescribed and administered according to pharmacologic principles and on a "timed" rather than an "as required" basis is essential for pain prevention and to minimize adverse effects. The aim of this multimodal approach to analgesia is early pain-free mobilization and restoration of function. Adequate rescue analgesia and options for breakthrough pain must be available.

Although it is important to employ a pain scale that has been validated, it is more important to utilize clinically useful scales with strong inter-observer reliability and a record of "user-friendliness" in the clinical environment. A pain assessment tool selected by physicians or senior administrative nurses that is not easy for the nurse caring for the patient to use and for the physician responding to that nurse's phone call to understand is useless, no matter how valid it is. If it is not easy to use in the clinical scenario, the nurse will not use it or record it. Most physicians are familiar with the Visual Analogue Scale, which uses a 0-10 scale for pain assessment. For that reason, the author believes that pain assessment tools based on a "0 is good, 10 is bad" format are superior to others, even if the others are scientifically more rigorous. It is more important to have the assessment performed, recorded, and acted upon at frequent intervals, using the assessment-intervention-reassessment cycle.

DIFFERENT TOOLS FOR DIFFERENT AGES

NEONATES AND INFANTS (LESS THAN 1 YEAR OLD)

As one might expect, the younger the child, the tougher the pain assessment. Both broad band and fine grained behavioral measure have been studied in infants. Among the fine grained measure, facial action scales appear to be most sensitive. This is a research tool that requires close-up videotaping of the face of the crying infant and coding of a number of facial parameters. At this time, cry measures are not developed to the point of being able to establish a pain cry (no matter what mothers might say!) (10).

As these little patients cannot communicate their pain, behaviors and physiologic variables are interpreted together. It may be difficult to differentiate between distress and pain in these infants; the clinical situation should be of some assistance here. Several assessment tools have been employed in neonates and infants. Not all are validated for neonates. Most tools were designed for use with occasional sharp pain such as heelstick. It is important to realize that infants who undergo repeated, similar sharp pains will begin to extinguish their behavioral responses to those pains. It is almost as if the infant, realizing that agitation and fighting will not save her from the heelstick, gives up expending useless energy on pain behaviors to conserve her strength.

One scale validated in neonates is the CRIES Score (11). This scale was validated in 24 infants from 32-60 weeks postconceptual age who had undergone major surgery. CRIES employs Crying, Requirement for oxygen, Increased vital signs, Expression and Sleepless as biobehavioral observations of pain. This tool illustrates some of the complexity of pain assessment in this age group. Following initial publication of the tool, the authors received many requests to provide clarification of the observed parameters and were forced to develop coding tips for other institutions to employ.

Common features of tools employed in this age group include observation of facial expression, body position and mobility, crying and response to comforting, blood pressure, heart rate, skin color or oxygen saturation, respiratory rate and sleeplessness. Obviously, all of these parameters can be influenced by nonpainful things. The age, maturity, and state of arousal will all affect the response to pain; the same infant may give widely varying responses depending on how recently she has eaten, whether she is gassy, or when she was last cuddled.

Dynamic pain assessment is more useful, where improvement in the behavioral and physiologic parameters are sought in response to comforting, analgesia or sedation. Most pain assessment tools are confounded in the intubated, ventilated patient.

OLDER INFANTS AND PREVERBAL CHILDREN (1-4 YEARS OF AGE)

Children in this group suffer from many of the problems noted in the neonatal group. They still cannot clearly self-report pain, and the younger members of this segment of the population may be sensitive to the effects of benzodiazepines and opioids. The older members of the group tend to be "all-or-none"—a toddler is either shrieking in anxiety/anger/pain or easily distracted. There is no middle-of-the road in toddler behavior.

Two physiologic-behavioral scales have been widely employed for postoperative pain in this age group. One, the Objective Pain Scale (OPS), was has been employed in postoperative children older than 3 months, while the other; the Children's Hospital of Eastern Ontario Pain Scale (CHEOPS) was employed in children suffering short, sharp pain, both perioperative and nonperioperative (12,13). Both suffer from the short-comings of observer-based pain assessment previously mentioned. In addition, there is good evidence that pain behaviors habituate when a child is in pain for several hours; the CHEOPS scale has been shown to be unreliable after the first several hours and there is no reason to believe that the OPS scale is any different (5). However, as also mentioned, it is most important to establish a standardized, reproducible, interobserver-reliable assessment that is easy to use and interpret for evaluating trends that are compatible with pain or comfort in an individual patient—or it will not be used at all.

These scales are very similar; however, the CHEOPS scale is a 4-13 scale, while the OPS is a 0-10 scale. Once again, it is clinically helpful for all caregivers to think, "0 is good, 10 is bad" for all age groups when it comes to pain assessment. Therefore, it is the author's opinion that although the CHEOPS is the better-validated scale, the OPS is the more practical to use in a busy hospital practice. This is particularly true if your hospital has chosen, as many have to use three different scales; one for infants and preverbal children (OPS), one for young children (FACES or OUCHER) and one for older children (VAS or Pain Ladder). It is important to note that many studies in the anesthesia literature use OPS or CHEOPS.

CHILDREN 4-7 YEARS OF AGE

Language skills develop at different rates in different children. Although toddlers may begin to use family-based pain terms at the age of 2 years, the process of cognitive development delays the capacity to provide good qualitative information until the age of 4 or 5 years. Most 4 year olds can differentiate the absence or presence of pain and can indicate pain intensity provided the number of choices of categories is limited to around 4. Many can speak well enough to be engaged in a dialogue to explain whether they have pain and to indicate how bad it is (mild, moderate or severe). However, they must use phrases they can understand; frequently family-specific phrases. They can understand the concept of "pieces of hurt" as used with the Poker Chip Tool (4 red poker chips are given to the child and she is asked to give back the number of chips that represent the 'pieces of hurt' she feels at that time) (14). Obviously this tool can suffer from a child's possessiveness.

The FACES scale can work, but the younger children may think they have to choose the happiest face and do not relate the faces to their own pain experience (15). Children at the younger end of this age group tend to be at extremes of the pain scale (all or nothing effect). A more detailed progression using faces of real children arranged vertically (OUCHER) may be useful, as can "pain ladders" (16). It is of interest to realize that Western children look at a line as going from left to right, while those whose language is read from right to left need their numerals to be rearranged accordingly. This is why a pain ladder, where the vertical emphasizes the difference between high and low can be helpful.

OLDER CHILDREN AND ADOLESCENTS

Visual Analogue Scales from 0-10 cm or 0-100 mm can be employed with this age group (17). Of course, instruction in the tool selected is still necessary. Children in this group as well as the prior group often relate their scores to other pain experiences. A variety of self-report tools including lines, words and pictures have been employed here.

CONCLUSION

As Thomas, commenting on Lord Kelvin's quote that opened this paper, has emphasized: "The task of converting observations into numbers is the hardest of all, the last task rather than the first thing to be done, and it can be done only when you have learned, beforehand, a great deal about the observations themselves. You can, to be sure, achieve a very deep understanding of nature by quantitative measurement, but you must know what you are talking about before you can begin applying the number for making predictions."

There are many ways to assess pain. Pain assessment is different at different times, in children of different ages, at different stages of maturity and development (18,19). As everything else in the pediatric population, ingenuity and a willingness to "think like a child" can be helpful. More important is selection of several clinically useful tools for different age groups, employed in a consistent manner with good inter-observer reliability. The author feels strongly that tools that can be reported as "0 is good, 10 is bad" are the most practical tools. Proactive pain management and assessment-intervention-reassessment are the cornerstones of pain management as we approach the next millennium.

REFERENCES

1. Thomas L: Late night thoughts on listening to Mahler's Ninth Symphony. New York, Viking, 1993
2. International Association for the Study of Pain, Subcommittee on Taxonomy. Pain terms: a list with definitions and notes on usage. Pain 6:249-252, 1979
3. Tyler DC, Tu A, Douthit J, Chapman DR: Toward validation of pain measurement tools for children: a pilot study. Pain 52:301-309, 1993
4. Chapman C, McGrath PJ: Pain Assessment in the Pediatric Patient.
5. In: The Management of Pain. Edited by Ashburn MA, Rice LJ. New York, Churchill Livingstone, 1997, pp 621-648.
6. Beyer JE, McGrath PJ, Berde CB: Discordance between self-report and behavioral pain measure in children aged 3-7 years after surgery. J Pain and Sympt Manage 5:350-356, 1990
7. Thompson KL, Varni JW: A developmental cognitive-biobehavioral approach to pediatric pain assessment. Pain 25:283-296, 1986
8. Manne SL, Jacobsen PB, Redd WH: Assessment of acute pediatric pain: do child self-report, parent ratings and nurse ratings measure the same phenomenon? Pain 48:45-52, 1992
9. Morton NS: Pain assessment in children. Paediatr Anaesth 7:267-272, 1997
10. Whaley L, Wong D: Nursing Care of Infants and Children, 4th ed. Philadelphia, Mosby-Year Book, 1991

11. Craig KD, Grunau RVE: Neonatal pain perception and behavioral measurement. In: Pain Research and Clinical Measurement (Vol 5): Pain in Neonates. Edited by Anand KJS and McGrath PJ. Amsterdam, Elsevier, pp 67-106, 1993

12. Krechel SW, Bildner J: CRIES: a new neonatal postoperative pain measurement score. Initial testing of validity and reliability. Paediatr Anaesth 5:53-61, 1995

13. Hannallah RS, Broadman LM, Belman BA, et al: Comparison of caudal and ilioinguinal/iliohypogastric nerve blocks for control of post-orchiopexy pain in pediatric ambulatory surgery. Anesthesiology 66:832-834, 1987

14. McGrath PJ, Johnson G, Goodman JT, et al: CHEOPS: A behavioral scale for rating postoperative pain in children. In: Advances in Pain Research and Therapy, Vol 9. Edited by Fields HL, Dubner R, Cevero F. New York, Raven Press, 1985, pp 395-401

15. Hester NO, Foster RL, Kristensen K: Measurement of pain in children: Generalizability and validity of the pain ladder and the poker ship tool. In: Advances in Pain Research and Therapy, Vol 15: Pediatric Pain. Edited by Tyler DC, Krane EJ, New York, Raven Press, 1990, pp 79-84

16. Wong D, Baker C: Pain in children: comparison of assessment scales. Pediatr Nurs 14:9-17, 1988

17. Beyer JE, Aradine CR: Content validity of an instrument to measure young children's perception of pain.. J Pediatr Nurs 1: 386-395, 1986

18. Savedra MC, Tesler MD: Assessing children's and adolescent's pain. Pediatrician 16:24-29, 1989

19. Porter F: Pain assessment in children: infants. In: Pain in Infants, Children and Adolescents. Edited by Schechter NL, Berde CB, Yaster M, Baltimore, Williams & Wilkins, 1993, pp 87-96

20. Mathews JR, McGrath PJ, Pigeon H: Assessment and measurement of pain in children. In: Pain in Infants, Children and Adolescents. Edited by Schechter NL, Berde CB, Yaster M, Baltimore, Williams & Wilkins, 1993, pp 97-111

APPENDICES

Table A. Cries neonatal postop pain assessment score.[a]

	0	1	2
Crying	No	High pitched	Inconsolable
Requires O_2 for Sat>95	No	<30%	>30%
Increased vital signs	HR and BP = or < preop	HR or BP ↑<20% preop	HR or BP ↑>20% preop
Expression	None	Grimace	Grimace/grunt
Sleepless	No	Wakes	Constantly at frequent awake intervals

[a]Krechel SW, Bildner J: CRIES: a new neonatal postoperative pain measurement score. Initial testing of validity and reliability. Paediatr Anaesth 5:53-61, 1995

Table B. Objective pain scale.[a]

Observation	Criteria	Points
Blood Pressure	± 10% preop	0
	± 10% preop	1
	± 20% preop	2
Crying	Not crying	0
	Crying but responds to tender loving care (TLC)	1
	Crying and does not respond to TLC	2
Movement	None	0
	Restless	1
	Thrashing	1
Agitation	Patient asleep or calm	0
	Mild	1
	Hysterical	2
Complaints of pain (where appropriate by age)	Asleep (or states no pain)	0
	Cannot localize	1
	Can localize	2

[a]Norden J, Hannallah R, Getson P, et al: Concurrent validation of an objective pain scale for infants and children. Anesthesiology 75:A934, 1991

182

Table C. Coding tips for using cries.

Crying | Characteristic cry of pain is high pitched.

If no cry or cry not high pitched, **score 0**

If cry high pitched but baby easily consolable, **score 1**

If cry high pitched and baby inconsolable, **score 2**

Requires O2 for Sat>95% | Look for changes. Babies experiencing pain manifest decreases in oxygenation as measured by TCO_2/SpO_2.

If no oxygen required, **score 0**

If <30% O2 required, **score 1**

If >30% O_2 required, **score 2**

Increased vital signs | *Note: Take BP last as this may wake child causing difficulty with other assessments. Use baseline preop parameters from a non-stressed period. Multiply baseline HR x 0.2 then add this to baseline HR to determine the HR which is 20% over baseline. Do likewise for mean BP.

If HR and BP are both unchanged or less than baseline, **score 0**

If HR or BP is increased but increase is <20% of baseline, **score 1**

If HR or BP is increased and increase is >20% of baseline, **score 2**

Expression | The facial expression most often associated with pain is a grimace. This may be characterized by: brow lowering, eyes squeezed shut, deepening of the nasolabial furrow, open lips and mouth

If no grimace is present, **score 0**

If grimace alone is present, **score 1**

If grimace and non-cry vocalization is present, **score 2**

Sleepless | This parameter is scored based upon the infant's state during the hour preceding this recorded score.

If the infant has been continuously asleep, **score 0**

If the infant has been awakened at frequent intervals, **score 1**

If the infant has been constantly, **score 2**

Table D. **Children's Hospital of Eastern Ontario pain scale.**[a]

Item	Behavior	Score	Definition
Cry	No cry	1	Child is not crying
	Moaning	2	Moaning or quiet vocalizing; silent cry
	Crying	2	Gentle crying or whimpering
	Screaming	3	Full-lunged cry, sobbing
Facial	Smiling	0	Score only if definite positive facial expression
	Composed	1	Neutral facial expression
	Grimace	2	Score only if definite negative facial expression
Child verbal	Positive	0	Child makes any positive statement or talks about other things without complaint
	None	1	Child not talking
	Other complaint	1	Child complains, but not about pain; e.g., "I want to see mommy" or "I'm thirsty"
	Pain complaints	2	Child complains about pain
	Both complaints	2	Child complains about pain and about other things, e.g., "It hurts; I want mommy"
Torso	Neutral	1	Body (not limbs) at rest; torso is inactive
	Shifting	2	Body in motion in a shifting or serpentine fashion
	Tense	2	Body is arched or rigid
	Shivering	2	Body is shuddering or shaking involuntarily
	Upright	2	Child is in vertical or upright position
	Restrained	2	Body is restrained
Touch	Not touching	1	Not touching or grabbing at wound
	Reaching	2	Reaching for but not touching wound
	Touching	2	Gently touching wound area
	Grab	2	Grabbing vigorously at wound
	Restrained	2	Child's arms are restrained
Legs	Neutral	1	Legs in any position but are relaxed; includes gentle swimming or serpentine movements
	Squirming/kicking	2	Definitive uneasy or restless movements in the legs and/or striking out with foot or feet
	Drawn up/tensed	2	Legs tensed and/or pulled up tightly to body and kept there
	Standing	2	Standing, crouching, or kneeling
	Restrained	2	Child's legs are being held down

[a]McGrath PJ, Johnson G, Goodman JT, et al: CHEOPS: A behavioral scale for rating postoperative pain in children. In: Advances in Pain Research and Therapy, Vol 9. Fields HL, Dubner R, Cevero F, eds. New York, Raven Press, 1985, pp 395-406

All Children's Hospital
St. Petersburg, Florida

PAIN ASSESSMENT TOOLS

These scales are to be used to assess pain and evaluate response to interventions.
Reassess at least every 4 hours, or more frequently as needed.

WONG-BAKER FACES PAIN RATING SCALE

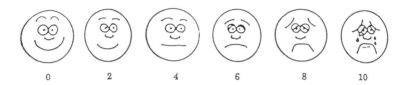

1. Explain to the child that each face is for a person who feels happy because
   he/she has no pain (hurt, or whatever word the child uses) or feels sad
   because he has some or a lot of pain
2. Point to the appropriate face and state, "This face is....
   - 0 - very happy because he doesn't hurt at all
   - 2 - hurts just a little bit
   - 4 - hurts a little more
   - 6 - hurts even more
   - 8 - hurts a whole lot
   - 10 - hurts as much as you can imagine, although you don't have to be
     crying to feel this bad
3. Ask the child to choose the face that best describes how he/she feels

Research reported in Wong, D., and Baker, C (1988) Pain in children: comparison
of assessment scales. Pediatric Nursing 14(1), 9-17. This tool may be reproduced
for use in the clinical setting.

NUMERIC SCALE FOR PAIN ASSESSMENT

No Pain   Worst Pain

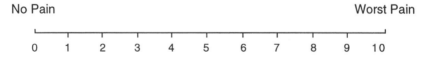

Explain to the person that at one end of the line is 0, wich means that a person feels
no pain (hurt). At the other end is a 10, which means the person feels the worst pain
imaginable. Ask the person to choose the number that best desribes his own pain.
Recommended for persons 7 years and older.

This tool may be reproduced for use in the clinical setting.

COMPLICATIONS AND RELATIVE SAFETY OF REGIONAL ANESTHESIA IN CHILDREN

L. M. Broadman

INTRODUCTION

The popularity of pediatric regional anesthetic techniques has been steadily increasing since the mid 1980's. A review of the literature concerning complications related to these techniques reveals four emerging themes: 1) single-injection caudal blocks are exceedingly safe, 2) caudal/epidural catheters have a low risk for infection, but may be more difficult to thread cephalad to a thoracic level than suggested by the original reports, 3) continuous epidural infusions with bupivacaine have led to some incidences of neurologic and cardiac toxicity, and 4) the recent use of spinal-axis opioids in children has produced many of the same problems found with adult usage.

Sang and colleagues recently published the results of a survey of pediatric regional anesthesia complications survey (1). Fourteen institutions with established pediatric pain services were asked to report all recorded complications that had occurred over the seven-year period from 1985 to 1992. In the 48,345 pediatric regional procedures reported (26,693 single-injection and 12,718 continuous infusions) there were a total of 34 critical complications (24 incidences of respiratory depression and 10 convulsions), and 16 noncritical but clinically significant complications (including three infections, one nerve root lesion, four heel sores, and one retained catheter). A more detailed analysis of the information contained in this study will be presented in a subsequent section of this manuscript.

Unfortunately, data from large controlled studies on these topics are limited. The vast majority of the information available for establishing safety and complication benchmarks either comes from pooled retrospective surveys derived from multiple centers or from single case reports.

T. H. Stanley et al. (eds.), Pain Management and Anesthesiology, 185–204.
© 1998 *Kluwer Academic Publishers. Printed in the Netherlands.*

SINGLE-INJECTION CAUDAL SAFETY AND COMPLICATIONS

LARGE SERIES, SURVEYS AND KEY CASE REPORTS

Although major advancements in clinical experience with the pediatric caudal block have been made in the last 10 to 15 years, only recently have reports of large series been published. In 1991 a survey by Gunter (2) involving 119 children's hospitals and anesthesiology residency programs reviewed the complications which had occurred during the performance of more than 150,000 caudal blocks. Gunter ascertained that the occurrence rate of catastrophic complications during the performance of single-injection caudal blocks was about 1:40,000. In the very large series at Children's National Medical Center which spanned the period from 1983-1995 and which involved over 7800 caudal blocks in infants and children resulted in only three noted complications: two recognized dural punctures and one high spinal in a former premature nursery graduate who received a caudal block following a failed spinal anesthetic (3). Hypotension and urinary retention have not been reported in either of these series. All authors stress that the key to safety with this procedure is knowledge of anatomy in children, meticulous attention to detail in selection and preparation of the site, and careful aspiration before drug injection. When these measures are taken, the single-injection caudal block is an exceedingly safe technique.

There appears to be an increased risk of unrecognized intravascular injection in infants weighing less than 10 kg. Veyckemans and others reported a series of 1,100 caudal blocks in children younger than seven years, 463 of which were performed in infants weighing less than 10 kg in weight (4). They noted 76 bloody taps, with eight recognized systemic reactions (systemic reactions were defined as an increase in heart rate greater than 20 beats per minute, usually with electrocardiographic changes, cutaneous vasoconstriction, and severe arterial hypertension). Epinephrine 1:200,000 was always added to the local anesthetic to act as an intravascular marker. The eight systemic reactions all occurred in infants weighing less than 10 kg; six were associated with negative aspirations for blood and were considered "concealed bloody taps." However, it is this author's impression that these "concealed bloody taps" may have actually been intraosseous injections. All episodes responded to hyperventilation with oxygen; there were no convulsions or episodes of cardiovascular collapse.

There have also been other recent reports of cardiac events in infants weighing less than 10 kg who received caudal blocks. Two infants weighing 4 and 8 kg who experienced episodes of ventricular tachycardia and brief cardiovascular collapse following attempted caudal blocks with bupivacaine-epinephrine solutions were recently reported by Ved and colleagues (5). There were negative aspirations in both circumstances and the authors believed that the malignant cardiac rhythms were due to epinephrine toxicity, and that slow fractional administration of local anesthetic solutions is an imperative.

Negative aspiration does not rule out the potential for a needle or catheter tip to lie within a blood vessel. McGown, in a series of 500 pediatric caudal blocks reported a 7% incidence of unintentional entry into a caudal epidural vessel (6), while Dalens and Hasnaoui reported a 10.6% incidence of blood return in their series of 750 caudal blocks when long needles were employed (7).

Intravenous injection can be prevented by repeated gentle aspiration after each needle movement. The use of excessive force during aspiration may fail to show blood if the suction force collapses the vein. Most bloody aspirates are due to intraosseous rather than intravenous placement of the needle. The cancellous mass of sacral bone is covered by a wafer-thin, brittle layer of cortex which can be easily damaged. This complication is best avoided by inserting the needle in the line of the sacral canal, avoiding excessive force, and keeping the bevel of the needle directed ventrally so that it slides over the anterior plate of the sacrum.

AIR LOSS OF RESISTANCE TO LOCATE EPIDURAL SPACE

Air loss of resistance techniques for caudal or epidural blockade should be avoided in pediatric patients. Reports indicate that children can develop a life-threatening venous air embolism from small quantities of air used during loss of resistance identification of the caudal epidural space (8). Schwartz and Eisenkraft (9) reported circulatory collapse in a 9-month-old infant who had 3.0 ml of air injected into the lumbar epidural space. In fact, children may be at more risk than adults because of their high incidence of probe-patent foramen ovale (up to 50% in children less than 5 years of age) (10).

Because of the lower extension of the dural sac, the risk of dural puncture theoretically is higher in infants and small children than in adults or older children. However, this complication is technique dependent and easily recognized if gentle aspiration is performed following placement of the needle and prior to the first injection of drug. If a dural puncture is noted, it would be prudent to abandon attempts at caudal blockade because of the risk of total spinal blocks (11).

THE RISK OF INFECTION FOLLOWING CAUDAL BLOCK PLACEMENT

Infection is frequently listed among the complications associated with both single-injection caudal blocks and caudal catheter techniques; however, post-caudal block infections have rarely been noted in clinical practice (1,2,12-15).

A very recent study by Strafford and colleagues (12) has substantiated the belief that epidural infections following the administration of protracted epidural analgesia via indwelling catheters is a very infrequent event in infants and children. These authors retrospectively reviewed the records of 1620 caudal/epidural catheter placements in infants and children over a six-year period. The catheters were left in place for as along as 14 days, median 2.4 days. Seventy catheters (3.7%) were placed via the caudal approach; the majority were lumbar epidural catheters (93%). A combination of bupivacaine and fentanyl was the most common perfusate. This study reported a zero percent incidence of clinically significant infections in postoperative patients, a rate which is not statistically different from the spontaneous abscess rate of 0.2 to 1.2 cases per 10,000 hospital admissions (16). Epidural abscess was not a reported complication in patients who received postoperative analgesia via a caudal/epidural catheter. One terminally ill child with a necrotic epidural tumor did develop candida colonization of her epidural space.

Strafford and colleagues emphasize that with aseptic catheter placement, daily inspection of the catheter and puncture site, and removal of the catheter at the first hint of difficulty continuous caudal/epidural analgesia in infants and children can be a very safe and efficacious technique for providing protracted analgesia (12).

Unfortunately, there are three very recent case reports (13-15) of infectious complications following the placement of indwelling epidural catheters in infants and children despite these catheters having been placed in accordance with the Strafford guidelines (12). Two of the reports deal with the development of skin pustules at the epidural catheter puncture site (13,14). The first report by Emmanuel (13) deals with a 4-year-old boy who received continuous caudal epidural analgesia for 29 hours following hypospadias repair. The catheter was placed under aseptic conditions, a bacterial filter was employed and a sterile transparent adhesive dressing covered the catheter puncture site throughout the infusion period. On the 10th postoperative day a small pustule was noted at the catheter insertion site, and on the 14th postoperative day a small extradural abscess was surgically incised and drained from the same area. The specimen and a small amount of pus were sent for culture, but no organism was ever isolated or identified. The child had an uneventful recovery.

More recently, Meunier and colleagues (14) reported two cases in which infants with biliary atresia developed localized skin infections at their lumbar epidural puncture sites. Both children had undergone Kasaï procedures and had received epidural analgesia for the first 48 postoperative hours at which time the catheters were removed. On the fifth postoperative day each child was noted to have an area of induration and a small pustule at the catheter entry site. In each case, the pus was evacuated and sent for culture. No organisms were isolated in the first case, so antibiotic therapy was not instituted. The second child was noted to have a recurrent collection of fluctuant subcutaneous material in the area of catheter insertion and underwent surgical incision and drainage of his subcutaneous abscess on postoperative days six and twelve. His *Staphylococcus aureus* infection was also treated with an appropriate course of oxacillin.

However, the most distressing case report is by Larsson and colleagues (15). These authors document the formation of an epidural abscess in a one-year old boy with severe visceral pain secondary to a rare condition, chronic intestinal pseudoobstruction. His pain could not be managed with parenteral narcotics and over a six month time span, from 7 months to one year of age, he had three lumbar epidural catheters placed for pain control. Each remained in place from 3 to 12 days. The child's third catheter had been deliberately placed more cephalad than previous ones in order to better target the area of non-operative chronic visceral pain and to minimize bupivacaine infusion requirements. It had been placed through a L1-L2 puncture site and the catheter tip had been threaded cephalad to T11-12. Eleven days after the placement of this third catheter the concentration of bupivacaine had to be increased from 0.125% to 0.375%. Despite the large dose of bupivacaine being infused (1.1 mg/kg/hr), the child's pain could not be adequately controlled and parenteral narcotics were administered. The next day (day 12) tender swelling was noted at the epidural catheter penetration site. The catheter was immediately removed. A bacterial culture from the epidural catheter tip revealed the growth of *Pseudomonas aeroginosa* which was sensitive to tobramycin. A Magnetic Resonance Imaging (MRI) confirmed the presence of an epidural abscess extending T5 to L5. The abscess was noted to be deforming and dislocating the medulla in this area. Surprisingly, the child had not developed any neurologic symptoms. He was treated non-surgically with intravenously administered antibiotics. The abscess could not be detected on a follow-up computed axial tomography study 11 days after the institution of antibiotic therapy. He survived this event without sequelae. These authors provide the following invaluable tip. When one notes a sudden and otherwise unexplained decrease in the of ability of previously effective epidural catheter to continue to provide adequate pain control, an epidural abscess should be included in the differential problem list (15).

Larsson and colleagues suggest that their patient's continuous bacteremia from his necrotizing enterocolitis may have led to the seeding of his epidural catheter and the subsequent development of his epidural abscess (15). Likewise, both children in the Meunier report were known to have congenital biliary atresia and a recent Kasaï procedure; and, as such, they probably had ascending cholangitis and bacteremia (14). It is this author's opinion that children with known or suspected bacteremia/septicemia are probably not suitable candidates to receive extradural analgesia.

Finally, it is this authors belief that extradural catheters can be safely used to provide prolonged and effective pain relief in properly selected pediatric patients. The widespread utilization of modern single-use needles, commercially prepared pediatric caudal/epidural catheter kits, aseptic techniques during caudal/epidural catheter placement, in-line bacterial filters, and the employment of occlusive transparent dressings to cover catheters and puncture sites have virtually eliminated many of the factors that could potentially lead to the development of post-block infections. Meunier and colleagues indicate that they have only had two infectious complications out of 2,000 extradural catheterizations performed over a ten year period (14). Likewise, this author and his associates have obtained similar results, in that they have not had a single infection during the placement of 3,500 in-dwelling pediatric caudal catheters.

PROBLEMS WITH TEST DOSING

There is no effective test dose or technique for the reliable detection of the intravascular injection of local anesthetic solutions during block placement in children simultaneously undergoing general anesthesia with volatile agents. Desparmet and colleagues (17) studied 65 children, ranging in age from 1 month to 11 years of age, and found that children who received an intravenous epinephrine-containing solution without atropine pretreatment did not demonstrate a consistent increase in their heart rates. Furthermore, 94% of children who received atropine premedication followed by intravenous epinephrine had only a brief heart rate increase of greater than 10 beats/min. (peaking at 45 seconds and lasting to 60 seconds post injection) (17). It must be emphasized that the atropine injection in this study was given to patients with a stable end-tidal halothane concentration of 1.0%. Increases in heart rate of 10 beats/min. or greater may be noted following needle placement in children who are not so deeply anesthetized. Perillo and colleagues (18) performed a similar study, comparing intravenous isoproterenol in doses of 0.05 µg/kg and 0.075 µg/kg. As in the epinephrine study by Desparmet (17), Perillo (18) was unable to show any consistent or predictable relationship between the infusion of the aforementioned test doses of isoproterenol and increases in heart rate.

As in adults, it is important to administer the local anesthetic in incremental doses rather than to rely completely upon a test dose. Even after needle replacement, the local anesthetic should be injected in small aliquots with careful monitoring for signs of systemic toxicity.

CAUDAL CATHETERS

THE ADVANTAGES OF CAUDAL CATHETERS

Lumbar and thoracic epidural anesthesia posses certain advantages over caudal anesthesia in infants and children undergoing upper abdominal and thoracic procedures. Both of the former techniques allow for the targeting of local anesthetic solutions at the site of surgery and therefore reduce the potential for toxic drug reactions and other morbidities. While these techniques, lumbar and thoracic epidural catheter placements, have been well described in children (19,20), both may be technically difficult and even hazardous to perform in infants and children. On the other hand, caudal catheters are very easy to place and the catheter tips may be threaded cephalad to the desired level (21,22); thereby, affording one the opportunity to provide thoraco-abdominal anesthesia/analgesia without the associated risk of spinal cord trauma and local anesthetic toxicity.

PRELIMINARY STUDIES ON THE PLACEMENT OF CAUDAL CATHETERS

In 1988 Bösenberg and colleagues (21) demonstrated in 20 neonates and older infants undergoing biliary tract surgery that it was possible to place a caudal epidural catheter and easily thread the catheter tip cephalad into the thoracic region. They used adult equipment (a 16-gauge intravenous catheter was used as the introducer and 18 gauge adult epidural catheter was employed). In all cases the epidural catheter tip was successfully passed into the thoracic region. In 19/20 cases the tip was passed within one vertebra of the desired level, the eighth thoracic vertebra. All tip placements were radiographically confirmed and all catheters were easily removed at the completion of surgery. There were no complications in any of their study patients.

In a subsequent study Gunter and Eng (22) studied the thoracic placement of epidural catheters by the caudal route in 20 children. They were able to correctly place 17 out of 20 styleted 24-gauge micro-catheters on the first attempt. All of the micro-catheters were advanced thorough a pediatric intravenous catheter which had been introduced into the children's caudal epidural space. Two other catheters were manipulated and finally came to rest in the proper position.

Bösenberg (21) and Gunter (22) have both shown that it is absolutely necessary to manipulate catheters in order to properly position them into desired lumbar and thoracic regions. In addition, both have demonstrated that it is technically easier and safer to gain access to either the lumbar and thoracic epidural space via the caudal route. While there is the potential for trauma to the spinal cord of infants and children during the direct placement of thoracic and lumbar epidural catheters, this risk is virtually eliminated by the use of the caudal approach

Gunter and Eng (22) offer several suggestions to improve the likelihood that one will be able to safely thread a pediatric epidural catheter into the thoracic region: 1) If resistance is encountered during the insertion of an epidural catheter, withdraw it a short distance and twist it prior to reinsertion. 2) If continued resistance is encountered, withdraw the catheter a short distance and flex the child's knees into their chest in order to manipulate the spine ever so slightly prior to attempting to reinsert the catheter. 3) **Never forcibly advance the catheter against resistance.**

PROBLEMS ENCOUNTERED DURING THE CEPHALAD ADVANCEMENT OF LUMBAR EPIDURAL CATHETERS

A very recent article by Blanco and colleagues (23) has demonstrated that it is very difficult and sometimes impossible to advance a catheter which has been placed in the lumbar epidural space cephalad to a thoracic level in infants and children older than one year of age. The Blanco group studied 39 infants and children who ranged in age from 0-96 months of age. They used an 18-gauge Touhy needle and air loss of resistance techniques to properly identify the epidural space at the L-4/L-5 interspace in all study patients. Unfortunately, only seven of the 19-gauge, unstyleted, polyethylene, multiorifice catheters could be advanced cephalad to the T-12 level. Twenty-three of the 39 catheters (60%) simply formed a loop at or about the L-4/L-5 region. Eight of the catheters were difficult to place. On the other hand, the fact that a catheter was easy to place did not positively correlate with the ability to advance the catheter tip cephalad. There were no inadvertent dural punctures and all catheters were removed without difficulty.

Why did the Blanco Group (23) encounter so much difficulty passing 19-gauge catheters cephalad, and Bösenburg (21) and Gunter (22) did not? Perhaps, it relates to the fact that Bösenburg placed his catheters in infants less than one year of age, and one would suspect that most of the infants in the Bösenburg study had not yet assumed upright posture. Therefore they had not developed lumbar lordosis and 19/20 of Bösenburg's catheters easily passed cephalad.

Gunter circumvented this problem in older infants and children by using wire styleted micro-catheters. The author has been using a wire styleted, open end, micro catheter for more than two years and coiling has not been a problem (Sims 20/24 Micro Catheter System®).

EPIDURAL INFUSIONS OF LOCAL ANESTHETICS

TOXICITY OF LOCAL ANESTHETICS

Bupivacaine is one of the most commonly used local anesthetic agents for pediatric caudal and epidural blocks. This agent can be used safely if maximum dosage guidelines are followed. However, complications relating to neurologic and cardiac toxicity have been reported.

While the toxic plasma bupivacaine level for adults is estimated to be 4.0 µg/ml (24), the level in infants and children is not known. Plasma levels which are less than 2.0 µg/ml are thought to be safe in children and have not been associated with neurologic or cardiac toxicity (25). However, a number of factors indicate caution in applying adult toxicity data to children. The metabolism of local anesthetics is greatly reduced in the neonate, because of both decreased plasma pseudocholinesterase and decreased hepatic microsomal activity (26,27). Also, alpha$_1$-acid glycoprotein (alpha$_1$-AGP) concentrations are quite low in infants less than two months of age and they do not reach adult levels until after the first year of life (28). Alpha$_1$-AGP is important as it is the primary binding substrate for cationic drugs such as local anesthetics. Albumin and other plasma proteins only play a very minor role in the binding of local anesthetic solutions. Reduced levels of alpha$_1$-AGP allow for more of the local anesthetic solution to remain in the unbound or free form, and it is only the unbound fraction of local anesthetics which can precipitate toxic reactions such as seizure activity and myocardial depression.

Children eliminate drugs faster than newborns and infants but more slowly than adults. This slower rate of elimination requires particular attention to continuous infusions of local anesthetic. The larger cardiac output of pediatric patients is a factor in the relatively rapid increase of local anesthetic blood levels, especially in the vessel-rich organs such as the brain and heart.

Other factors that have been noted to potentially increase susceptibility to bupivacaine toxicity include concomitant administration of volatile agents (29), acidosis (30), hypoxia (31), and hyponatremia and hyperkalemia (32), as well as rapid increases in plasma bupivacaine levels (33).

Several studies have evaluated bupivacaine plasma levels following single bolus doses. Following lumbar epidural administration of 0.25% bupivacaine (3.0 mg/kg), Eyres and colleagues (34) noted that plasma levels peak at 20 minutes and ranged from about 1.0-2.0 µg/ml. Ecoffey (35) studied ten infants who ranged in age from 3-36 months of age. Six of the infants had thoracic epidural catheters and four lumbar catheters. All were injected with 0.5% bupivacaine (3.75 mg/kg). Peak plasma levels occurred in 20 minutes, and with the exception of one child with a plasma level of 2.2 µg/ml, all values were less than 1.8 µg/ml (35). Eyres and coworkers (36) found plasma bupivacaine concentrations after caudal injection of 0.25% bupivacaine (3 mg/kg) ranged from 1.2 to 1.4 µg/ml in children. Mazoit and colleagues (27) studied infants receiving 2.5 mg/kg of bupivacaine for caudal analgesia, and found that serum and plasma levels were both in the range of 0.5-1.9 µg/ml. Stow and colleagues (37) noted that peak plasma concentrations were reached at around 20 minutes after caudal administration. In each study, the peak plasma levels of bupivacaine were less than those that are considered to be toxic in adults, and peak plasma levels occurred 20 minutes after administration by caudal, lumbar and thoracic injections.

Desparmet (38) evaluated plasma bupivacaine levels in six children who were given a loading dose of 0.25% bupivacaine (0.5 ml/kg) without epinephrine injected into the lumbar epidural space, followed in thirty minutes by an infusion of the same drug at a rate of 0.08 ml/kg/hr. Plasma bupivacaine levels were assayed from specimens obtained at four hour intervals between 24 and 48 hours after the start of the infusion, and then every two hours until 10 hours had elapsed following termination of all infusions. Plasma levels in these six children were highly variable, ranging from 0.2 to 1.2 µg/ml. No increase was noted in plasma levels between 24 and 48 hours. However, research on adults has shown that continuous epidural infusions of bupivacaine produce constant plasma levels until approximately 50 hours after the start of infusion when a dramatic increase occurs (39).

McIlvaine et al. evaluated plasma bupivacaine levels in children receiving intrapleural infusions at rates of 0.5-2.5 mg/kg/h (40). Plasma bupivacaine levels ranged from 1.0 to 7.0 µg/ml. None of these children were noted to experience any signs of toxicity; however, this may be due either to the small number of patients in the series, or to the fact that some of the children received diazepam within the first 24 hours following surgery.

Agarwal and colleagues (41) reported two cases of neurotoxicity related to continuous bupivacaine infusions. Both patients received 0.25% bupivacaine with 1:200,000 of epinephrine. The first case involved a 9.4-kg three year old girl with chronic interstitial lung disease who was scheduled for a right middle lobe lung biopsy. During the procedure, an intrapleural catheter was placed. It should be noted that systemic absorption of local anesthetic agents is far greater in the intrapleural space than in either the intercostal or caudal space. One hour after a bolus of 0.66 mg/kg was given, an infusion of 0.25 mg/kg/h was begun. Five hours later the infusion was increased to 0.5 mg/kg/h owing to complaints of increased discomfort. Twenty-one hours after the start of the infusion the patient had two tonic-clonic seizures which were treated with intravenous phenobarbital (100 mg). The patient's bupivacaine level was 5.6 µg/ml at the time of her seizures. The second patient to develop seizures from systemic accumulation of bupivacaine was a 26-kg nine-year-old with cerebral palsy. She was a former premature infant, but at the time of the report she was an otherwise healthy child, scheduled for selective dorsal rhizotomy. After a bolus of bupivacaine (1.25 mg/kg) was injected into her caudal epidural catheter, an infusion at the rate of 1.25 mg/kg/hr was started. Fifty-six hours after the start of the infusion, the patient had three tonic-clonic seizures that were successfully treated with phenobarbital. The patients bupivacaine level at the time of the first seizure was 5.4 µg/ml.

Of interest in the report by Agarwal and colleagues (41) is the absence in both cases of prodromal warning signs, which might have alerted caregivers the impending onset of acute bupivacaine neurotoxicity. Both patients were reported to be calm, cooperative, and restful. The only unusual complaint was from the second patient, who reported a "falling" or "tumbling" sensation several hours prior to the onset of seizure activity (41). Early central nervous system manifestations of toxicity may not be apparent in children because they are less likely to articulate their symptoms. In awake infants and toddlers these symptoms may be misinterpreted as irritability or "fussiness." The first signs of local anesthetic toxicity in a pediatric patient may be dysrhythmia or cardiovascular collapse (5,42).

McCloskey and colleagues (43) reported three cases of children who experienced toxic side effects from continuous epidural infusions of bupivacaine. Bupivacaine 0.25% with 1:200,000 of epinephrine was used for all three patients. The first child was a 3.89 kg one day old infant scheduled for direct closure of exstrophy of the bladder. Local anesthetic solution in bolus doses of, 2.5, 1.87, and 1.87 mg/kg, was administered at hours 0, 1.5, and 3.0, respectively. At hour 4.5, a bupivacaine infusion was begun at the rate of 2.5 mg/kg/h. Ten hours after the start of the infusion, the patient developed bradycardia and hypotension. The infusion was discontinued and the infant was quickly intubated. Bag and mask ventilation with oxygen was instituted and epinephrine (10 μg/kg) was given intravenously. The sinus bradycardia suddenly changed to ventricular tachycardia, which partially responded to three boluses of lidocaine (1.0 mg/kg) and one dose of sodium bicarbonate (1.0 meq/kg). Normal sinus rhythm was established through the intravenous infusion of phenytoin (5.0 mg/kg). However, two hours later the patient's rhythm reverted once again to ventricular tachycardia and generalized tonic-clonic seizures occurred. Both were treated successfully with intravenous diazepam, 0.25 mg/kg and serially administered phenytoin for a total dose of 7.0 mg/kg. The plasma bupivacaine level at the time the infusion was discontinued was 5.6 μg/ml, and 12 hours later it dropped to 3.7 μg/ml. The child had no neurologic sequelae as a result of the aforementioned events and enjoyed an uneventful recovery.

The second patient reported by McCloskey and colleagues (43) was a 45-kg eight-year-old child scheduled for bladder augmentation. Boluses of 1.40, 0.83, 0.55, and 1.00 mg/kg were given at 0, 1.5, 3.5, and 5.5 hours, respectively. An infusion of 1.67 mg/kg/h was begun at hour 9.5. After another 25 hours, the patient experienced two generalized tonic-clonic seizures which responded to diazepam. The plasma bupivacaine level shortly after the seizure was 6.6 μg/ml. The third patient was a 12-kg four year old girl with bilateral knee trauma resulting from a motor vehicle accident. There were no signs of head trauma. The patient received bupivacaine boluses during surgery of 2.50, 1.67, 1.67, and 1.67 mg/kg at hours 0, 2.0, 4.0, and 5.5, respectively. A bupivacaine infusion was begun 3.0 hours after the last intraoperative dose at the rate of 1.67 mg/kg/h. At hour 26, the patient's level of analgesia decreased from T-10 to L-2. A leak at the catheter insertion site was noted, and the catheter was replaced. A 0.42 mg/kg bolus was given and the infusion was re-instituted at 2.0 mg/kg/h. Eight hours later, the patient experienced a generalized tonic clonic seizure which resolved with diazepam. The patient's plasma bupivacaine level was 10.2 µg/ml at the time of her seizure. Neurologic examinations of all three patients after seizure activity resolved were normal.

The infusion rates for all three patients in the aforementioned case report were excessively high. This led McCloskey and colleagues (43) to develop infusion guidelines based on extrapolations from linear pharmacokinetic projections for bolus caudal and epidural bupivacaine levels. They suggested 0.4 mg/kg/h for infants less than six months old and 0.75 mg/kg/h for older children (43). However, lower infusion rates, which provide adequate analgesia yet pose less potential for toxic complications, have been established by Berde (44). His recommended dosage guidelines for epidural bupivacaine infusions include a loading dose of 2.0-2.5 mg/kg and an infusion rate not in excess of 0.4-0.5 mg/kg/h in older infants, toddlers, and children and less than 0.2-0.25 mg/kg/h in neonates. Of the ten convulsions noted in the survey by Sang (1), eight occurred after either repeated bolus doses of bupivacaine or infusion rates greater than O.5 mg/kg/h.

The second complication related to bupivacaine toxicity is cardiac dysrhythmia. This is perhaps a more serious complication since it may be refractory to conventional treatment. Maxwell and colleagues (42) have successfully employed phenytoin in the treatment of two neonates with bupivacaine-induced cardiac toxicity. The first infant is the same 3.89 kg one day old with exstrophy of the bladder presented by McCloskey (43). The second patient was a 4.4 kg full term infant, also with exstrophy of the bladder, who received three caudal bolus doses of bupivacaine, 2.50, 1.25, and 1.75 mg/kg, at 0, 2.5, and 4.5 hours, respectively. Five minutes after the third dose was administered, the patient developed wide-complex tachydysrythmia. All anesthetic agents were discontinued, and 100% oxygen was administered. After bretylium 5.0 mg/kg was administered, the patient's heart rate increased from 120 to 240 beats per minute and his blood pressure decreased from 90/60 to 65/40 torr. Normal sinus rhythm was established after phenytoin was administered in divided doses for a total dose of 7.0 mg/kg.

If inadequate analgesia persists after the maximum dose of bupivacaine has been administered and incorrect needle placement and technical problems have been ruled out, it is unwise to administer additional bupivacaine. Either an epidural or systemic opioid can be added in conjunction with the epidural infusion, or the epidural may be discontinued in favor of systemic opioids or other analgesics.

Some practitioners prefer continuous infusions of caudal or epidural lidocaine (42) to bupivacaine because of the ability to rapidly and easily monitor plasma concentrations of the former agent in most hospital laboratories.

EPIDURAL/CAUDAL OPIOIDS

Probably no other aspect of pediatric postoperative pain management has shown more growth and development in the past decade than the use of spinal axis opioid and local anesthetic infusions. However, delayed respiratory depression is always possible, whether the opioid is administered via the caudal, epidural, or spinal route, especially in young infants. This is particularly true with concomitant administration of systemic opioids. Of the 24 incidents of respiratory depression in the survey by Sang and colleagues (1), 22 of the patients had received neuraxial opioids and 12 of the 24 had received supplementary intravenous sedation.

The pharmacokinetic parameters observed after epidural morphine administration in older children have been found to be similar to those previously measured in adults, including a significant decrease in the minute ventilatory response to breathing an end-tidal CO_2 pressure of 55 torr. Breathing such a mixture caused a significant shift in the CO_2 response curve for more than 22 hours following epidural morphine administration (45). Krane and colleagues (46) demonstrated that caudal morphine in a dose of 33 µg/kg provides excellent analgesia with a lower incidence of the delayed respiratory depression. Such delayed respiratory depression was previously reported by Krane when a larger dose of 100 µg/kg was administered to a 2.5-year-old boy (47). Valley and Bailey (48) reported the use of caudal morphine 70 µg/kg diluted with normal saline in 138 children undergoing major abdominal, thoracic and orthopedic surgery. Children weighing less than 5 kg received 3.0 ml of solution, while those weighing 5-15 kg received 5.0 ml and those weighing over 15 kg received 10 ml of solution. Of note is the high incidence of respiratory depression which occurred in 11 children in this study (48). Of these 11 children, 10 were under one year of age and most had received concomitant systemic opioids along with the extradural opioids. The mean time from the administration of caudal morphine until the onset of respiratory depression in this group was 3.8 hours; no respiratory depression occurred in any child later than 12 hours after the last dose. All episodes of respiratory depression were successfully managed with naloxone, 5-20 µg/kg followed by infusions of 2-10 µg/kg/h.

Bailey and colleagues (49) compared the efficacy of caudal, epidural, and intravenous butorphanol in reducing the incidence of adverse side effects associated with epidural morphine. They found that there was no difference in the incidence of adverse side effects between the children who had received butorphanol and those who had not. Lawhorn and Brown (50) found a decreased incidence of opioid-related complications when butorphanol (40 μg/kg) was added to epidural morphine (80 μg/kg).

The addition of clonidine to epidural morphine appears to provide prolonged analgesia without increasing the incidence of adverse side effects (51).

SPINAL ANESTHESIA

POST DURAL PUNCTURE HEADACHE

The incidence of postdural puncture headaches (PDPH) in children following spinal anesthesia or inadvertent "wet taps" during placement of epidural blocks, is quite low (52) and the problem rarely occurs in children less than 12 years of age (53). Lumbar puncture with a 20 or 22-gauge needle is a frequent diagnostic procedure in pediatric patients, and is often used to provide chemotherapy in children. Even under these circumstances, PDPH is infrequent and rarely requires treatment (52). An epidural blood patch provides effective treatment for PDPH in pediatric patients when the child has not responded to conventional therapy and symptoms persist for more than a week (54). Sedation and EMLA® cream may be beneficial adjuncts to reduce the pain and emotional trauma of blood patch therapy. Practitioners should consider the child's age and level of maturity when determining whether conscious or deep sedation will be required. The volume of autologous blood recommended varies from 0.5-0.75 ml/kg, and should be injected slowly (54).

SPINAL OPIOIDS

Nichols and colleagues (55) studied the disposition and respiratory effects of subarachnoid morphine in ten infants and children undergoing craniofacial surgery. All these children required cerebrospinal fluid (CSF) drainage as part of the surgical procedure; this was accomplished by placing a subarachnoid catheter at the L4-L5 interspace. The same catheter was used to administer subarachnoid morphine (2.0 μg/kg) prior to the conclusion of surgery, and then to sample and measure the CSF concentration of morphine at 6, 12, and 18 hours. Corresponding plasma concentrations of morphine were determined by radioimmunoassay. Subarachnoid morphine produced a reduction in both the slope and the intercept of the ventilatory response curve; this reduction was greatest 6 hours after morphine administration, and the ventilatory response only partially recovered 12 and 18 hours later. This study documents that infants and children may experience respiratory depression for at least 18 hours following subarachnoid morphine administration and that appropriate monitoring and safeguards are essential.

CONCLUSIONS

1.   Single-shot caudal blocks are safe in infants and children as long as one follows these simple guidelines: monitor the children, be familiar with the anatomy, and limit the dose of bupivacaine to 2.5-3.0 mg/kg.

2.   Test dosing is not reliable in infants and children and neither is gentle aspiration. One must limit the dose of bupivacaine and use basic precautions in order to prevent potentially catastrophic complications. The author suggests that bupivacaine 0.125% be used in all caudal blocks and that the volume be limited to 1.0 ml/kg. Finally, it is imperative that one administer the local anesthetic solution slowly and that it be delivered in small, divided doses.

3.   Air embolism has occurred in infants and children during the use of air-loss-of-resistance techniques. Air should not be used while attempting to identify the caudal or lumbar epidural spaces in infants and children. Saline should be used instead.

4. Continuous infusions of bupivacaine can provide prolonged and effective analgesia, but they can also lead to convulsions, dysrhythmias, and other disastrous complications. By limiting the bolus dose of the local anesthetic as well as the infusion rate, one can make continuous techniques both safe and efficacious. Berde (43) suggests that loading doses not exceed 2.0-2.5 mg/kg. Infusion rates for older infants, toddlers, and children should not exceed 0.4-0.5 mg/kg/h and for infants and neonates infusion dosages should not be greater than 0.2- 0.25 mg/kg/h.

5.   Epidural and spinal axis opioids can provide excellent postoperative analgesia with minimal side effects. Lower doses of epidurally administered morphine, such as 33 µg/kg, can provide analgesia that is just as effective as large doses such as 80-100 µg/kg but may be associated with far fewer adverse side effects. Respiratory depression has not been observed in any child later than 12 hours following a single bolus injection of epidural morphine. Therefore, twelve hours may be the benchmark to use when establishing postoperative monitoring and nursing care guidelines for children who have received spinal axis opioids.

REFERENCES

1. Sang CN, Berde CB, and the Safety in Regional Analgesia Study Group: A multicenter study of safety and risk factors in pediatric regional anesthesia. Anesthesiology 81:A1386, 1994.
2. Gunter J: Caudal anesthesia in children: A survey. Anesthesiology 75:A936, 1991.
3. Broadman LM, Rice LJ: Neural blockade for pediatric surgery. In: Neural blockade in clinical anesthesia and management of pain (3rd ed). Edited by: Cousins MJ and Bridenbaugh PO. Philadelphia: J. B. Lippincott, 1996. (in press).
4. Veyckemans F, Van Obbergh LJ, Gouverneur JM: Lessons from 1100 pediatric caudal blocks in a teaching hospital. Reg Anesth 17:119-125, 1992.
5. Ved SA, Pinosky M, Nicodemus H: Ventricular tachycardia and brief cardiovascular collapse in two infants after caudal anesthesia using a bupivacaine-epinephrine solution. Anesthesiology 79:1121-1123, 1993.
6. McGown RG: Caudal analgesia in children: five hundred cases for procedures below the diaphragm. Anaesthesia 37:806-818, 1982.
7. Dalens B, Hasnouai A: Caudal anesthesia in pediatric surgery: success rate and adverse effects in 750 consecutive patients. Anesth Analg 68:83-89, 1989.
8   Guinard J-P, Borboen M: Probable venous air embolism during caudal anesthesia in a child. Anesth Analg 76:1134-1135, 1993.
9. Schwartz N, Eisenkraft JB: Probable venous embolism during epidural placement in the infant. Anesth Analg 76:1136-1138, 1993.
10. Nora JJ: Etiologic aspects of heart disease. In: Heart disease in infants, children and adolescents (3rd ed). Edited by: Adams FH, Emmanouilides CG. Baltimore: Williams and Wilkins, 1983: p14.
11. Desparmet J: Total spinal anesthesia after caudal anesthesia in an infant . Anesth Analg 70:665-667, 1990.
12. Strafford MA, Wilder RT, Berde CB: The risk of infection from epidural analgesia in children: a review of 1620 cases. Anesth Analg 80:234-238, 1995.
13. Emmanuel ER: Post-sacral extradural catheter abscess in a child. Br J Anaesth 73:548-549, 1994.
14. Meunier JF, Noorwood P, Dartayet B, Dubousset AM, Ecoffey C: Skin abscess with lumbar epidural catheterization in infants: is it dangerous? Report of two cases. Anesth Analg 84:1248-9, 1997.
15. Larsson BA, Lundberg S, Olsson GL: Epidural abscess in a one-year old boy after continuous epidural analgesia. Anesth Analg 84:1245-7, 1997.
16. Baker AS, Ojemann RG, Swartz MN, Richerdson EJ: Spinal epidural abscess. N Engl J Med 293:463-468, 1975.
17. Desparmet J, Mateo J, Ecoffey C, Mazoit X: Efficiency of an epidural test dose in children anesthetized with halothane. Anesthesiology 72:249-251, 1990.

18. Perillo M, Sethna NF, Berde CB: Intravenous isoproterenol as a marker for epidural test-dosing in children. Anesth Analg 76:178-181, 1993.
19. Ecoffey C, Dubousset A-M, Samii K: Lumbar and thoracic epidural anesthesia for urologic and upper abdominal surgery in infants and children. Anesthesiology 65:87-90, 1986.
20. Ruston FG: Epidural anaesthesia in infants and children. Can Anaesth Soc J 1:37-40, 1954.
21. Bösenberg AT, Bland BAR, Schulte-Steinberg O, Downing JW: Thoracic epidural anesthesia via caudal route in infants. Anesthesiology 69:265-269, 1988.
22. Gunter JB, Eng C: Thoracic epidural anesthesia via the caudal approach in children. Anesthesiology 76:935-938, 1992.
23. Blanco D, Llamazares J, Rincón R, Ortiz M, Vidal F. Thoracic epidural anesthesia via the lumbar approach in infants and children. Anesthesiology 84:1312-1316, 1996.
24. Tucker GT: Pharmacokinetics of local anaesthetics. Br J Anaesth 58:717-731, 1986.
25. Sethna NF, Berde CB: Pediatric Regional Anesthesia. In: Pediatric Anesthesia (3rd ed). Edited by: Gregory G. New York: Churchill Livingstone, 1994: 281-317
26. Morgan D, McQuillan D, Thomas J: Pharmacokinetics and metabolism of the anilide local anesthetics in neonates. Eur J Clin Pharmacol 13:365-371, 1978.
27. Mazoit JX Denson DD, Samii K: Pharmacokinetics of Bupivacaine following caudal anesthesia in infants. Anesthesiology 68:387-391, 1988.
28. Lerman J, Strong HA, Le Dez KM, Swartz J, Rieder MJ, Burrows FA: Effects of age on serum concentration of alpha$_1$-acid glycoprotein and the binding of lidocaine in pediatric patients. Clin Pharmacol Ther 46: 219-245, 1989.
29. Eyres RL, Kidd J, Oppenheimer R, Brown TCK: Local anaesthetic plasma levels in children. Anaesth Intens Care 6:243-247, 1978.
30. Rosen MA, Thigpen JW, Shnider S, Foutz SE, Levinson G, Koike M: Bupivacaine- induced cardiotoxicity in hypoxic and acidotic sheep. Anesth Analg 64:1089-1096, 1985.
31. Heavner JE, Dryden CF, Sanghani V, Huemer G, Bessire BS, Badgwell JM: Severe hypoxia enhances central nervous system and cardiovascular toxicity of bupivacaine in lightly anesthetized pigs. Anesthesiology 77:142-147, 1992.
32. Timour Q, Freysz M, Mazze R, Couzon P, BertrixL, Faucon G: Enhancement by hyponatremia and hyperkalemia of ventricular conduction and rhythm disorders caused by bupivacaine. Anesthesiology 72:1051-1056, 1990.
33. Scott DB: Evaluation of clinical tolerance of local anesthetic agents. Br J Anaesth 47:328-333, 1975.

34. Eyres, RL, Hastings C, Brown TCK, Oppenheim R C: Plasma bupivacaine concentrations following lumbar epidural anesthesia in children. Anaesth Intens Care 14:131-134, 1986.
35. Ecoffey C, Dubousset AM, Samii K: Lumbar and thoracic epidural anesthesia for urologic and upper abdominal surgery in infants and children. Anesthesiology 65:87-90, 1986.
36. Eyres RL, Bishop W, Oppenheim RC, Brown TCK: Plasma bupivacaine concentrations in children during caudal epidural analgesia. Anesth Intens Care 11:20-26, 1983.
37. Stow PJ, Scott A, Phillips A, White JB: Plasma bupivacaine concentrations during caudal analgesia and ilioinguinal-iliohypogastric nerve block in children. Anaesthesia 43:650-653, 1988.
38. Desparmet J, Meistelman C, Barre J, Saint-Maurice C: Continuous epidural infusion of bupivacaine for postoperative pain relief in Children. Anesthesiology 67:108-110, 1987.
39. Richter O, Klein K, Abel J, Ohnesorge FK, Wust HJ, Theissen FMM: The kinetics of bupivacaine plasma concentrations during epidural anesthesia following intraoperative bolus injection and subsequent continuous infusion. Int J Clin Pharmacol Ther Toxicol 22:611-617, 1984.
40. McIlvaine WB, Knox RF, Fennessey PV, Goldstein, M: Continuous infusion of bupivacaine via intrapleural catheter for analgesia after thoracotomy in children. Anesthesiology 69:261-264, 1988.
41. Agarwal R, Gutlove DP, Lockhart CH: Seizures occurring in pediatric patients receiving continuous infusion of bupivacaine. Anesth Analg 75:284-286, 1992.
42 Maxwell LG., Martin LD, Yaster M: Bupivacaine-induced cardiac toxicity in neonates: successful treatment with intravenous phenytoin. Anesthesiology 80:682-686, 1994.
43. McCloskey JJ, Haun SE, Deshpande JK: Bupivacaine toxicity secondary to continuous caudal infusion in children. Anesth Analg 75:287-293, 1992.
44. Berde CB: Convulsions associated with pediatric regional anesthesia. Anesth Analg 75:164-166, 1992.
45. Attia J, Ecoffey C, Sandouk P, Gross JB, Samii K: Epidural morphine in children: pharmacokinetics and CO_2 sensitivity. Anesthesiology 65:590-594, 1986.
46. Krane EJ, Tyler DC, Jacobson LE: The dose response of caudal morphine in children. Anesthesiology 71:48-52, 1989.
47. Krane EJ: Delayed respiratory depression in a child after caudal epidural morphine. Anesth Analg 67:79-82, 1988.
48. Valley RD, Bailey AG: Caudal morphine for postoperative analgesia in infants and children: a report of 138 cases. Anesth Analg 72:120-124, 1991.
49. Bailey AB, Valley RD, Fried EF, Sellman GS, Calhoun P: Epidural morphine combined with epidural or intravenous butorphanol for postoperative analgesia. Anesthesiology 79:A1136, 1993.

50. Lawhorn CD, Brown RE: Epidural morphine with butorphanol in pediatric patients. J Clin Anesth 6:91-94, 1994.
51. Jamail S, Monin S, Begon C, Dubousset AM, Ecoffey C: Clonidine in pediatric caudal anesthesia. Anesth Analg 78:663-666, 1994.
52. Bolder PM: Postlumbar puncture headache in pediatric oncology patients. Anesthesiology 65:696-698, 1986.
53. Verneau D: Spinalini anestezie v pediatrike chirurgii. Cas Lek Cesk 40:1206-1209, 1962.
54. Kumar V, Maves T, Barcellos W: Epidural blood patch for treatment of subarachnoid fistula in children. Anaesthesia 46:117-118, 1991.
55. Nichols D, Yaster M, Lynn A, Helfaer M, Deshpande JK, Mason P, Carson BS, Bezman M, Maxwell LG Tobias J, Grochow LB: Disposition and respiratory effects of intrathecal morphine in children. Anesthesiology 79:733-738, 1993.

PEDIATRIC SEDATION CHALLENGES OUTSIDE THE OPERATING ROOM

L. J. Rice

Many medical interventions require adults to cause physical or emotional discomfort to a child. A common defense toward this need to cause pain is denial by the health care worker that the child has pain; "Let's get this lumbar puncture over as fast as we can. The needle will only hurt for a few seconds. He doesn't need anything for that brief pain." There may be an assumption that infants and young children cannot really feel pain because of incomplete development of their nervous system. The fact that newborns cry with heel puncture is interpreted as "reflexive"; thinking not unlike that of 18th century partygoers who would stick pins in dogs and cats in order to be amused by the "reflexive" pain behavior; comfortable in their belief that this withdrawal of the affected limb was "merely a reflex" and not a symptom of "real pain."

Pain has both physical and emotional components (1). Since children have such an exaggerated fear of needles, simply removing the sharp pain is often not enough to alleviate the pain. A double-blind study comparing intravenous fentanyl and midazolam to premedicate 25 children and adolescents undergoing lumbar punctures (LP) and bone marrow aspirations (BMA) indicated that while 100% of the children and their parents preferred these agents to any other premedication, 72% of the children chose midazolam over fentanyl (2). This preference for amnesia is certainly substantiated by the need to sedate children to ensure cooperation during procedures where there is no physical pain, such as magnetic resonance imaging or nuclear medical therapy.

In the last 20 years, anesthesiologists have been asked to provide sedation, analgesia, or general anesthesia for non-surgical procedures. Our presence is increasingly requested for cardiac catheterizations, MRI examinations, invasive radiology procedures, lumbar punctures and bone marrow evaluations, among others (3). The anesthesiologist's expertise in patient evaluation, monitoring, and drug selection, as well as a unified approach to the needs of sedated/anesthetized patients can improve

205

T. H. Stanley et al. (eds.), Pain Management and Anesthesiology, 205–216.

patient care, as well as increase "throughput" and "cost-efficient use of facilities."

In addition, the Joint Commission on Accreditation of Healthcare Organizations (JCAHO) includes regulations that are pertinent to the practice of sedation. The 1996 regulations state that: 1) there must be "protocols for care of patients receiving sedation that carries the risk of loss of protective reflexes." Protocols must include appropriate equipment, monitoring, documentation and outcome monitoring. 2) sedation which "may be reasonably expected to result in the loss of protective reflexes" is considered anesthesia and must follow the same standards as anesthesia care given in the operating room.

Conscious sedation is a medically controlled state of depressed consciousness in which 1) protective reflexes are maintained; 2) the patient retains the ability to maintain a patent airway independently and; 3) there is an appropriate response to physical stimulation or verbal command ("open your eyes").

Deep sedation is a medically controlled state of depressed consciousness in which 1) protective reflexes may not be maintained; 2) the patient may not maintain a patent airway independently and; 3) the patient is unable to appropriately respond to physical stimulation or verbal command ("open your eyes"). The deeply sedated patient can easily move to a state of general anesthesia.

OVERALL CONSIDERATIONS

As the "pediatrician (and internist) of the operating room", the anesthesiologist integrates overall perianesthetic patient care including. preanesthetic evaluation, fasting status, proper medication selection, monitoring, postanesthetic care and followup.

Many nonanesthetic practitioners are not experienced in a systematic approach to patients requiring attention to patient selection, extensive monitoring, recording of vital signs during sedation, and evaluation before discharge. In addition, titration of medications to a sedated/anaesthetic endpoint, the balance of multiple medications/techniques for a goal of amnesia, analgesia, depression of noxious reflexes, and the need to demonstrate recovery from this therapeutic milieu are also unfamiliar to nonanesthesiologists.

The involvement of anesthesiologists outside the operating room provides a high level of experienced care for deeply sedated or anesthetized patients. In addition, the faceless anesthesiologist becomes more visible and other healthcare workers become aware of the approach that we take to these situations. This exposure outside the operating suite provides an opportunity to communicate principles and methods that we use daily to other physicians who can then employ these principles successfully for patients when the anesthesia service is not directly involved.

THE DEVIL IS IN THE DETAILS

Guidelines to consider: As in all other area of practice, there are many places to look to assist in developing required protocols. Regulations, guidelines and protocols abound (4). The JCAHO Handbook is an important place to look. In addition, the Standards and Guidelines of the American Society of Anesthesiologists (ASA) includes multiple Standards that should be consulted when planning to provide frequent sedation/anesthesia for a specific area of the hospital, as well as Guidelines for Nonoperating Room Anesthetizing Locations (5).

In 1992, the Committee on Drugs of the American Academy of Pediatrics (AAP) updated its policy on Guidelines for Monitoring and Management of Pediatric Patients During and After Sedation for Diagnostic and Therapeutic Procedures (6). These guidelines were directed towards nonanesthesiologists who provide sedation outside of the operating room, and were established with the consultation of the Committee on Standards, the Committee on Pediatric Anesthesiology of the ASA, and the Society for Pediatric Anesthesia. These guidelines were meant to establish <u>uniform</u> standards of care throughout all subspecialties providing pediatric sedation. The AAP guidelines emphasize selection of candidates for sedation, medical evaluation, facilities, equipment, fasting, monitoring, documentation, personnel and post sedation requirements.

The AAP guidelines particularly emphasize the risk of escalation of care and vigilance of personnel for the deeply sedated child, and the need for escalation of care should the "consciously sedated child" become deeply sedated. Although Guidelines are meant to be suggestions rather than commandments, the imprimatur of the specialty society (AAP, ASA or other) puts a practitioner on notice that his/her professional society has thoughtfully considered a topic and evaluated the literature to set forth these suggestions.

How about for my institution? Protocols developed by the anesthesia, nursing, physician and other involved professional staff should be developed for each anesthetizing location. Patient selection, time and method of scheduling patients for the anesthesia service, appropriate number of cases per day, required laboratory work and required history and physical evaluation should be established in a multidisciplinary planning stage. The anesthesia service must decide if ASA physical status III or IV patients should be anesthetized in these outlying areas, and what consultations and laboratory work is required. Appropriate "triggers" for individual patient consultation should be identified and a pathway worked out clearly stating who is responsible for the phone call to the anesthesia service.

In addition to fasting guidelines, a protocol for chronic medication use should be set—e.g., all asthmatics should receive their usual medications the day of the procedure. This protocol should conform with that used for patients cared for in the operating room or the protocol should clearly state why these patients can be treated differently.

Fasting guidelines should be similar to those employed in the operating room. At All Children's Hospital (ACH), relatively healthy infants less than 1 year of age are often sedated with chloral hydrate or Nembutal for radiology with monitoring by a specially trained sedation nurse, and NPO of 4 hours for solids and clear liquids. NPO guidelines may be different for the 2 services.

These same sedation nurses provide postanesthesia care in a room adjacent to the MRI unit or CT scanner in addition to instructing parent pre- and post procedure, calling the family the day before and after the procedure, and providing quality assurance monitoring. In addition, there is a "minor procedure" area with sedation protocols and specially trained nurses in another area of the hospital for gastroenterology, oncology and other invasive procedures at ACH. This area is limited to "conscious sedation" only, and the anesthesia service virtually never goes there. If a child needing a procedure usually performed in that area does not qualify for sedation by virtue of his/her medical problems, the child is booked into the operating room block time and the procedure is performed there or in an induction room with a dedicated anesthesia team.

The JCAHO requires that written policies be in place in any area where sedation is employed. Documentation of pre-procedure evaluation (such as telephone interviews), as well as provision of written instructions for fasting times and recovery information are also important parts of good patient care. All health care providers involved in sedation should be knowledgeable with regard to the drugs employed, interpretation of the monitored parameters (especially pulse oximetry) and basic airway management.

NONPHARMACOLOGIC TOOLS

Behavioral, or noninvasive methods have been employed with good effect for children undergoing painful procedures. These techniques have been particularly helpful for children who face repeated painful procedures, such as oncology patients (7,8). Behavioral methods enhance the child's ability to cope by allowing him or her to gain some control of the situation and participate actively in treatment. These methods also recognize the child's dignity, and acknowledge both the fear and discomfort of cancer or other painful states. They may be termed relaxation techniques or coping techniques. Distraction is also helpful.

Parents are the most important people in a child's life. They represent security and safety. During times of stress and pain, young children want to be with their parents, expecting to be protected, or at least comforted (9). Most experiences with parental presence are positive, although a very anxious parent can increase the distress of a child.

It is important to realize that parents need to be "coached" as to how they can best help their child; many parents sit silent for fear of disrupting the procedure. "Coaching" the parent and reinforcing helpful actions during the procedure will allow the parent some ability to assist his/her child. This will also aid the parent in coping; many parents are very frustrated at their helplessness and inability to assist their sick child. Even if the parents are not present during the procedure, education as to how best to support their child before and after the procedure are also important.

PHARMACOLOGIC TOOLS

If pharmacologic intervention is planned, then an anxious child about to undergo a procedure expected to produce minimum pain may require an anxiolytic alone (10). An analgesic should be included for more invasive procedures. If repeated procedures are planned, the intervention for the first should be maximized so that anticipatory anxiety does not develop. A child who has a history of significant anxiety should be referred prior to the first planned procedure for psychological intervention in addition to the use of pharmacology.

Choice of drugs and dosages, and selections of routes of administration will depend upon the setting in which the child will undergo the painful procedure; emergency room, treatment room, or clinic. Avoidance of intramuscular injections is preferable; however there may sometimes be no alternative due to lack of patient cooperation. The availability of trained personnel, the invasiveness of the procedure, the patient's clinical and psychological status and the equipment available will also have an impact.

It is also important to remember that combinations of medications can have a much more potent respiratory depressant effect than single medications. Most of the serious or fatal problems that have occurred in ambulatory pediatric patients undergoing sedation have occurred with a combination of opioid and benzodiazepine. Some of these untoward incidents have occurred on the trip home, underscoring the need for proper recovery from these potent medications prior to discharge. If possible, local anesthetics should be administered prior to a painful procedure, in addition to appropriate sedation and/or analgesia.

TOPICAL MEDICATIONS

Since children hate needles, preparations that remove the pain of the needle are of benefit. Injection of local anesthetic not only stings, but is also a needle procedure. Topical anesthetics can remove the pain of the needle without themselves requiring a needle (11). Recognition of this by the appropriate-aged child can decrease anticipatory anxiety; however the child will have to learn that topical anesthetics "make the skin sleepy." Few children will simply believe what they are told without experiencing the analgesia for themselves.

Both Eutectic Mixture of Local Anesthetics (EMLA cream) and NumbyStuff (iontophoresis of lidocaine) have been employed. EMLA is an emulsion of the solid pure bases of lidocaine and prilocaine. A concentration of 80% lidocaine-prilocaine is achieved by a cream that has only a 5% concentration of local anesthetic. The high concentration of lidocaine and prilocaine in an unionized form in this high-water-content medium stimulates transdermal spread.

NumbyStuff is a patch and apparatus combination that causes lidocaine to penetrate to a depth of 8-11 mm by iontophoresis. This requires a small electrical current, and a cooperative child for at least 10 minutes. Some children find the electrical current "buzz" to be troublesome and will not use it. Children who are using a topical local anesthetic for the first time will still be afraid of the needle.

MIDAZOLAM

Midazolam is a short acting, water soluble benzodiazepine devoid of analgesic properties. The drug has become particularly popular because of its short duration, predictable onset, and lack of active metabolites. Although originally formulated for intravenous use, the same medication used orally has proven very successful in producing light sedation and amnesia (12). Unfortunately, the drug has a very bitter taste that is difficult to disguise. Several strategies including dilution in cola syrup, apple juice with sweeteners, ibuprofen syrup, or liquid acetaminophen have been described. Allowing self administration through a prefilled syringe in a comforting environment (parent's arms) has met with the most success in these authors' experience.

Respiratory depression is rare with oral administration of midazolam. As a general rule, this medication and mode of administration comes the closest of any of the current sedatives available to providing true conscious sedation—providing a sedated yet arousable and cooperative patient at the indicated doses.

The recommended oral dose is 0.5-0.75 mg/kg, with onset of sedation in approximately 20-30 minutes, with a rapid offset approximately 30 minutes after the peak effect is noted. Intravenous midazolam can be titrated to effect in doses of 0.05-0.1 mg/kg, while intramuscular midazolam has been employed in doses of 0.3 mg/kg. Nasal midazolam, while used by some as a premedication, both stings the nasal mucosa and tastes bad as it drips into the back of the throat. The dose is 0.2 mg/kg; most kids will only accept it one time. Administration of local anesthetic often provides the analgesia necessary to allow a painful procedure to be performed.

PROPOFOL

Propofol is a 2,6-diisopropylphenol compound that has potent sedative and hypnotic properties. Because it is only slightly soluble in water, the drug is dissolved in a solution of soybean oil. The nature of this solution requires the drug be handled in a sterile manner and used quickly once it is opened. Onset of action is extremely rapid and *induction of anesthesia* may be achieved with 2-3 mg/kg in 95% of patients within 60-90 seconds. Sleep may be induced by as little as 1.5 mg/kg and maintenance of sedation is usually accomplished through the use of an intravenous infusion at 50-150 μg/kg/minute. Recovery from the drug is faster than with any other intravenous sedative (2-3 minute redistribution time) and the incidence of prolonged sedation or vomiting is extremely low (13,14). A dose related decrease in blood pressure is noted that is similar to that found with other anesthetics. Propofol causes pain on injection—this may be prevented by administering a small dose of lidocaine (1 mg/kg) through the IV catheter prior to administration of the drug or administering the drug through a fast-flowing intravenous line into a large vein such as an antecubital vein.

Because anesthesia, with its complete loss of airway reflexes, respiratory depression, and cardiovascular depression can be induced so rapidly with propofol, many hospitals limit its use to anesthesia personnel. The role of this drug in the ICU and emergency department remains to be defined—clearly only individuals skilled in airway management should be administering the drug.

Propofol is an ideal agent for brief periods of deep sedation. Minimal adverse effects and rapid awakening are unique among currently available agents. Extreme caution is advised in using this drug as general anesthesia is induced rapidly—may be limited to use by anesthesia personnel and in the intensive care environment.

KETAMINE

Ketamine is a unique medication of the phencyclidine class that binds to opioid receptors and possesses intense analgesic, sedative, and amnestic qualities. It has a long track record of safety as a sedative for painful procedures in children, particularly those undergoing burn debridement or tubbing (15,16). A functional dissociation is created between the cortical and limbic systems of the brain. Spontaneous respirations and airway reflexes are maintained. The eyes remain open with a slow nystagmic gaze with intact corneal and light reflexes. Patients may exhibit random tonic movements of the extremities.

Ketamine generally causes an increase in heart rate, blood pressure, cardiac output and intracranial pressure. The drug should be used with caution (or not at all) in patients with suspected increased intracranial pressure or open globe injuries. Oral secretions are mildly increased with oral ketamine although administration of an antisialogogue is rarely required. This drug also has bronchodilator qualities. Ketamine causes hyperactive airway reflexes, with a risk of laryngospasm. It has been documented to cause an incompetent gag reflex and should be administered with caution to patients with a full stomach or with gastroesophageal reflux. Prolonged emergence may occur, but postsedation emesis and dysphoria are rare with sedative doses of ketamine.

The oral dose recommendation is 5-6 mg/kg (17). Onset of sedation occurs in 15-30 minutes and effects may be prolonged with this route—lasting 3 to 4 hours. Intramuscular ketamine in doses of 3-4 mg/kg allow for start of an intravenous and lasts about 20 minutes, with recovery time of up to an hour, while intravenous ketamine can be titrated in doses of 0.5-1 mg/kg. All side effects are dose-dependent and more likely to occur with intravenous doses.

FENTANYL

Fentanyl is a powerful synthetic opioid which is 100 times more potent than morphine. It has a very high degree of fat solubility that allows for very rapid penetration of the blood brain barrier (12). The sedation effects are relatively brief as the offset of the drug is dependent on redistribution rather than elimination.

Respiratory depression is a significant risk and may outlast opioid effects by as much as 60-90 minutes. Strict adherence to monitoring standards is mandatory. Respiratory depression is *markedly* increased when the drug is combined with midazolam or other sedative and increased vigilance for possible airway management requirements should be made when the drugs are administered together.

The IV dose recommendation is 0.5-1 µg/kg/dose, titrated to a total dose of 4-5 µg/kg. Fentanyl as a sole agent offers excellent pain relief with mild sedation at these doses. Maximal effect occurs within 5 minutes when administered intravenously. Opioid effects last for 30-40 minutes.

Oral transmucosal fentanyl (OTFC) is available as a sweetened lozenge on a plastic stick of various strengths (200 µg, 300 µg and 400 µg). The recommended dosage is 15-20 µg/kg orally (18). Generally there is excellent and rapid uptake of the drug from the oral mucosa although the effectiveness of a given dose varies with how much of the drug is swallowed by the patient rather than allowed to absorb transmucosally. Drug that reaches the stomach for absorption may be responsible for prolonged serum concentrations. Sedation reliably occurs within 15-30 minutes. Note: Awareness may be maintained even when the patient appears asleep.

Adverse effects of this form of the drug are those commonly associated with mu receptor agonists. Pruritus occurs in 44%. Nausea and vomiting occurs in approximately 15-20% of patients and is not prevented by the administration of antiemetics. Respiratory depression with oxygen desaturation to less than 90% has been reported in 5% of children but usually resolves with verbal prompting. Other adverse effects including chest wall and glottic rigidity are possible but much more common with the IV form of the drug.

Careful respiratory and cardiac monitoring is mandatory especially when the drug is combined with other sedatives

SUCROSE PACIFIER

Before the advent of modern pediatric anesthesia, sugar-dipped pacifiers or "whiskey nipples" were used in conjunction with restraints for surgical operation such as pyloromyotomy in neonates. A recent study evaluated sterile water and three different concentrations of sucrose in infants 1-6 days of age prior to undergoing heel prick sampling (19,20). There was a significant reduction in crying time with the use of this maneuver, with a greater reduction in those infants who received the highest concentration of sucrose. Perhaps this simple maneuver should be employed more frequently in infants undergoing brief painful procedures.

NITROUS OXIDE

Nitrous Oxide (N_2O) is a colorless, odorless gas that has both analgesic and anxiolytic effects. The drug must be delivered with oxygen to avoid a hypoxic gas mixture. This may be accomplished though the use of flow meters from separate sources or through the delivery of a fixed 50% mixture of N_2O/oxygen (Entonox). The drug may be delivered alone at concentrations of 30-50% for moderately painful procedures or in combination with a mild sedative at lower concentrations for similar effect (21, 22). Onset of sedation and analgesia occurs in minutes and is terminated rapidly when the gas is discontinued. Nitrous oxide has minimal cardiovascular and respiratory effects when not combined with a potent sedative or opioid. Studies in large groups of patients (some with mild IV sedation) have failed to show any significant risk of cardiopulmonary depression when nitrous oxide is used at the concentrations cited here.

If any inhalational agent is to be used, Occupational Safety and Health Administration (OSHA) guidelines for scavenging and room air turnovers must be met. This requirement may make the use of N_2O impractical except in dedicated rooms where such equipment is present.

Nitrous oxide is useful for brief painful procedures and may be combined with a mild sedative. Expensive equipment and ventilation apparatus required for delivery will limit its widespread use.

CONCLUSIONS

Painful procedures cause not only pain, but fear in pediatric patients. This occurs prior to the anticipated procedure as well as during the procedure. It is always important to maximize the intervention for the first procedure so that anticipatory anxiety does not increase with each procedure. Whether to add pharmacologic intervention to the psychologic and behavioral tools employed for every patient should be determined by the level of anxiety and context of the procedure. Parental education is always valuable, and parental presence is frequently an aide to the child's coping and ability to cooperate.

Psychologic intervention and local anesthesia may be sufficient for pain control and enhancing the child's mastery and feelings of self-esteem. However, if the procedure is expected to be very painful, prolonged, or repeated, pharmacologic adjuncts should be considered. The goals of procedure-related pain management are to make the procedure as non-threatening and comfortable as safely possible. This will limit the child's fear of future procedures, enhance cooperation, encourage mastery and a feeling of control, and involve the parents in an intervention that is supposed to, after all, help the child to get well.

REFERENCES

1. Anderson CTM, Zeltzer LK, Fanurik D. Procedural pain. In Schechter NL, Berde CB, Yaster M (eds): Pain in Infants, Children and Adolescents. Williams & Wilkins, Baltimore, pp 435-451, 1993
2. Sandler ES, Neyman C, Connor K: Midazolam vs fentanyl premedication for painful procedures in children with cancer. Pediatrics 89:631-634, 1992
3. Management of Childhood Pain: New Approaches to Procedure-Related Pain. J Pediatrics 122(suppl), 1993
4. Holzman RS, Cullen DJ, Eichhorn JH, Philip JH: Guidelines for sedation by nonanesthesiologists during diagnostic and therapeutic procedures. J Clin Anesth 6:265-276, 1994
5. American Society of Anesthesiologists. Practice guidelines for sedation and analgesia by non-anesthesiologists. Anesthesiology 84:459-468, 1996
6. American Academy of Pediatrics, Committee on Drugs. Guidelines for monitoring and management of pediatric patients during and

after sedation for diagnostic and therapeutic procedures. Pediatrics 89:1110-1112, 1992

7. Ellis JA, Spanos NP: Cognitive-behavioral interventions for children's distress during bone marrow aspirations and lumbar punctures: a critical review. J Pain Sympt Manag 9:98-112, 1994

8. Patterson KL, Ware LL: Coping skills for children undergoing painful medical procedures. Iss Comp Pediatr Nurs 11:113-117, 1988

9. Bauchner H: Procedures, pain and parents. Pediatrics 87:563-566, 1991

10. Yaster M, Krane EJ, Kaplan RF et al: Pediatric Pain Management and Sedation Handbook, Mosby-Year Book, 1997

11. Freeman JA, Doyle E, Im NT, Morton NS: Topical anaesthesia of the sin: a review. Paediatr Anaesth 3, 129-139, 1993

12. Coté CJ: Sedation for the pediatric patient. Pediatr Clin North Am 41:31-51, 1994

13. Martin TM, Nicolson SC, Bargas MS: Propofol anesthesia reduces emesis and airway obstruction in pediatric outpatients. Anesth Analg 76:144-149,1993

14. Frankville DD, Spear RM, Dyck JB: The dose of propofol required to prevent children from moving during magnetic resonance imaging. Anesthesiology 79:953-958, 1993

15. Rice LJ: Ketamine--from "star wars" to dinosaur in 25 years? In Stanley TH, Shafer PG (eds): Pediatric and Obstetrical Anesthesia. Kluwer Academic Publishers, Dordrecht, the Netherlands, p 345-361, 1995

16. Green SM, Nakamura R, Johnson NE: Ketamine sedation for pediatric procedures: part 2 review and implications. Ann Emerg Med 19:1033-1042 1990

17. Gutstein JB, Johnson KL, Heard MB et al: Oral ketamine preanesthetic medication in children. Anesthesiology 76:28-34, 1992

18. Ashburn MA, Streisand JB: Oral Transmucosal fentanyl: Help or hinderance?. Drug Safety 11:295-298,1994

19. Haouari N, Wood C, Griffiths G, Levene M: The analgesic effect of sucrose in full term infants: a randomised, controlled trial. Br Med J 310:1498-1502, 1995

20. Editorial: Pacifiers, passive behaviour, and pain. Lancet 339:275, 1992

21. Wattenmaker I, Kasser JR, McGravey A: Self-administered nitrous oxide for fracture reduction in children in an emergency room setting. J Orthoped Trauma 4:35-39, 1990.

22. Litman RS, Berkowitz RJ, Ward DS: Levels of consciousness and ventilatory parameters in young children during sedation with oral midazolam and increasing concentrations of nitrous oxide. Anesthesiology 83:A1182, 1995

SPINAL OPIOIDS: CLINICAL APPLICATIONS FOR ACUTE AND CHRONIC PAIN

S.M. Walker, M.J. Cousins, D.B. Carr

INTRODUCTION

Spinal delivery of analgesic agents is widely utilized in clinical practice, and the concept of "selective spinal analgesia" is well accepted. The safety and efficacy of spinal opioid analgesia has been established, although questions appropriately arise concerning selection of this technique versus systemic medication (1). Significant advances have been made in opioid pharmacology (including understanding of the "plasticity" of opioid mechanisms, and the recent discovery of new endogenous opioid peptides), and the pharmacology of the primary afferent synapse in the dorsal horn (with identification of multiple receptor mechanisms which can modulate pain transmission).

OPIOID PHARMACOLOGY

EFFICACY OF SPINAL OPIOIDS

It is necessary to show that the spinal route is more efficacious and at least as safe, but preferably safer than existing methods, as more invasive procedures can be associated with increased complications. Comparative efficacy data are beginning to emerge, but often studies are not conducted in an adequate double blind, double dummy crossover design (2) with use of appropriate equivalent doses and optimally effective regimens for the alternative routes. In addition, it is important to accurately see the effects of the stated route. High doses of lipid soluble agents will result in significant plasma concentrations. Epidural infusion of alfentanil was shown to result in similar plasma concentrations as the same dose administered intravenously, and there was no significant improvement in the analgesia provided by the epidural route (3). In many cases, correct placement of the epidural catheter has not been confirmed prior to commencement of the study. Therefore, the integrity of the thera-

T. H. Stanley et al. (eds.), Pain Management and Anesthesiology, 217–236.
© 1998 Kluwer Academic Publishers. Printed in the Netherlands.

peutic procedure under investigation cannot be verified (4), and the effectiveness of "epidural" administration will be inadequately assessed.

PHARMACOKINETICS OF SPINAL OPIOIDS

The onset of analgesia after spinal opioid administration is earlier with more lipid soluble agents. Compared to the intrathecal route, epidural opioid administration is further complicated by pharmacokinetic (dural penetration, fat deposition, systemic absorption) and pharmacodynamic aspects (larger doses of opioid result in blood concentrations that cannot be ignored). Phenylpiperidine derivatives (meperidine, fentanyl, lofentanil) are highly lipid soluble and have a rapid onset of analgesia after epidural dosing that coincides with an early peak drug concentration in CSF (5-7). Lipid-soluble epidural opioids enter spinal fluid by way of the arachnoid granulations in the dural cuff region in addition to diffusion across the dura (8). Unionized drug will rapidly be transferred to CSF, into spinal radicular arteries, and into epidural veins. In the presence of brisk spinal artery blood flow and slow epidural venous flow, transfer of the drug to the spinal cord will predominate while the concentration gradient is high. Morphine has low lipid solubility and the slowest onset of action. A somewhat quicker onset of analgesia for hydromorphone than morphine after lumbar epidural administration despite comparable lipophilicity and similar blood and CSF pharmacokinetics may reflect more rapid supraspinal action of the former compound (9).

Duration of analgesia is inversely related to lipid solubility but is also influenced by the rate of dissociation from receptors and accumulation in epidural fat (1). Intrathecal injection of an ionized, lipid soluble drug results in low residual concentrations in CSF (6) owing to rapid systemic uptake. Hence, less drug is carried in the CSF to the brain. Egress of lipid soluble opioids will also be hastened by rapid uptake into epidural veins. Intrathecal injection of a highly ionized and hydrophilic drug such as morphine produces high CSF concentrations (10,11). Because it has low lipid solubility, morphine diffuses slowly from CSF to opioid receptors, nonspecific binding sites and clearance sites (arachnoid granulations). Slower efflux from spinal cord and CSF result in a long duration of analgesia, and greater migration to the brain (12). Cephalad CSF flow which carries drug remaining in the CSF to the brain, may be hastened by Valsalva maneuver or intermittent positive pressure ventilation.

Pharmacodynamics of Spinal Opioids

Opioid receptors are found throughout the spinal gray matter but are most prominent in the substantia gelatinosa, and are predominantly of the mu subtype (70% mu, 20% delta and 10% kappa) (13,14). In the dorsal horn, opioids act both at presynaptic sites to reduce release of primary afferent transmitter release, and at postsynaptic sites to inhibit dorsal horn neurons by activation of potassium channels and hyperpolarization (13).

Of all opioids studied in the postoperative period, morphine has the greatest dosage-sparing effect for epidural versus intravenous administration (15). The quality of morphine analgesia is superior when this drug is given epidurally than when it is given systemically (16,17), and the analgesic effect of epidural morphine correlates poorly with blood morphine concentration (1). Epidural fentanyl is second only to morphine in the degree of dosage sparing achieved by epidural versus intravenous drug delivery (15). Analgesia from epidural fentanyl, alfentanil and sufentanil may be evident in patients whose plasma opioid concentrations are below analgesic levels (18). However, epidural administration of lipophilic opioids alone may offer little advantage over the intravenous route (3) if the catheter tip is placed distant from the required area of blockade and large doses are used. Meperidine is the only currently available opioid that has significant local anesthetic actions when applied to individual dorsal root axons or that is effective when used as a sole intrathecal agent for surgery (19,20). Sameridine, a novel molecule with both local anesthetic and opioid properties, is being tested in clinical trials as a new spinal anesthetic that offers prolonged postoperative pain control (21).

Spinal opioids have been shown to be effective against nociceptive, visceral and neuropathic pain. However, in many cases, improved analgesia may be achieved by combination with other agents. Spinal opioids alone may be only partially effective in severe visceral pain (e.g., during labour); and the control of neuropathic pain is enhanced by combination with non-opioid spinal analgesics such as clonidine.

Combination with Other Agents

Epidural infusion of a combination of local anesthetic and opioid is now well established as a safe and effective means of providing analgesia after major surgery or trauma. The value of such mixtures, particularly in managing incident or movement-related pain in addition to pain at rest, has led to their adoption outside the acute pain setting for chronic management of cancer pain. Keeping the concentration of bupivacaine below 0.1% minimizes the incidence of sensorimotor block during both acute and chronic infusion (1).

Alpha-2 agonists significantly shift the opioid dose-response curve to the left when they are coadministered intrathecally (22), and thus have a synergistic analgesic action . Addition of clonidine to intrathecal infusions of morphine (23) and hydromorphone has successfully controlled previously intractable cancer pain, and clonidine may be more effective for neuropathic pain (24,25). Clonidine can also benefit sympathetically maintained pain, that is often a component of chronic neuropathic pain due to cancer or nonmalignant causes. Clonidine does not produce respiratory depression (26,27), and nausea was less marked in one study with the combination of epidural clonidine and morphine compared to morphine alone (24). Dexmedetomidine, a second generation alpha-2 agonist is currently in clinical trials as a preoperative medication for perioperative sympatholysis and analgesia (27), but may have a role as a spinal analgesic in the future.

As knowledge of the physiology and pharmacology of spinal sensory processing increases, non-opioid receptor systems are being modulated with the aim of improving analgesia and reducing side-effects (13,29). Potential agents include NMDA antagonists, GABA agonists such as midazolam, neostigmine, N-type calcium channel antagonists such as SNX 111, nonsteroidal antiinflammatory drugs, amitriptyline, and chromaffin cell implants (29). Analgesic efficacy, as well as systemic and local toxicity, of potential spinal analgesics must be carefully evaluated prior to clinical use. The clinical role of many non-opioid spinal analgesics and their interactions with spinal opioids remains to be determined.

PLASTICITY OF OPIOID MECHANISMS

Opioid actions are subject to changes within the nervous system ("plasticity"), and also modulation by a number of other transmitters, which may decrease or enhance the action of exogenous opioids (13,14). Opioid analgesia may be decreased by anti-opioid peptides such as CCK and F8a, or by activity of excitatory amino acids on the NMDA receptor. Alternatively, opioid activity may be synergistically enhanced by alpha-2 agonists acting via descending inhibitory noradrenergic pathways. Pathological changes may also affect opioid receptors. In the presence of inflammation, increased peripheral opioid receptors may provide further sites of action for opioids. By contrast, degeneration and loss of presynaptic receptors following nerve damage will reduce opioid responsiveness; but this should be overcome by dose escalation as supraspinal sites of action will not be affected by primary afferent damage. Morphine has only minor effects on A-fiber activity and therefore pain such as allodynia which may be mediated by A-fiber activity, is likely to be poorly responsive to opioids (14).

Differences in drug metabolism and elimination and the level of active metabolites may also account for side-effects and some of the individual variation noted in the effective analgesic dose of morphine. Morphine is metabolized in the liver to morphine-3-glucuronide (M3G) and morphine-6-glucuronide (M6G). M6G has similar affinity for mu receptors to morphine but is ten times as potent an analgesic (14). M3G has no affinity for the mu receptor, may antagonize the action of morphine at supraspinal sites, and has been postulated to cause paradoxical pain in patients receiving very high doses of morphine (30). Intracerebroventricular administration of M3G causes agitation (14). Chronic morphine administration, impaired renal function, and age greater than 70 years have all been associated with higher ratios of morphine metabolites to morphine (14,31,32).

TOLERANCE TO OPIOIDS

The development of tolerance is only one factor involved in declining analgesic effects or requirements for increased opioid dose, in chronic pain patients (33,34). Increased activity in nociceptive pathways from disease progression, evolution of neuropathic pain, changes in pharmacokinetic factors, as well as plasticity of opioid mechanisms will all influence opioid responsiveness (34). Rapid escalation early during opioid therapy may be evidence less of tolerance than of either a behavioral issue or of pain mechanism(s) that are intrinsically insensitive to opioid analgesia (1). Tolerance is a greater issue in intact animals or normal volunteers than during opioid therapy for chronic experimental or clinical pain. Tolerance and dose escalation are not inevitable consequences of prolonged treatment, and therapeutic effectiveness is usually sustained (35,36).

Tolerance to one opioid may not confer complete tolerance to another opioid drug. Changing from epidural morphine to buprenorphine (a kappa and mu agonist) improved analgesia in 32% of patients and reduced side-effects; and changing from buprenorphine to morphine improved analgesia in a further 46% of patients (35). Intrathecal DADL (D-Ala2-D-Leu5)enkephalin, a moderately selective delta receptor agonist, has been used to provide analgesia in patients tolerant to morphine (36,37). More selective and potent delta-selective opioids are becoming available (38) but as they require high doses for epidural and systemic use, their clinical application may be predominantly for intrathecal use (1). Animal studies have shown a dosage-sparing effect when mu and delta selective opioids are combined (39,40).

Morphine exposure increases the ED50 for morphine analgesia. This could result from downregulation (decreased receptor number) and desensitization (decreased receptor-effector coupling) (41) . However, some studies suggest that tolerance is unrelated to receptor changes (42), and intracellular processes are involved. Similar excitatory amino acid receptor-mediated cellular and intracellular mechanisms have been implicated in the development of neuronal plastic changes which lead to central sensitization and hyperalgesia (43), and also morphine tolerance (44). Manipulations which prevent NMDA receptor activation, calcium influx, or the intracellular consequences of NMDA receptor activation may inhibit the induction of tolerance and dependence (45). Many of the excitatory amino acid NMDA receptor interactions are mediated through the intracellular second messenger nitric oxide (NO). The NO synthase inhibitor, NG-nitro-L-arginine (NorArg) , attenuates the development of morphine tolerance (46). A further intracellular consequence of NMDA receptor activation is translocation of protein kinase C (PKC). GM1 ganglioside inhibits the translocation of PKC, and when coadministered with morphine reduced the development of tolerance (45). Increased knowledge of the cellular changes associated with tolerance may lead to agents which can be coadministered with opioids, to reduce the development of tolerance.

In animal studies, repeated administration of the NMDA receptor non-competitive antagonist MK-801 and the competitive antagonist LY274614, has been shown to inhibit the development of tolerance to the analgesic effect of morphine (45-47). Clinically, NMDA receptor antagonists may have a role in patients who have inadequate analgesia or unacceptable side-effects with high intrathecal doses of opioids, as a continuous low dose intravenous ketamine infusion facilitated rapid reduction in intrathecal morphine dosage (48). Dextromethorphan, a widely used anti-tussive drug (49), is also an NMDA antagonist, which has been shown to attenuate and reverse morphine tolerance in animal studies (50). As dextromethorphan is available in an oral form and has few side-effects, it may have a role in patients requiring long term opioids (51). The effects of combinations of an NMDA antagonist and chronic opioids on respiratory mechanisms requires further study.

NEW OPIOID PEPTIDES

Endorphins, enkephalins and dynorphins bind with low to moderate specificity to the mu, delta and kappa opioid receptors. Recently, two peptides (endomorphin-1 and endomorphin-2) have been identified in mammalian brain which have the highest specificity and affinity for the mu receptor of any endogenous substance so far described (52). Nociceptin (orphinan FQ), a 17 amino acid peptide, acts as a potent endogenous agonist of the opioid receptor-like 1 (ORL1) receptor and has been shown in animal studies to have analgesic actions following intrathecal adminis- tration (53,54). The clinical applications of these new agents is unclear at this stage, but they may provide tools for further dissecting the endoge- nous opiate pathways in the brain and spinal cord (55).

EFFECTS OF SPINAL OPIOIDS OTHER THAN ANALGESIA

RESPIRATORY SYSTEM

Respiratory depression is a rare but potentially serious side-effect of spinal opioid administration, particularly in opioid-naive patients treated for acute pain. Early onset (within two hours) respiratory depression has been attributed to blood borne drug quickly reaching the brain (such as after rapid absorption of lipophilic opioid given epidurally); whereas delayed respiratory depression (6 to 24 hours) may result from slow rostral migration of hydrophilic drug such as morphine within the CSF. Risk fac- tors for respiratory depression after intrathecal opioid administration include advanced age; poor general condition; use of hydrophilic opioid i.e., morphine; high doses; marked changes in thoracoabdominal pressure, including artificial ventilation; lack of tolerance to opioids; and concomi- tant administration by other routes of opioids or other CNS depressant drugs (1). Large surveys yield incidence estimates of respiratory depression after epidural morphine ranging from 0.09 to 0.25%. These estimates com- pare favorably with incidences of 1% for respiratory depression after parenteral morphine whether given by conventional injection or patient- controlled analgesia (1). Analgesia can be preserved during reversal of spinal opioid-induced respiratory depression by titrated doses or infusions of naloxone 5 µg/kg/hr (56). Respiratory depression has not been seen in cancer patients already receiving opioids who then receive spinal opioids, unless complications such as liver failure supervene, or if intrathecal pump refills are inadvertently injected subcutaneously or directly into the catheter via a side-port (57).

Although individual trials are conflicting and often fall short of statistical significance, meta-analysis of published data has shown a benefit of epidural over systemic opioid analgesia in decreasing postoperative pulmonary complications (58). Epidural opioids alone have a less advan- tageous effect on postoperative parameters of pulmonary function when compared to epidural local anesthetics or combinations of local anesthetic and opioids (59).

GASTROINTESTINAL TRACT

The occurrence of postoperative vomiting is multifactorial, and pain itself has been implicated as a cause of postoperative nausea. Nausea and vomiting occur in approximately one quarter of postoperative patients treated with spinal opioids, but most studies include too few patients or are inadequately controlled to confirm a difference in the incidence of postoperative nausea and vomiting related to different routes of administration. Nausea and vomiting following epidural morphine has been observed 6 hours after administration, which coincided with other evidence of rostral spread of morphine in CSF to intracerebral structures (60). Epidural use of lipid soluble opioids such as pethidine, fentanyl and sufentanil (61-63) may be associated with the lowest incidence of nausea and vomiting, but comparison between different agents is still inadequate. Treatment may include conventional anti-emetics such as droperidol (64), 5HT3 antagonists (65), or even low dose propofol (66). The incidence of nausea and vomiting seems to be less with repeated epidural dosing and is low in patients who require long-term spinal opioid therapy (1).

Opioids given systemically or epidurally delay gastric emptying and decrease gastrointestinal motility. Epidural morphine may be associated with a decrease in times to pass flatus and feces postoperatively, when compared to intramuscular morphine (67). Spinal opioids are unlikely to have positive effects on postoperative ileus, while local anesthetics which inhibit gastrointestinal inhibitory reflexes may be of advantage (59). In a single dose post-cholecystectomy study, epidural morphine delayed gastric emptying in contrast to no detrimental effects after epidural bupivacaine (68). Combination of opioid with epidural bupivacaine may reduce some of the beneficial effect on postoperative gastrointestinal paralysis (59).

CARDIOVASCULAR SYSTEM

Cardiovascular effects of opioids differ between basal, pain-free subjects and those studied perioperatively or while in pain. During noxious stimuli in awake or anesthetized animals and humans, parasympathetic outflow decreases and sympathetic activity increases, as do levels of circulating catecholamines (18,69). Increases in heart rate, blood pressure, myocardial oxygen consumption, systemic vascular resistance, and ventricular vulnerability to fibrillation result. Opioid analgesia by spinal or systemic routes decreases all these parameters (70). Clinical effects of spinal analgesia on myocardial function have been most evident when local anesthetics, alone or supplemented with opioids, are administered via the thoracic epidural space (71,72). In both experimental and clinical studies, spinal opioid analgesia has not been clearly proven to benefit cardiovascular morbidity and mortality beyond what may be attributed to effective analgesia alone (73).

STRESS RESPONSE

Tissue injury, the inflammatory response and afferent stimuli conducted through somatosensory and sympathetic pathways all play a role in precipitating the stress response to surgery. Epidural or intrathecal opioid administration is less effective in reducing the surgical stress response than neural blockade techniques with local anesthetics (59). This is in accordance with the lack of effect of intrathecal morphine on sympathetic nerve activity compared to the pronounced sympathetic blockade during spinal anesthesia with local anesthetics (74). Combinations of local anesthetic and opioid may improve pain relief and reduce surgical stress response. Addition of epidural opioid to local anesthetic may further reduce the stress response in lower limb orthopedic surgery (75,76), but epidural local anesthetic and opioid does not block the cortisol response to upper abdominal or thoracic surgery (77,78). The effect of epidural opioid on postoperative nitrogen balance is also less than observed with epidural local anesthetic (59).

URINARY RETENTION AND PRURITUS

Spinal morphine in humans produces a naloxone-reversible inhibition of the volume-evoked micturition reflex (79) to a greater degree than is seen after systemic administration of equianalgesic doses. Anecdotal reports suggest that bladder dysfunction may be less with spinal fentanyl (80), pethidine (61) and methadone (81) than with morphine, but conclusive comparative studies are not available. The incidence of pruritus varies markedly, is as high as 70% after epidural morphine in some studies, but does not appear to be related to dose (82). The incidence of severe pruritus that troubles the patient appears to be close to 1% (83). Patients requiring long term spinal opioids become tolerant to these effects, and the incidence of ongoing urinary retention and/or pruritus is low.

OUTCOME

The greatest benefit associated with epidural techniques have been shown in high risk patients undergoing major surgery in whom epidural anesthesia (+/- general anesthesia) was followed by adequate epidural analgesia for several days postoperatively (84). Most commonly a combination of local anesthetic and opioid is used. Currently insufficient numbers have been studied with adequate standardization of patient groups, type of surgery, site of catheter insertion, type and duration of analgesic agent delivered, to clearly determine the risk-benefit analysis of epidural or intrathecal analgesia in low risk patients who have a low incidence of complications.

Improved pain relief with epidural analgesia is unlikely to improve outcome and reduce hospital stay in isolation. Modification of surgical and nursing protocols to ensure early enteral feeding, improved nutrition and active mobilization is required to maximize the effects of neural blockade on pain, perioperative stress responses and organ dysfunction. A combined approach which incorporates all aspects of postoperative rehabilitation is likely to offer the best chance to improve outcome, reduce hospital stay and ensure cost-benefit advantages (59).

CHRONIC PAIN

Neuraxial drug delivery should be considered when severe pain cannot be controlled with systemic drugs because of dose-limiting side-effects or toxicity (85,86). Outpatient management of refractory cancer pain is possible with implanted catheters and pumps for spinal drug delivery (13,87,88). Increasingly, these techniques are also being utilized for chronic noncancer pain which can be 'malignant' in terms of its effect on quality of life. The site of drug delivery (epidural, intrathecal or intracerebroventricular) and choice of system (tunneled catheter, fully implanted system, internal or external infusion device) will depend on: the site and nature of the pain; the expected duration of therapy; local expertise in invasive techniques; the availability of ongoing outpatient care; cost; and perceived risk to benefit ratios.

Data on the long term efficacy of spinal opioids is emerging but interpretation of different studies is difficult due to variation in inclusion criteria, outcome parameters and duration of follow up. Adequate diagnostic testing with temporary catheters should be performed prior to implantation to ensure that pain is opioid responsive (89). Frequently pain relief alone is assessed, but is not reported in a uniform manner (e.g., proportion of patients achieving "good" or "excellent" relief; or overall degree of pain relief across all patients). Particularly in patients with chronic non-cancer pain, improvement in functional capabilities rather than analgesia alone should be considered. Independent assessment of outcome is ideal, and a reduction in side-effects or improved efficacy over systemic treatments without an increase in complications needs to be confirmed (90,91). As with the use of oral opioids for chronic noncancer pain (92,93), the use of spinal opioids should be part of a multimodal and interdisciplinary pain management plan.

Comparative data of epidural, subarachnoid and intracerebroventricular opioids in patients with cancer pain suggest similar efficacy with 58 to 75% of patients achieving excellent pain relief (87). In a retrospective survey of patients receiving intraspinal morphine for cancer and non-cancer pain the mean percent relief was 61% (94); whereas study of 18 patients with intraspinal opioids for failed back surgery syndrome or arachnoiditis only four patients were reported to have objective evidence of benefit at 2 year follow up (95). Clinical trials of opioids as single agents for neuraxial delivery in chronic pain have questioned whether this technique offers advantages over systemic infusion (96). Spinal delivery may be most desirable for patients likely to require multidrug neuraxial infusion for the control of neuropathic or incident pain.

COMPLICATIONS OF LONG-TERM ADMINISTRATION

NEUROTOXICITY

Neurotoxicity may relate to: spinally administered compounds themselves; preservatives; compatibility of drug solutions with CSF; direct trauma and inflammatory reactions provoked by intraspinal catheters. In experimental animals with chronically implanted catheters mild deformation and local demyelination has been reported to occur where the catheter contacted the spinal cord. The same changes were seen in animals given saline or opioids (97). However, evaluation of therapy induced damage is difficult to distinguish from disease related changes; compression and infiltration by malignant tissue, or previous radiotherapy and antineoplastic drugs may cause substantial damage to the spinal cord and nerve roots. The potential roles of insertion trauma, catheter material, analgesic solution, drug preservatives, and treatment duration are difficult to delineate (98,99). Safety during chronic epidural or intrathecal infusions of morphine, alfentanil and sufentanil have been reported.

HYPERALGESIA

High concentrations of intrathecal morphine are associated with hyperalgesia in rats. This appears to be non-opiate receptor mediated, as the hyperalgesia is exaggerated rather than reversed by naltrexone (100). A patient with advanced cancer requiring 40-80 mg/day intrathecal morphine developed hyperalgesia and myoclonus (101). Hyperalgesia with segmental allodynia at the level of the catheter tip also occurred in a patient receiving high dose epidural morphine (15 mg/hr) and resolved with decrease in the morphine dose. A combination of morphine and bupivacaine 0.125% was subsequently used to control pain (102).

COMPLICATIONS OF DELIVERY SYSTEMS

Complications of spinal delivery systems include:
1) Infection. The highest incidence of superficial infections (i.e., involving the catheter site, but not resulting in epidural abscess or meningitis) is seen with percutaneous catheters. Tunneling catheters for a short distance does not appear to improve infection rates (103), but use of a long subcutaneous tunnel and a fibrous cuff or external filter is associated with fewer superficial infections (104,105). Implanted systems with a subcutaneous portal have a lower incidence of catheter related problems, with reported infection rates of 8 to 12% (36,103). If treated early, superficial infections can be limited to the subcutaneous tissues and are not associated with epidural abscess formation or meningitis. Central nervous system infection is a serious potential complication related to spinal therapy, but appears to be infrequent. The true incidence of infectious complications is difficult to determine as cases are often reported in isolation, and the number of patients undergoing invasive treatments is unknown and continuing to change. Spinal delivery system infection must be treated aggressively and usually requires removal of the system. In some cases intrathecal reservoirs and catheters have been retained, and used to sample CSF and administer intrathecal aminoglycoside antibiotics (106).
2) Epidural fibrosis. Formation of a fibrous capsule around the tip of chronically implanted epidural catheters can result in pain on injection, loss of analgesia and limitation of duration of effective drug delivery by this route (36).
4) Dislodgment of catheter. The incidence of catheter dislodgment is highest for percutaneous epidural catheters (up to 40%) (102,107) and reduced by use of a subcutaneous portal (36,103) or an implanted intrathecal system.

5) Mechanical failure of implanted infusion device. Newer pro-grammable models require battery replacement, but have an expected life span of 3-5 years.

CONCLUSION

Treatment of acute pain has been changed forever by the application of spinal analgesia to relieve pain after operation or trauma. Early randomized prospective studies (108) provided clear evidence of superiority of epidural opioids and local anesthetics over opioids given intramuscularly, and of patient preference for epidural opioids. However, pain relief with spinal opioids as single agents is similar, in a small number of studies to carefully tuned intravenous infusion of opioids or meticulously maintained somatic nerve blocks (109). Yet clinical trials of single opioids given spinally or systemically have diminishing relevance to today's practice of spinal analgesia, that relies increasingly upon drug combinations to suppress activity-related pain and to hasten postoperative rehabilitation (1,59).

Continuation of established trends to consider pain control an integral part of medical care in general, and to allocate increasing resources to palliative care, will help those with chronic pain from cancer and non-malignant disease. Although spinal analgesia is necessary for only a minority of patients with cancer pain, the power of spinal analgesia to relieve refractory cancer pain has advanced the field as a whole. Recent success with spinal drug combinations and novel intrathecal analgesics, and increasing use of outpatient spinal analgesia, have altered the context and results of therapy. Current debates concerning patient, device, and infusate selection require further comparative trials. In light of growing numbers of patients receiving opioids systemically or by neuraxial infusion for chronic noncancer pain, separate trials that assess somewhat different outcomes are needed.

Several aspects of spinal administration of opioids require further study:

1.   improvement in outcome compared to other analgesic routes needs to be confirmed in adequately controlled trials and/or accurate meta-analysis, as there is now an increased emphasis on evidence based medicine in clinical practice;

2.   prospective randomized controlled clinical studies are required to establish the efficacy and incidence of side-effects related to long term spinal opioid administration;

230

3.   optimal timing for the use of spinal delivery is currently difficult to determine as referral practices and indications for more invasive
pain management strategies vary between different centers;

4.   the efficacy, dose-response relationships, side-effect profile,
toxicity and drug interactions of analgesic agents should be determined
before spinal administration and adoption into routine clinical practice;

5.   the cost-effectiveness of spinal delivery requires further
investigation. As the costs of health care and the pressure for cost con-
tainment increase, it becomes necessary to provide "pharmacoeconomic"
data along with efficacy and outcome data (1).

REFERENCES

1. Carr DB, Cousins MJ: Spinal route of analgesia, opioids and future
    options, Neural Blockade in Clinical Anaesthesia and Management
    of Pain. Vol III. Edited by Cousins MJ, Bridenbaugh PO. JB Lippincott
    Philadelphia (in press)
2. Cousins MJ, Plummer JL: Design of studies of spinal opioids in acute
    and chronic pain, The Design of Analgesic Clinical Trials. Edited by
    Max M, Portenoy RK, Laska EM. New York, Raven Press, 1990
3. van den Nieuwenhuyzen MC, Burm AG, Vletter AA, et al: Epidural
    vs intravenous infusion of alfentanil in the management of post-
    operative pain following laparotomies. Acta Anaesthesiol Scand
    40:1112-1118, 1996
4. Bromage PR: Fifty years on the wrong side of the reflex arc. Reg
    Anesth 21:1-4, 1996
5. Cousins MJ, Mather LE, Glynn CJ, et al: Selective spinal analgesia.
    Lancet 1:1141, 1979
6. Glynn CJ, Mather LE, Cousins MJ, et al: Peridural meperidine in
    humans: analgetic response, pharmacokinetics and transmission into
    CSF. Anesthesiology 55:250, 1981
7. Sjostrom S, Hartvig P, Persson P, Tamsen A: Pharmacokinetics of
    epidural morphine and meperidine in man. Anesthesiology 67:877,
    1987
8. Moore RA, Bullingham RSJ, McQuay HJ, et al: Dural permeability to
    narcotics: in vitro determination and application to extra-dural
    administration. Br J Anaesth 54:1117, 1982
9. Brose WG, Tanelian DL, Brodsky JB, et al: CSF and blood
    pharmacokinetics of hydromorphone and morphine following
    lumbar epidural administration. Pain 45:11, 1991
10. Nordberg G, Hedner T, Mellstrand T, Dahlstrom B. Pharmacokinetic
    aspects of epidural morphine analgesia. Anesthesiology 58: 545-51,
    1983
11. Tung A, Maliniak K, Tenicela R, Winter PM: Intrathecal morphine
    for intraoperative and postoperative analgesia. JAMA 244:2637, 1980

12. Gourlay GK, Cherry DA, Cousins MJ: Cephalad migration of morphine in CSF following lumbar epidural administration in patients with cancer pain. Pain 23:317, 1985

13. Yaksh TL: Intrathecal and epidural opiates: a review, Pain 1996 - An Updated Review. Edited by Campbell JN. Seattle, IASP Press, 1996, pp.381-393

14. Dickenson AH: Where and how do opioids work, Progress in Pain Research and Management Vol 2, Proceedings of the 7th World Congress on Pain, Seattle. Edited by Gebhart GF, Hammond DL, Jensen TS. Seattle, IASP Publications, 1993, pp 525-552.

15. Chrubasik J, Chrubasik S, Mather L: Postoperative Epidural Opioids. Germany, Springer-Verlag, 1993

16. Brown DV, McCarthy RJ: Epidural and spinal opioids. Curr Opin Anesthesiol 8:337, 1995

17. Eriksson-Mjoberg M, Svensson JO, Almkvist A, et al: Extradural morphine gives better pain relief than patient-controlled i.v. morphine after hysterectomy. Br J Anaesth 78:10-16, 1997

18. Coda BA, Brown MC, Schaffer R, et al: Pharmacology of epidural fentanyl, alfentanil and sufentanil in volunteers. Anesthesiology 81:1149-1161, 1994

19. Sangarlangkarn S, Klaewatanong V, Jonglerttrakool P, Khankaew V: Meperidine as a spinal anesthetic agent: a comparison with lidocaine-glucose. Anesth Analg 66:235, 1987

20. Acalovschi I, Bodolea C, Manoiu C: Spinal anesthesia with meperidine. Effects of added a-adrenergic agonists: epinephrine versus clonidine. Anesth Analg 84:1333-1339, 1997

21. Carpenter RL: Future epidural or subarachnoid analgesics: local anesthetics. Reg Anesth 21 (6S):75, 1996

22. Yaksh TL, Reddy S: Studies in the primate on the analgetic effects associated with intrathecal actions of opiates, alpha adrenergic agonists and baclofen. Anesthesiol 54:451-467, 1981

23. Van Essen EJ, Bovill JG, Ploeger EJ, Beerman H: Intrathecal morphine and clonidine for control of intractable cancer pain. A case report. Acta Anaesth Belg 39:109-112, 1988

24. Eisenach JC, DuPen S, Dubois M, et al: The epidural clonidine study group: Epidural clonidine analgesia for intractable cancer pain. Pain 61:391-399, 1995

25. Lee Y-W, Yaksh TL: Analysis of drug interaction between intrathecal clonidine and MK-801 in peripheral neuropathic pain rat model. Anesthesiol 82:741-748, 1995

26. Eisenach J, Detweiler D, Hood D. Hemodynamic and analgesic actions of epidurally administered clonidine. Anesthesiol 78:277-287, 1993

27. Filos KS, Goudas LC, Patroni O, Polyzou V: Hemodynamic and analgesic profile after intrathecal clonidine in humans. Anesthesiol 81:591-601, 1994

28. Goudas LC: Clonidine. Curr Opin Anesth 8:455, 1995

29. Yaksh TL, Malmberg AB: Interaction of spinal modulatory receptor systems, Pharmacological Approaches to the Treatment of Chronic

Pain: New Concepts and Critical Issues, Progress in Pain Research and Management, Vol I. Edited by Fields HL, Liebeskind JC. Seattle, IASP Press, 1994, pp.151-171

30. Morley JS, Watt J, Wells C, et al: Paradoxical and other pain uncontrolled by morphine, in Gebhart GF, Hammond DL, Jensen TS (eds): Progress in Pain Research and Management Vol 2, Proceedings of the 7th World Congress on Pain, Seattle, IASP Publications, chap 41, 1993, pp 621-630

31. McQuay HJ, Carroll D, Faura CC, et al: Oral morphine in cancer pain: influences on morphine and metabolite concentration. Clin Pharmacol Ther 48:236-244, 1990

32. Portenoy RK, Foley KM, Stulman J, et al: Plasma morphine and morphine-6-glucuronide during chronic morphine therapy for cancer pain: plasma profiles, steady-state concentrations and the consequences of renal failure. Pain 47:13-19, 1991

33. Portenoy RK, Foley KM, Inturissi CE: The nature of opioid responsiveness and its implications for neuropathic pain: new hypotheses derived from studies of opioid infusions. Pain 43:273-286, 1990

34. Portenoy RK: Opioid tolerance and responsiveness: research findings and clinical observations, Progress in Pain Research and Management Vol 2, Proceedings of the 7th World Congress on Pain. Edited by Gebhart GF, Hammond DL, Jensen TS. Seattle, IASP Publications, chap 40, 1993, pp 595-619

35. Onofrio BM, Yaksh TL: Long term pain relief produced by intrathecal morphine infusion in 53 patients. J Neurosurg 72:200, 1990

36. Krames ES, Wilkie DJ, Gershow J: Intrathecal D-Ala2-D-Leu5-enkephalin (DADL) restores analgesia in a patient analgetically tolerant to intrathecal morphine sulfate. Pain 24:205-209, 1986

37. Moulin DE, Max MB, Kaiko RF, et al: The analgesic efficacy of intrathecal D-Ala2-D-Leu5-enkephalin in cancer patients with chronic pain. Pain 23:213-221, 1985

38. Dooley CT, Chung NN, Wilkes BC, et al: An all D-amino acid opioid peptide with central nalgesic activity from the combinatorial library. Science 266:2019, 1994

39. Adams J, Tallarida R, Geller E, Adler M: Isobolographic super-additivity between delta and mu opioid agonists in the rat depends on the ratio of compounds, the mu agonist and the analgesic assay used. J Pharmacol Exp Ther 266:1261, 1993

40. Traynor JR, Elliot J: Opioid receptor subtypes and cross-talk with mu receptors. TIPS, 14:18, 1993

41. Fleming WW, Taylor DA: Cellular mechanisms of opioid tolerance and dependence, The Pharmacology of Opioid Peptides. Edited by Tseng LF. Langhorn, PA, Harwood Academic Press, 1995 pp.463

42. Lutfy K, Yoburn BC: The role of opioid receptor density in morphine tolerance. J Phar Exper Ther 256:575-580, 1991

43. Woolf CJ, Chong MS: Pre-emptive analgesia - treating postoperative pain by preventing the establishment of central sensitization. Anesth Analg 77:362-379, 1993

44. Mao J, Price DD, Mayer DJ: Mechanisms of hyperalgesia and morphine tolerance: a current view of their possible interactions. Pain 62:259-274, 1995

45. Mayer DJ, Mao J, Price DD: The development of morphine tolerance and dependence is associated with translocation of protein kinase C. Pain 61:365-374, 1995

46. Elliot K, Minami N, Kolesnikov YA, Pasternak GW, Inturissi CE: The NMDA receptor antagonists, LY274614 and MK-801, and the nitric oxide synthase inhibitor, NG-nitro-L-arginine, attenuate analgesic tolerance to the mu-opioid morphine but not to kappa opioids. Pain 56:69-75, 1994

47. Mao J, Price DD, Mayer DJ: Experimental mononeuropathy reduces the antinociceptive effects of morphine: implications for common intracellular mechanisms involved in morphine tolerance and neuropathic pain. Pain 61:353-364, 1995

48. Walker SM, Cousins MJ: Reduction in hyperalgesia and intrathecal morphine requirements by low-dose ketamine infusion. J Pain Symptom Manage (in press)

49. Bem JL, Peck R: Dextromethorphan - an overview of safety issues. Drug Safety 7:190-199, 1992

50. Elliot K, Hyansky A, Inturissi CE: Dextromethorphan attenuates and reverses analgesic tolerance to morphine. Pain 59:361-368, 1994

51. Lipton SA: Prospects for clinically tolerated NMDA antagonists: open-channel blockers and alternative redox states of nitric oxide. Trends Neurosci 16:527-532, 1993

52. Zadina JE, Hackler L, Ge LJ, Kastin AJ: A potent and selective andogenous agonist for the m-opiate receptor. Nature 386:499-501, 1997

53. Yamamoto T, Nozaki-Taguchi N, Kimura S: Effects of intrathecally administered nociceptin, an opioid receptor-like1 (ORL1) agonist, on the thermal hyperalgesia induced by unilateral constriction injury to the sciatic nerve in the rat. Neurosci Lett 224:107-110, 1997

54. King MA, Rossi GC, Chang AH, et al: Spinal analgesic activity of orphinan FQ/nociceptin and its fragments. Neurosci Lett 223:113-116, 1997

55. Julius D: Another opiate for the masses? Nature 386:442, 1997

56. Rawal N, Schott U, Dahlstrom B et al: Influence of naloxone on analgesia and respiratory depression following epidural morphine. Anesthesiology 64:194-201, 1986

57. Coombs DW, Maurer LH, Saunders RL, Gaylor M: Outcomes and complications of continuous intraspinal narcotic analgesia for cancer pain control. J Clin Oncol 2:1414-1420, 1984

58. Ballantyne JC, Carr DB, Chalmers TC, et al: Comparative effects of postoperative analgesic therapies upon respiratory function: meta-analysis of initial randomized control trials. Anesth Analg (in press)

59. Kehlet H. Modification of responses to surgery by neural blockade: clinical implications, Neural Blockade in Clinical Anaesthesia and Management of Pain. Vol III. Edited by Cousins MJ, Bridenbaugh PO. JB Lippincott, Philadelphia (in press)

60. Bromage PR, Camporesi EM, Durant PAC, Nielsen CH: Rostral spread of epidural morphine. Anesthesiology 56:431-436, 1982

61. Brownridge P: Epidural and intrathecal opiates for postoperative pain relief. Anaesthesia 38:74, 1983

62. Donadoni R, Rolly G, Noorduin H, Vanden Bussche G: Epidural sufentanil for postoperative pain relief. Anaesthesia 40:634, 1985

63. Welchew EA: The optimum concentration for epidural fentanyl. A randomised double-blind comparison with and without 1:200000 adrenaline. Anaesthesia 38:1037-1041, 1983

64. Horta M L; Horta BL: Inhibition of epidural morphine-induced pruritus by intravenous droperidol. Reg Anesth 18:118-120, 1993

65. Pitkšnen MT, Niemi L, Tuominen MK, Rosenberg PH: Effect of tropisetron, a 5-HT3 receptor antagonist, on analgesia and nausea after intrathecal morphine. Br J Anaesth 71:681-684, 1993

66. Tšrn K, Tuominen M, Tarkkila P, Lindgren L: Effects of sub-hypnotic doses of propofol on the side effects of intrathecal morphine. Br J Anaesth. 73: 411-2, 1994

67. Rawal N: Neuraxial administration of opioids and nonopioids, Regional Anesthesia and Analgesia. Edited by Brown DL. Philadelphia, WB Saunders Co, 1996, pp.208-231

68. Thorn SE, Wattwil M, Naslund I: Postoperative epidural morphine, but not epidural bupivacaine, delays gastric emptying on the first day after cholecystectomy. Reg Anesth 17:91-94, 1992

69. Kehlet H: The modifying effect of general and regional anaesthesia on the endocrine metabolic response to surgery. Reg Anaesth 7(S):538, 1982

70. Cozian A, Pinaud M, Lapage, et al: Effects of meperidine spinal anesthesia on hemodynamics, plasma catecholamines, angiotensin I, aldosterone, and histamine concentrations in elderly men. Anesthesiology 64:815, 1986

71. Reiz S, Bennett S: Cardiovascular effects of epidural anaesthesia. Curr Opin Anaesth 6:813, 1993

72. Chaney MA: Intrathecal and epidural anesthesia and analgesia for cardiac surgery. Anesth Analg 84:1211-1221, 1997

73. Bode RH, Lewis KP, Zarich SW, et al: Cardiac outcome after peripheral vascular surgery: comparison of general and regional anesthesia. Anesthesiology 84:3, 1996

74. Kirno K, Lundin S, Elam M: Effects of intrathecal morphine and spinal anaesthesia on sympathetic nerve activity in humans. Acta Anaesth Scand 37:54, 1993

75. Moore RA, Paterson GMC, Bullingham RES, et al: Controlled comparison of intrathecal cinchocaine with intrathecal cinchocaine and morphine. Br J Anaesth 56:847, 1984

76. Nielsen TH, Nielsen HK, Husted SE, et al: Stress response and platelet function in minor surgery during epidural bupivacaine and general anaesthesia: effect of epidural morphine addition. Eur J Anaesthesiol 6:409, 1989

77. Zwarts SJ, Hasenbos MAMW, Gielen MJM, Kho HG: The effect of continuous epidural analgesia with sufentanil and bupivacaine during and after thoracic surgery on the plasma cortisol concentration and pain relief. Reg Anesth 14:183, 1989

78. Liem TH, Booij LHDJ, Gielen MJM et al: Coronary artery bypass grafting using two different anesthetic techniques: Part 3: adrenergic responses. J Cardiothor Vasc Anesth 6:162-167, 1992

79. Reiz S, Westberg M: Side-effects of epidural morphine. Lancet 2:203, 1980

80. Naulty JS, Johnson M, Burger GA, et al: Epidural fentanyl for post cesarean delivery pain management. Anesthesiology 59:A415, 1983

81. Evron S, Samueloff A, Simon A et al: Urinary function during epidural analgesia with methadone and morphine in post-cesarean section patients. Pain 23:135, 1985

82. Ballantyne JC, Loach AB, Carr DB: Itching after epidural and spinal opiates. Pain 33:149, 1988

83. Bromage PR, Camporesi EM, Chestnut D: Epidural narcotics for postoperative analgesia. Anesth Analg 59:473, 1980

84. Liu S, Carpenter RL, Neal JM. Epidural anesthesia and analgesia. Their role in perioperative outcome. Anesthesiol 82:1474-1506, 1995

85. Ferrante FM, Bedder M, Caplan RA et al: Practice guidelines for cancer pain management. Anesthesiology 84:1243, 1996

86. Krames ES: Intraspinal opioid therapy for chronic nonmalignant pain: current practice and clinical guidelines. J Pain Symptom Manage 11:333, 1996

87. Ballantyne JC, Carr DB, Berkey CS, et al: Comparative efficacy of epidural, subarachnoid, and intracerebroventricular opioids in patients with pain due to cancer. Reg Anesth 21:542-556, 1996

88. Chrubasik J, Chrubasik S: Meta-analysis in the efficacy of intrathecal and epidural opiates, Cancer Pain Management. Edited by Parris W. Boston, Butterworth-Heinemann, 1997, pp. 207-214

89. Jadad, AR, Popat MT; Glynn CJ, McQuay HJ: Double-blind testing fails to confirm analgesic response to extradural morphine. Anaesthesia 46:935-937, 1991

90. Hassenbusch SJ: Epidural and subarachnoid administration of opioids for nonmalignant pain: technical issues, current approaches and novel treatments. J Pain Symptom Manage 11:357-362, 1996

91. Bedder MD: Epidural opioid therapy for chronic nonmalignant pain: critique of current experience. J Pain Symptom Manage 11:353-356, 1996

92. Molloy AR, Nicholas MK, Cousins MJ: Role of opioids in chronic non-cancer pain. Med J Aust 167:9-10, 1997

93. Stein C: Opioid treatment of chronic nonmalignant pain. Anesth Analg 84:912-914, 1997

94. Paice JA, Penn RD, Shott S: Intraspinal morphine for chronic pain: a retrospective, multicenter study. J Pain Symptom Manage 11:71-80, 1996

95. Yoshida GM, Nelson RW, Capen DA, et al: Evaluation of continuous intraspinal narcotic analgesia for chronic pain from benign causes. Am J Orthop 25:693-694, 1996

96. Kalso E, Heiskanen T, Rantio M et al: Epidural and subcutaneous morphine in the management of cancer pain: a double-blind cross-over study. Pain 67:443-449, 1996

97. Yaksh TL, Noueihed RY, Durant AC: Studies of the pharmacology and pathology of intrathecally administered 4-anilinipiperidine analogues and morphine in the rat and cat. Anesthesiol 64:54-66, 1986

98. Sjoberg M, Karlsson P-A, Nordborg C, et al: Neuropathologic findings after long-term intrathecal infusion of morphine and bupivacaine for pain treatment in cancer patients. Anesthesiol 76:173-186, 1992

99. Coombs DW, Fratkin JD, Meier FA et al: Neuropathologic lesions and CSF morphine concentrations during chronic continuous intraspinal morphine infusion. Pain, 22:337, 1985

100. Yaksh TL, Harty GJ, Onofrio BM: High doses of spinal morphine produce a nonopiate receptor-mediated hyperesthesia: clinical and theoretic implications. Anesthesiol 64:590-597, 1986

101. De Conno F, Caraceni A, Martini C, et al: Hyperalgesia and myoclonus with intrathecal infusion of high-dose morphine. Pain 47:337-339, 1991

102. Hogan Q, Haddox JD, Abram S, et al: Epidural opiates and local anesthetics for the management of cancer pain. Pain 46:271-279, 1991

103. De Jong PC, Kansen PJ: A comparison of epidural catheters with or without subcutaneous injection ports for treatment of cancer pain. Anesth Analg 78:94-100, 1994

104. DuPen SL, Peterson DG, Bogosian AC, et al A new permanent exteriorized epidural catheter for narcotic self-administration to control cancer pain. Cancer 59:986-993, 1987

105. Ohlsson L, Rydberg T, Eden T, et al: Cancer pain relief by continuous administration of epidural morphine in a hospital setting and at home. Pain 48:349-353, 1992

106. Schoeffler P, Pichard E, Ramboatiana R, et al: Bacterial meningitis due to infection of a lumbar drug release system in patients with cancer pain. Pain 25:75-77, 1986

107. Hicks F, Simpson KH, Tosh GC: Management of spinal infusions in palliative care. Palliative Med 8:325-332, 1994

108. Modig J, Paalzow L: A comparison of epidural morphine and epidural bupivacaine for postoperative pain relief. Acta Anaesthesiol Scand 25:437-441, 1981

109. Gauthier-Lafaye P, Muller A: Anesthesie loco-regionale et traitment de la douleur. 3rd Ed. Paris, Masson, 1996

EPIDURAL STEROIDS

A. P. Winnie

INTRODUCTION

Injection into various parts of the peridural space has been advocated for the management of sciatica since 1930 (1), but with the findings of Mixter and Barr (2) in 1934, linking the signs and symptoms of sciatica with a herniated nucleus pulposus, surgery has continued to be the definitive therapy for this problem. However, over the years except in patients with a rapidly progressive neural deficit, surgery has provided disappointing therapeutic results, so efforts to find a non-surgical therapeutic approach have continued. From a theoretical point of view, two approaches to the problem of non-surgical therapy have been developed, one aiming to remove the etiologic mechanism and the other aiming to modify the response to that mechanism.

CHEMONUCLEOLYSIS

The approach which attempts to remove the disc without surgery was first described by Lyman Smith (3), who in 1963 reported a procedure which he termed "chemonucleolysis," in which chymopapain was injected percutaneously into the involved disc. By depolymerizing the cementing protein of the chondromucoid complex, chymopapain was said to reduce the molecular size and viscosity of the nucleus pulposus, resulting in chemical decompression. While Smith was able to provide complete relief in slightly over 80% of his patients (4), not all reports indicated similar success rates (5). Though chemonucleolysis appeared to be a simple procedure in expert hands, it was a painful one that required the administration of a general anesthetic, and for the first 12-36 hours following the injection, there was a significant incidence of severe lumbar muscle spasm. Most importantly, there was a 1-2% incidence of anaphylaxis associated with this procedure (6).

T. H. Stanley et al. (eds.), Pain Management and Anesthesiology, 237–245.
© 1998 *Kluwer Academic Publishers. Printed in the Netherlands.*

EPIDURAL AND INTRATHECAL STEROIDS

The other approach to non-surgical therapy seeks not to treat the etiologic mechanism itself but rather the radiculopathy which results. This was the approach of Lievre and his associates (7), who in 1953 reported on the beneficial effect of hydrocortisone injected into the epidural space in 20 patients. Subsequently others began to try this technique in selected cases. Cappio (8) reviewed the early literature abroad and reported that good results were obtained in 67% of the first 80 of these cases, and later in this country Goebert and his co-workers at the Cleveland Clinic treated 113 patients with painful radiculopathies with hydrocortisone and procaine injected caudally and obtained good results in 72% of the patients (9).

After first determining its safety in laboratory animals (10), the Cleveland Clinic group then went on to record an improved success rate following the injection of 40 mg of methylprednisolone and 40 mg of procaine intrathecally (11), and reported no complications following the injection of steroids with procaine into either the extradural or intradural compartments.

In spite of the simplicity of this therapeutic approach to the management of discogenic pain and its freedom from side effects and complications, the present author, like many others, was initially skeptical of its efficacy. Therefore in 1968 we initiated a preliminary study to evaluate the efficacy of methylprednisolone as a therapeutic modality for discogenic pain and to compare the result obtained when the drug was injected epidurally with the result obtained when the drug was injected intrathecally, with both injections consisting of methylprednisolone alone (without local anesthetic) and both injections being made as close to the level of the lesion as possible. The data obtained in that study indicated that methylprednisolone is an effective therapeutic modality in the management of discogenic pain in about 80% of the patients so treated, and that the success rate is almost identical regardless of whether the drug is injected intrathecally or epidurally, as long as the injection is made as close to the level of the disc as possible (12).

Following publication of this study in 1972, we have continued to obtain a high degree of success using this therapeutic regimen. Unfortunately, most of the patients with sciatica are referred first to surgeons, so there has been little data available indicating the success rate of epidural and/or intrathecal steroids as a primary course of therapy, since most surgeons consider it a "last resort" in the management of discogenic pain in patients in whom laminectomy, with or without fusion, has failed to provide relief. As a result, much of the published data has been obtained in a mixture of patients consisting of a few who refused surgery and many who had failed to obtain relief following surgery.

Therefore, in the mid 1970's we undertook a study of 30 patients with discogenic pain in whom only intrathecal and/or epidural Depo-Medrol was utilized as the primary form of therapy (13). This study indicated three important findings: First, that of the 30 patients receiving only epidural and/or intrathecal Depo-Medrol, 29 obtained complete and apparently permanent relief. The one patient who did not obtain relief underwent surgery and no disc was found. Second, in the majority of the cases (14 out of 30), one injection of Depo-Medrol was insufficient. Thirteen required two injections and 3 required three. And finally, contrary to the report of Abram, if one route of injection fails to provide relief, the other route of injection may provide success. Such was the case in 8 of the 30 patients in that particular study.

MECHANISM OF ACTION OF EPIDURAL/ INTRATHECAL STEROIDS

When Mixter and Barr first demonstrated the relationship between disc protrusion and radicular pain (2), they believed that the signs and symptoms of sciatica were due to the mechanical compression of the nerve root by the protruded disc; and this mechanical explanation of sciatica is what prompted surgeons to consider laminectomy to be curative. However, the results of surgery failed to support this hypothesis.

More recently Olsson (14) experimentally produced cervical disc protrusion in dogs and found that the size of the disc and the amount of compression were less important in the production of symptomatology than the accompanying inflammation. The etiologic role of inflammation in sciatica is supported by the observation during lumbar laminectomy under local anesthesia that inflamed spinal nerves adjacent to a prolapsed disc are very sensitive to minor manipulations, whereas uninflamed nerves can be manipulated with very little discomfort (15). Inflammation of nerve roots in patients with low back pain has been demonstrated myelographically (16) and visually at the time of surgery (17) and has been confirmed on histological examinations of biopsy specimens taken from nerve roots during surgery (18-20). Indeed, improvement in clinical symptoms has been shown to coincide with the resolution or diminution of nerve root edema in the presence of persistent herniated intervertebral disc (16).

A landmark study in establishing the premise that inflammation is a key in radiculopathy was the work of McCarron who injected autologous nucleus pulposus material into the epidural space of dogs (21). Those animals that receive an epidural injection of nuclear material daily for five days showed biochemical and histological evidence of intense inflammation on gross inspection and microscopic analysis of the spinal cord, dural sac, and nerve roots as compared with control animals that had only saline injection, indicating that a very small amount of nuclear material can cause a marked inflammatory response. The clinical correlate may be that the leak of a small amount of nuclear material that cannot be detected by routine laboratory studies obtained in the patient's evaluation for radiculopathy does cause significant symptoms. In other words, in spite of the fact that x-rays studies indicate "a mildly bulging disc unlikely to be causing the patient's symptoms," in reality, the patient has a clinically significant, chemical radiculopathy. Saal and his co-workers (22) have crystallized our understanding that inflammation of the nerve roots is the pathological process in patients with radiculopathy by identifying phospholipase A-2 (PLA-2) as the offending substance. PLA-2, which is present in a high concentration in nuclea material is an enzyme that liberates arachidonic acid from cell membranes. A toxic spill of PLA-2 can occur when either leakage or herniation occurs, and provokes an intense inflammatory reaction in the surrounding neural tissue that causes the symptoms of radicular pain (23). Saal and his co-workers reported that the concentration of PLA-2 was 20 to 100,000 times that of normal tissue when samples were obtained from patients at the time of disc surgery. Steroid, then, can prevent the action of PLA-2 on cell membranes (that of releasing arachidonic acid), which further generates substances such as prostaglandins that are operative in the inflammatory cascade.

Thus it would appear that a disc degeneration is at first an anatomical event with an associated loss of elasticity of the annular fibers and the creation of fissures within the annulus as it dries with age and is subjected to deforming pressures (22). These changes allow variable amounts of nuclear material to leak out when poorly distributed pressures are applied to the spinal segment. The exact interaction of many biochemical and enzymatic substances involved (proteoglycan, PLA-2, arachidonic acid products, interleukins, etc.) is not clearly defined, but the reality is that inflammation causes pathology that escapes identification with the routine and customary laboratory studies of the patient with low back pain.

The concept that "sciatica" is the result of an inflammatory process of the involved nerve root(s), gives a rational basis to the use of cortico-steroids in the vicinity of the inflamed nerve root(s) to counteract the inflammation. As already pointed out, our own studies, which simply applied this information clinically by treating discogenic pain with intrathecal and epidural steroids supports the "inflammatory" hypothesis (12,13). Furthermore, understanding that the acute phase of discogenic pain is inflammatory provides insight into the positive relationship between the time of treatment in relation to the onset of symptoms: the earlier epidural steroids are injected, the greater the possibility of success, since the entire process is inflammatory. With the passage of time, the process of healing begins with resultant intra- and extra-neural fibrosis, which causes fixation of the nerve roots within the intervertebral foram-ina, neural ischemia, and progressively diminishing responsiveness to anti-inflammatory agents. Many studies demonstrate the relationship of success to the time of treatment with steroids: Brown, for example, treated 56 consecutive patients with 80 mg of Depo-Medrol and experienced a 100% success rate when the epidural steroids were injected in less than three months and a 20% success rate when utilized thereafter (24). Though our success rate was similar with both approaches, because of the increasing concerns of anesthesiologists about the litigious state of medicine, intrathecal steroid injections gave way to epidural injections in spite of the fact that there have been no complications reported in the literature following intrathecal steroid injections, provided (1) reasonable dosages were administered; (2) the number of injections was reasonable; and (3) the patient was free of central nervous system disease, i.e., multiple sclerosis.

CONTROVERSIAL ASPECTS OF EPIDURAL STEROIDS

Other investigators have been unable to reduplicate our high success rates. Carron has challenged the credibility of our reports; but we are convinced that the success rate will depend, to a large degree, upon the accuracy of the diagnosis. If the patient has truly and only discogenic pain, then the chances of success are great. Our studies have also been criticized for not providing concurrent controls and/or randomization, and this is true. However, Dilke and his co-workers (25) had already reported on a randomized study of 100 consecutive patients with low back pain and radicular pain in the lower extremity, in which 10 ml of normal saline and 80 mg of methylprednisolone were injected epidurally in the study group, while the control group received an injection of 1 ml of sterile saline in the intraspinous ligament in the lumbar area. Of the patients who received Depo-Medrol, 46% reported complete pain relief one week after the injection, compared with 11% of the control group. More recently Cuckler (26) and his co-workers have carried out a prospective, randomized, and double-blind study comparing methylprednisolone and saline in patients with radicular pain due to a herniated nucleus pulposus or due to spinal stenosis. They detected no statistically significant difference between the control and experimental groups, whether the pain was due to acute disc herniation or spinal stenosis.

The problem with both of these studies is the fact that only a single dose of steroid was utilized and the success or failure of the technique was based on this one therapeutic intervention. Our studies have shown rather conclusively that two and in many cases three injections are necessary, and that for some reason, in certain patients one route of injection (intrathecal or epidural) succeeds where the other has failed. In view of the simplicity and safety of this technique, with the virtual absence of significant side effects, it would appear that in patients with an acute herniated nucleus pulposus, this form of therapy should be carried out prior to any other. The early use of epidural/intrathecal steroids could markedly reduce the loss of income resulting from prolonged bed rest and traction, and may even save the expense of a CAT scan if the therapy is successful.

As a matter of fact, there is good evidence that the earlier this treatment is initiated the greater will be the chance of success. Brown (24) was the first to report that the success rate was related to the duration of symptoms at the time of treatment, noting 100% efficacy in those patients treated within the first three months, and only 20% when treated later. Ryan and Taylor (27) tried to make an even more precise correlation between the time of treatment and success therefrom, finding in their study of 108 patients the following results: patients who were treated within the first two weeks of symptoms achieved a 77% success rate, from 2-4 weeks a 72% success rate, from 4-6 weeks a 60% success rate, and over 6 weeks a 43% success rate. However, unlike their predecessors, the latter investigators actually injected 40 mg of methylprednisolone intrathecally, followed by 40 mg epidurally. Nonetheless, these two investigators felt that their data and the obvious relationship between time of treatment and incidence of success provided clinical support for the theory that epidural steroids are effective in disc protrusion with "irritative" [inflammatory] neuropathy, but not "compressive neuropathy". In other words, they felt that the reason for the progressive decrease in success with time was due to the fact that as time progresses, the continued inflammatory response produced progressively increasing intraneural fibrosis and ischemic changes that become irreversible, and that will not be affected by steroids.

Finally, while most anesthesiologists dilute their depo-steroid with local anesthetic (usually up to 10 cc), we do not do so for very definite reasons: first of all, the large volume of the diluted solution causes it to spread and to bathe many normal nerves. We want to deposit the steroid on the inflamed nerve only. Secondly, the solution that does bathe the inflamed nerve is diluted 5- to 10-fold, so less steroid gets to the targeted nerve root. Thirdly, the local anesthetic stops the pain, but the pain returns before the steroid has become effective, and this has a definite negative psychological effect. And finally, in reviewing over thirty epidural steroid treatments that resulted in litigation, I encountered four patients who died because of the addition of the local anesthetic. In view of the fact that the local anesthetic added to the steroid has no therapeutic effect, the risk/benefit rate of adding it is unacceptable. And in addition, I feel that our high success rate is a result of the fact that we do not dilute the steroid.

However, there are specific indications for injecting local anesthetic BEFORE injecting Depo-Medrol into the epidural space: first, if a patient is in such pain he cannot cooperate, a few cc's of local anesthetic will allow him/her to do so. Furthermore, in a patient with a previously operated back, such an injection of local anesthetic (prior to the injection of steroid) will verify whether the needle is in the epidural space and whether there is sufficient scarring to prevent the local anesthetic from reaching the nerve roots. Obviously, if interference with the spread of the local anesthetic results from old scarring, it must be anticipated that the spread of the Depo-Medrol will be obstructed as well. And finally, from a medico-legal point of view, the use of such a test-dose will indicate definitively that the needle (and the subsequent injection) is in the epidural space.

CONCLUSIONS

In short, for optimal results with epidural steroids, it is critically important that the diagnosis be correct, i.e. (that one is dealing with an inflammatory neuropathy), that the treatment is instituted early (while the process is predominantly inflammatory) and that the sequence and timing of the injections are appropriate. The use of the proper steroid is equally important, if not for success, for preventing complication: We have only utilized Depo-Medrol, since Gardner showed this to be the safest agent when used intrathecally, though others have achieved results similar to ours using dexamethasone. Hydrocortisone should never be utilized, as it is irritating to the meninges and can cause grand-mal seizures (28,29). The beauty of this form of therapy is that if it does not provide the expected relief, other therapeutic modalities can still be carried out. However, if this therapeutic approach were followed routinely in patients having their first acute herniated disc, it is this author's opinion that very few would ever need to undergo a laminectomy and discectomy.

REFERENCES:

1. Evans W: Intrasacral epidural injection in the treatment of sciatica. Lancet 1930;2:1225-1229.
2. Mixter WJ and Barr JS: Rupture of the intervertebral disc with involvement of the spinal canal. J Neurosurg 1934;21:74-81.
3. Smith L: Enzyme dissolution of the nucleus pulposus in humans. JAMA 1964;187:137-140.
4. Smith L: Chemonucleolysis. Clin Orthop 1969;67:72-80.
5. Ford LT: Clinical use of chymopapain in lumbar and dorsal disc lesions. Clin Orthop 1969;67:81-87.
6. Massie WK: Editorial comment. Clin Orthop 1969;67:2-5.
7. Lievre JA, Block-Michel H and Attali, P: L'injection trans-sacree. Etude clinique et radiologigue. Bull et Mem Soc Med Hop Paris 1957;73:1110-1118.
8. Cappio M: Il trattamento idrocortisonico per via epidurole sacrole delle lombroscaitalgie. Reumatismo 1957;9:60-70.
9. Goebert HW Jr, Jallo SJ, Gardner WJ et al: Painful radiculopathy treated with epidural injections of procaine and hydrocortisone acetate: Results in 113 patients. Anesth Analg 1961;40:130-134.
10. Sehgal AD, Tweed DC, Gardner WJ et al: Laboratory studies after intrathecal corticosteroids. Arch Neurol 1963;9:64-68.
11. Gardner WJ, Goebert HW Jr, Sehgal AD: Intraspinal corticosteroid in the treatment of sciatica. Trans Am Neurol Assoc 1961;86:214-215.
12. Winnie AP, Hartman JT, Meyer HL Jr, Ramamurthy S and Barangan V: Pain Clinic II: Intradural and extradural corticosteroids for sciatica. Anesth Analg 1972;51:990-999.
13. Winnie AP and Ramamurthy S: Steroids for discogenic pain. Paper presented at the VI World Congress of Anesthesiology, Mexico City, Mexico, April 1976.
14. Olsson SE: The dynamic factor in spinal cord compression. A study of dogs with special reference to cervical disc protrusion. J Neurosurg 1958;15:308-321.
15. Murphy RW: Nerve roots and spinal nerves in degenerative disc disease. Clin Orthop 1977;129:40-46.
16. Berg A: Clinical and myelographic studies of conservatively treated cases of lumbar intervertebral disc. Acta Chir Scand 1958;104:124-129.

17. Roaf J: Some observations regarding 905 patients operated upon for protruded lumbar intervertebral disc. Am J Surg 1959;97:388-399.
18. Lindahl O, Rexed B: Histologic changes in spinal nerve roots of operated cases of sciatica. Acta Orthop Scand 1950;20:215-225.
19. Irsigler FJ: Nikroskopische Befunde in den Ruckenmarkswurzeln beim lumbalen und lumbosakrolen (dorsolateralen) Diskusprolaps. Acta Neurrochir (Wien) 1951;1:478-516.
20. Marshall LL, Trethwie ER: Chemical irritation of nerve root in disc prolapse. Lancet 1973;2:230.
21. McCarron RF, Wimpee MW, Hudkins PG, et al: The inflammatory effect of nucleus pulposus; a possible element in the pathogenesis of low back pain. Spine 1987;12:760-764.
22. Saal JA, Franson RC, Dobrow R, et al: High levels of inflammatory phospholipase A-2 activity in lumbar disc herniations. Spine 1990;15:674-678.
23. Marshall LL, Trethewie ER, Curtain CC: Chemical radiculitis: a clinical, physiological and immunological study. Clin Orthop 1987;129:61-67.
24. Brown FW: Management of diskogenic pain using epidural and intrathecal steroids. Clin Orthop 1977;129:72-78.
25. Dilke TFW, Burry HC and Grahame R: Extradural corticosteroid injection in the management of lumbar nerve root compression. Br Med J 1973;2:635-637.
26. Cuckler JM, Bernini PA, Wiesel SW, Booth RE Jr, Rothman RH and Pickens GT: The use of epidural steroids in the treatment of lumbar radicular pain. J Bone Joint Surg 1985;67-A:6366.
27. Ryan MD and Taylor KF: Management of lumbar nerve-root pain by intrathecal and epidural injections of Depo Methylprednisolone Acetate. Med J Aust 1981;2:532-534.
28. Oppelt WW and Rall DP: Production of convulsions in the dog with intrathecal corticosteroids. Neurol 1961;11:925-927.
29. Ildirim I, Furcolow ML et al: A possible explanation of posttreatment convulsions associated with intrathecal corticosteroids. Neurol 1970;20:622-625.

MECHANISMS AND TREATMENT OF SPINAL CORD INJURY PAIN: AN UPDATE

P. J. Siddall, D. A. Taylor and M. J. Cousins

INTRODUCTION

Pain following spinal cord injury (SCI) is a well recognized clinical problem and increasing use of animal models of SCI has led to advances in our understanding of basic mechanisms (for reviews see 1,2). However, there is still much that we do not understand about basic mechanisms and SCI pain continues to present as a difficult management problem.

While some advances have recently been made in this area, there are several major issues which need to be addressed if further progress is to be made. First, there is little agreement as to which epidemiological factors are responsible for the development of pain. Secondly, there is no consensus on a classification system of SCI pain. Thirdly, the mechanisms of SCI pain, including psychological factors, are poorly understood. Lastly, there are few controlled studies which clearly indicate a rational and effective approach to treatment in this group.

EPIDEMIOLOGY

PREVALENCE

There remains a need for further studies on the prevalence of pain following SCI. The figures obtained vary and depend to a large extent on the types of pain that were included, how long after injury the subjects were interviewed and the severity of pain that qualified for inclusion. The most comprehensive summary remains the analysis by Bonica which demonstrated that an average of 69% of people with SCI reported experiencing pain at any time following their injury (3). In nearly one third of these people, the pain was severe.

T. H. Stanley et al. (eds.), Pain Management and Anesthesiology, 247–262.
© 1998 *Kluwer Academic Publishers. Printed in the Netherlands.*

The factors involved in the development of SCI pain are unclear. Evidence from past studies has been contradictory and there is still no clear correlation between factors such level of injury, completeness and the presence of pain.

It has been variously reported that cervical (4), thoracolumbar (5) and conus medullaris and cauda equina (6-8) injuries are most likely to be associated with the presence of pain. However, other studies have found that there was no significant relationship between the presence or severity of pain and the level of injury (9,10).

It is also not clear whether completeness of the spinal cord lesion is more or less likely to result in pain. Evidence from autopsy studies of people with SCI has suggested that pain is more likely to be associated with incompleteness (11). It has also been proposed from clinical observation that neuropathic pain is more common in people with incomplete lesions (12,13). However, with the findings regarding level of injury, there are studies that demonstrate no significant relationship between completeness and the presence or severity of pain (9,10). It was concluded from these latter two studies that psychosocial rather than physiological factors are more closely associated with the experience or severity of pain following SCI (9,10).

A recent study by our own group investigated the relationship between surgery and the presence of pain following SCI. A significantly higher number of people in the surgically managed group had musculoskeletal pain 1 month following their injury. However, beyond this time point, there was no significant relationship between pain and the presence of musculoskeletal, neuropathic or visceral pain up to 12 months following injury (14).

CLASSIFICATION

The disparate findings regarding the prevalence and factors that may be involved in the development of pain following SCI are in large part due to the lack of an agreed upon classification system of SCI pain. The lack of a taxonomy continues to be one of the fundamental problems that hinders both SCI pain research and management.

Many classification systems have been used in the past and this has led to confusion in the interpretation of results obtained in different studies. After examination of classification systems that have been used previously, we have proposed a system that seeks to provide a simple but comprehensive method of classifying the different types of pain that occur following SCI (15) (Table 1).

Table 1. Classification system for spinal cord injury pain.

AXIS 1 (System)	AXIS 2 (Region)	AXIS 3 (Source)
MUSCULOSKELETAL		
VISCERAL		
NEUROPATHIC	- AT LEVEL*	- RADICULAR
		- CENTRAL
	- BELOW LEVEL*	
OTHER (e.g., syringomyelia, complex regional pain syndromes, overuse syndromes, headache associated with dysreflexia compressive mononeuropathies)		

*Level refers to the neurological level of the spinal cord lesion, i.e., the lowest segment with normal spinal cord function.

We have identified several symptom/sign constellations which have been described by previous authors in an attempt to classify these into separate categories which can then be labeled. These constellations generally fall into five broad categories. The five categories are: 1) musculoskeletal; 2) visceral; 3) neuropathic pain at the level of the lesion (neuropathic I); 4) neuropathic pain below the level of the lesion (neuropathic II); and 5) other types of pain.

It seems logical to assign pains to these five categories as it appears from previous reports that these pains are distinguishable in terms of descriptors and/or site. Presumably the categories also have different mechanisms. Several authors have mentioned other types of pain such as psychological or psychogenic (16-18) headache associated with dysreflexia(19), "sympathetic" (16), reflex sympathetic dystrophy (3,20), pain associated with spasticity (16) and compressive neuropathies (3). The question of the inclusion of psychological or psychogenic pain will be dealt with later but in our opinion psychological pain should not be included as a separate category.

MUSCULOSKELETAL PAIN

Musculoskeletal pain arises from damage or overuse in structures such as bones, ligaments, muscles, intervertebral discs and facet joints.

Musculoskeletal pain also includes mechanical pain due to damage to spinal structures, e.g., the acute pain that occurs prior to spinal stabilizing operations. Musculoskeletal pain can be identified by location (at or above lesion level in those with complete spinal cord lesions) and by pain features (dull, aching, worse with activities, eased by rest).

VISCERAL PAIN

Visceral pain can be identified by location (abdomen) and by pain features (dull, poorly localized, cramping, related to visceral function or pathology). If investigations fail to find evidence of visceral pathology, and if blockade of peripheral inputs from visceral structures fails to alleviate pain, then consideration must be given to classifying the pain as neuropathic rather than visceral.

NEUROPATHIC PAIN

Neuropathic pain can be identified by location (region of sensory disturbance) and by features (sharp, shooting, electric, burning, stabbing). Neuropathic pain can be further divided into neuropathic at level pain and neuropathic below level pain.

NEUROPATHIC AT LEVEL PAIN

For the first type of neuropathic pain, we propose the term "neuropathic at level pain". This includes people who have pain in a region of sensory disturbance in a segmental pattern within 2 segments above or below of the level of injury and with neuropathic features (burning, stabbing, electric, shooting).

Neuropathic at level pain can be further divided according to the source of pain, i.e., Axis 3 (radicular or central). However, this can only be done where there is definitive evidence which allows this division to be made. It is recognized that some patients with neuropathic pain at the level of the lesion will have pain of nerve root origin. Pain arising from nerve root damage may be suggested by neuropathic features (e.g., burning, stabbing, shooting, electric descriptors, presence of allodynia) with characteristics such as increased pain in relation to spinal movement. The pain may be due to direct damage to the nerve root during the initial injury or it may be secondary to spinal column instability and impingement by facet or disc material. In the past, pain that occurs at the level of the lesion and has features of nerve root pain in the absence of definitive evidence of nerve root damage has often been classified as radicular. However, pain with features which are suggestive of nerve root damage may occur in the absence of root damage and may be due to spinal rather than nerve root pathology. Therefore, the term "radicular" to describe this type of pain should be used with caution.

It is also possible that neuropathic SCI pain in a segmental distribution at the level of injury is due to pathology within the spinal cord or other parts of the central nervous system. Some previous classification systems included this type of pain as a separate category and distinguished it from pain due to nerve root pathology (8,19,21,22). The only distinguishing feature of central pain appears to be that the pain is bilateral in distribution (19,21). We propose, therefore, that this type of pain be referred to as neuropathic at level central pain.

Therefore, pain which occurs at the level of spinal cord injury in a segmental pattern with neuropathic features may be termed either "neuropathic at level radicular pain", i.e., pain due to nerve root pathology or "neuropathic at level central pain", i.e., pain due to changes within the spinal cord or possibly supraspinal structures. While recognizing that neuropathic at level radicular and central pains form separate entities, we propose that, unless there is definitive evidence of nerve root damage (e.g., imaging evidence of intervertebral foraminal compression), no further classification can be made beyond neuropathic at level pain.

NEUROPATHIC BELOW LEVEL PAIN

For the second type of neuropathic pain, we propose the term "neuropathic below level pain". "Below level" is a term that has been used by others (23,24), is easy to identify and is consistent with the terminology used to identify neuropathic at level pain. Terms used by others either have a similar meaning to below level (e.g., remote, below lesion) or use descriptors that can be confused with other types of neuropathic pain (e.g., dysesthetic, burning). "Central pain" is another term that has been used. This is also misleading because, as discussed above, neuropathic at level pain may also have central mechanisms. "Deafferentation pain" has also been used but fails to distinguish between the two types of neuropathic pain, both of which are the result of deafferentation. We propose that neuropathic below level pain should include pain that is described by the words burning, tingling, aching, shooting, stabbing. However, in distinction to neuropathic at level pain, neuropathic below level pain is present at least three segments below the level of injury and is more likely to be diffuse.

OTHER PAIN TYPES

The last category in our proposed classification system includes other specific types of pain which several authors mention but are not included in the categories listed above. These types of pain are specific pains that are a consequence of SCI. These include such pains as syringomyelia, headache associated with dysreflexia, compressive mononeuropathies and reflex sympathetic dystrophy. It should also be noted that the recent IASP Classification of Chronic Pain has replaced the terms "reflex sympathetic dystrophy and causalgia" with the terms "complex regional pain syndrome, types I and II" respectively (25). This terminology should be used instead of other terms such as "shoulder-hand syndrome", which are often used to describe complex regional pain syndrome, type I.

Regarding the issue of psychological pain, several authors include this category when describing pain categories following SCI (16-18), while other authors specifically exclude it (3,26,27). We agree with the views of Britell and Mariano (26) that inclusion of psychological pain as a separate category implies a dualistic approach to pain which is inconsistent with current thinking. There is no doubt that psychological issues have tremendous importance in the experience and expression of pain (28). It should be recognized that psychological factors will interact with physiological factors to affect any of the pains described above.

MECHANISMS

POSSIBLE MECHANISMS OF SCI PAIN

The mechanisms of SCI pain are still largely unknown. While the mechanisms of musculoskeletal pain are more obvious, the mechanisms of neuropathic pain are poorly understood. A variety of mechanisms have been proposed (for reviews see 2,29). These include: 1) Local irritation at the site of injury; 2) Activation of alternative pathways inside or outside the spinal cord (30); 3) Biochemical changes such as those affecting N-methyl-D-aspartate (NMDA) receptors and calcium flux; 4) Abnormal firing and/or reorganization of spinal (31) and supraspinal (32) deafferented neurons (33); and 5) Loss of descending spinal inhibitory or intraspinal glycinergic and/or GABAergic mechanisms (34,35); and 6) the concept of a "pattern generating mechanism" or "neuromatrix" which is responsible for the generation or perception of pain (36,37). Some of these proposed mechanisms are inferred from studies using other models of neuropathic pain. However, the majority of these studies use models of peripheral nerve injury and there have been relatively few studies which investigate pain mechanisms in a SCI model.

ANIMAL STUDIES

Three models are currently in use in animal studies of SCI pain. One model uses laser irradiation to produce an ischemic injury to the spinal cord (38,39). One uses intraspinal injections of an excitatory amino acid to produce an excitotoxic lesion (40). Another model uses a weight drop to produce a contusive lesion of the spinal cord (41). All models produce a condition in which there is increased sensitivity to light touch (allodynia) in the dermatomes corresponding to the level of injury. They therefore appear to model neuropathic at level SCI pain. Both the ischemic model (42) and the excitotoxic model (43) of SCI pain have demonstrated hyperexcitability of spinal cord neurons to mechanical stimuli following damage to the spinal cord.

CLINICAL STUDIES

Neurophysiological studies in humans have indicated that SCI is associated with two major changes in the properties of cells in the principal sensory nucleus of the thalamus (44). First, these cells demonstrate somatotopic reorganization with a mismatch between receptive and projected fields. This means that stimulation of a cell in the thalamus that has inputs from the SCI border zone results in a sensation which is perceived to arise from the anesthetic region. Secondly, cells in the thalamus that have lost inputs demonstrate abnormal bursting activity. Therefore it may be that these changes occur in sensory neurons in the higher central nervous system following SCI and that these neurons act as a spontaneous pain generating mechanism.

MANAGEMENT

ANIMAL PHARMACOLOGICAL STUDIES

A number of studies have investigated the effectiveness of different agents in reducing allodynia in the ischemic model of SCI pain (45). Chronic allodynia in the ischemic SCI model is not affected by morphine, clonidine, baclofen and carbamazepine (45). In the same model, chronic allodynia is relieved by a cholecystokinin (CCK) type B antagonist and this effect is reversed by naloxone (45). Interestingly, systemic naloxone also induced allodynia in animals which had not previously exhibited this feature. Therefore, it may be that one factor in the development of chronic allodynia following SCI is a result of the loss of opioidergic control following the upregulation of endogenous CCK.

The most recent studies by this group demonstrate that systemic administration of nitric oxide synthase inhibitors (46) and excitatory amino acid antagonists, including dextromethorphan (47), relieved spinal cord injury induced allodynia. Intrathecal but not systemic administration of clonidine was also found to be effective in relieving chronic allodynia in rats with an ischemic SCI (48).

CLINICAL PHARMACOLOGICAL STUDIES

A variety of agents and procedures are used in the management of SCI pain. However, their use is largely empirical or based on anecdotal evidence and there is still a general lack of controlled studies. Several of the studies that have used controls have not demonstrated any effect of the agent being assessed.

Simple analgesics and opioids are helpful in the short term for the management of musculoskeletal pain but are largely ineffective in the management of neuropathic SCI pain. A variety of medications has been used for management of neuropathic pain with limited success. Traditionally anticonvulsants, tricyclic antidepressants and local anesthetics and their congeners such as mexiletine have been used alone or in combination for the management of SCI pain with neuropathic features.

A case study suggests that people who have spasticity and pain following SCI may benefit from oral administration of the anticonvulsant divalproex sodium (49). However, a double-blind cross-over study investigating the effectiveness of sodium valproate in relieving "central" pain in 20 people with SCI found no statistically significant difference between valproate and placebo (50). A placebo controlled trial examining the effectiveness of mexiletine in neuropathic SCI pain found no significant effect on the level of pain (51).

Other less "traditional" agents have also been used with some success. Evidence from a recent case series suggests that propofol may be beneficial in some people with central pain including neuropathic SCI pain (52). In keeping with evidence from animal studies, it has been found that systemic administration of the N-methyl D-aspartate receptor antagonist ketamine reduced both spontaneous and evoked neuropathic pain following SCI (53).

SPINAL ADMINISTRATION OF AGENTS

Epidural and intrathecal administration of morphine, clonidine and baclofen are used for the management of SCI pain and spasticity. Several recent reports have described the response of SCI pain to intrathecal administration of baclofen. While some report an improvement in pain (54), a recent case series found that while intrathecal administration of baclofen was useful for pain associated with spasticity, it was of little benefit for chronic neuropathic SCI pain (55).

The use of spinal clonidine may provide a more hopeful alternative either singly or in combination with other agents. As described above it was found to be effective in an animal model, and some reports confirm this clinically. Two case reports have described the effectiveness of intrathecal clonidine combined with either morphine (56) or baclofen (57) when morphine or baclofen alone was ineffective for the treatment of neuropathic below level SCI pain. Trials of other agents that are currently being investigated for the management of other types of neuropathic pain, such as NMDA antagonists, and drugs acting at adenosine and opioid receptors, may also prove beneficial in SCI pain.

STIMULATION TECHNIQUES

Both transcutaneous nerve stimulation (TENS) and epidural spinal cord stimulation (ESCS) have been used with limited effectiveness in the management of SCI pain and previous reports suggest that they are more beneficial in those with incomplete lesions. A recent survey of 25 people who received ESCS for treatment of SCI pain found that over 40% of people reported a mean 65% pain relief at the end of the stimulation test period. However, the percentage of people with 50% pain relief had fallen to less than 20% after the average follow up time of 3 years (58). The best response was obtained in those with incomplete thoracic lesions and those with neuropathic at level pain. Stimulators are now available with dual systems and eight electrodes which provide better and more reliable coverage of the area to be stimulated. It is hoped that use of these devices will result in better pain relief.

SURGICAL PROCEDURES

Although results are often disappointing, two procedures continue to have a prominent place in the surgical management of SCI pain. These are DREZ lesions and cordotomy.

Previous work has suggested that DREZ lesions are most effective for the management of radicular rather than diffuse neuropathic below level SCI pain (59). A retrospective review of 39 SCI people with pain associated with cauda equina and conus medullaris lesions found that 54% of people were pain free after DREZ lesions without medications and 20% only required nonopioid analgesia (60). Better results were associated with incomplete lesions and pain that had an electrical quality. It should be noted however that 21% had complications which included weakness bladder or sexual dysfunction, cerebrospinal fluid leak and wound infection (60). Another recent case series also suggested that DREZ lesions may be effective in people with neuropathic SCI pain (61).

A recently described operation of cordomyelotomy which aims to preserve descending inhibitory tracts has been claimed to produce significant relief of paroxysmal pain in those with complete paraplegia. Although the operation has only been performed on three people, two had excellent relief after more than ten years (62).

PSYCHOLOGICAL ISSUES

The study of the psychology of pain following SCI has been neglected. Indeed, little has been published since the valuable series of five articles edited by Elliott and Wegener in 1992 (63). In a letter to *Pain*, Cohen (64) argued that Summers et al., (10) had misquoted an earlier paper by Cohen et al (65). This letter, and a reply by Summers and Rapoff (66), led to an agreement that: 1) Pain was a major problem in adjustment for many people with SCI; 2) The psychological concomitants of SCI pain are poorly understood; and that 3) Instruments used to measure psychological variables in normal or in chronic pain populations, may not necessarily be valid with people with SCI.

Recent reviews on SCI continue to give little attention to the importance of psychological processes in SCI pain, although Calodney (67), Ditunno and Formal (68) and Segatore (69) offered useful comments. There have been no recent studies on environmental (including treatment environment) influences on SCI pain and pain behavior, although Yoshida (70) presented a relevant analysis of environmental influences on self-concept following SCI, and Spencer et al. presented a study on the socialization of SCI patients to the culture of a rehabilitation hospital. Both studies have relevance for the study of pain following SCI (71).

Psychological instruments, such as the State-Trait Anxiety Inventory, and more particularly, the Beck Depression Inventory, which confound the physical effects of injury and treatment with the psychological consequences of SCI, continue to be used (72). Emphasis is still being given to identifying psychological pathology following SCI, or to interpreting normal reactions to an abnormal event (SCI), or pathology, rather than to understanding patient experience following SCI (73). However, Taylor presented a study on the increases which occur in psychological strength and positive affect following SCI. This study was based in part on a qualitative analysis of patient experience, including pain following injury (74).

In otherwise heuristically useful studies, Stensman (75) suggested conclusions about SCI pain based on a sample of four and Craig et al. (73) suggest a relationship between depression and SCI pain, and offer recommendations for treatment, although Craig et al. (73) used an affective measure of pain, that does not measure pain intensity. Miller and Eggerth (76) usefully discuss SCI as a traumatic event, Maurer (77) discussed the principles necessary in the design of SCI pain management programs, and Cundiff, Blair and Puckett (78) describe a successful group SCI pain management program.

Recent studies which emphasize patient experience following SCI, rather than attempts to identify pathology, are particularly interesting, and could usefully be supplemented by similar studies on patient experience of SCI pain. Further studies on treatment and other environmental influences on SCI pain would also be valuable. One recent study which examines the relationship between pain and depression suggest that a relationship develops over time and is not present on admission (79). Although it is difficult to assess, the conclusion from the study was that change in pain affected depression more than a change in depression affected pain.

CONCLUSIONS

Several advances in our understanding of pain following SCI have been made in recent years that may lead to improvements in clinical management. A classification system has been proposed that will hopefully engender debate and lead to an agreed taxonomy of SCI pain. This is a fundamental and yet much needed step. The increased use of animal models of SCI pain is providing further information on mechanisms and providing direction for treatment. The demonstration of the effectiveness of dextromethorphan may be useful in treating chronic allodynia following SCI, but has yet to be followed up clinically. The development of suitable nitric oxide synthase inhibitors may also provide a novel approach to treatment.

Although there is a need for controlled studies, clinical reports have suggested that combined spinal administration of clonidine and morphine or clonidine alone provide an effective alternative for the management of neuropathic SCI pain. These reports await substantiation by controlled trials. Most recently it has been announced that the International Association for the Study of Pain is instituting a Task Force to address the problem of pain associated with spinal cord injury. The formation of such a Task Force recognizes the problem that exists and the combined effort that such a group can initiate will hopefully lead to significant new advances in this field.

ACKNOWLEDGMENTS

This work was supported by the Motor Accidents Authority, N.S.W., WorkCover's Injury Prevention, Education and Research Grants Scheme, the Spinal Research Fund, Royal North Shore Hospital, Sydney, Australia and the National Health & Medical Research Council, Australia.

REFERENCES

1. Siddall PJ, Taylor DA, Cousins MJ: Pain associated with spinal cord injury. Curr Opin Neurol 8:447-450, 1995.
2. Yezierski RP: Pain following spinal cord injury: the clinical problem and experimental studies. Pain 68:185-194, 1996.
3. Bonica JJ: Introduction: semantic, epidemiologic, and educational issues, Pain and Central Nervous System Disease: The Central Pain Syndromes. Casey KL (ed). New York, Raven Press, 1991, pp.13-29.
4. Holmes G: Pain of central origin, Contributions to medical and biological research, Vol. 1. New York, P.B. Hoeber, 1919, pp. 235-246.
5. Davis L, Martin J: Studies upon spinal cord injuries. J Neurosurg 4:483-491, 1947.
6. Botterell EH, Callaghan JC, Jousse AT: Pain in paraplegia: clinical management and surgical treatment. Proc R Soc Med 47:281-288, 1953.
7. Burke DC: Pain in paraplegia. Paraplegia 10:297-313, 1973.
8. Nashold BS: Paraplegia and pain, Deafferentation Pain Syndromes: Pathophysiology and Treatment. Edited by Nashold BS, Ovelmen-Levitt J. New York, Raven Press, 1991, pp. 301-319.
9. Richards JS, Meredith RL, Nepomuceno C, Fine PR, Bennett G: Psycho-social aspects of chronic pain in spinal cord injury. Pain 8:355-366, 1980.
10. Summers JD, Rapoff MA, Varghese G, Porter K, Palmer RE: Psychosocial factors in chronic spinal cord injury pain. Pain 47:183-189, 1991.
11. Kakulas BA, Smith E, Gaekwad U, Kaelan C, Jacobsen PF: The neuropathology of pain and abnormal sensations in human spinal cord injury derived from the clincopathological data base at the Royal Perth Hospital, Recent Achievements in Restorative Neurology, Vol. 3, Altered Sensation and Pain. Edited by Dimitrijevic MR, Wall PD, Lindblom U. Basel, Karger, 1990, pp. 37-41.

12. Davidoff G, Roth E, Guarracini M, Sliwa J, Yarkony G: Function-limiting dysesthetic pain syndrome among traumatic spinal cord injury patients: a cross-sectional study. Pain 29:39-48, 1987.

13. Beric A, Dimitrijevic MR, Lindblom U: Central dysesthesia syndrome in spinal cord injury patients. Pain 34:109-116, 1988.

14. Sved P, Siddall PJ, McClelland J, Cousins MJ: Relationship between surgery and pain report following spinal cord injury. Spinal Cord 1997 [In Press].

15. Siddall PJ, Taylor DA, Cousins MJ: Classification of pain following spinal cord injury. Spinal Cord 35:69-75, 1997.

16. Kaplan LI, Grynbaum BB, Lloyd KE, Rusk HA: Pain and spasticity in patients with spinal cord dysfunction. JAMA 182:918-925, 1962.

17. Bedbrook GM: Pain and phantom sensation, The Care and Management of Spinal Cord Injuries. Edited by Bedbrook GM. New York, Springer-Verlag, 1981, pp. 224-229.

18. Donovan WH, Dimitrijevic MR, Dahm L, Dimitrijevic M: Neurophysiological approaches to chronic pain following spinal cord injury. Paraplegia 20:135-146, 1982.

19. Burke DC, Woodward JM: Pain and phantom sensation in spinal paralysis, Handbook of Clinical Neurology. Edited by Vinken PJ, Bruyn GW. New York, Elsevier, 1976, pp.489-499.

20. Gallien P, Nicolas B, Robineau S, Lebot MP, Brissot R: The reflex sympathetic dystrophy syndrome in patients who have had a spinal cord injury. Paraplegia 33:715-720, 1995.

21. Riddoch G: The clinical features of central pain. Lancet 234:1150-1156, 1938.

22. Tunks E: Pain in spinal cord injured patients, Management of Spinal Cord Injuries. Edited by Bloch RF, Basbaum M. Baltimore, Williams and Wilkins, 1986, pp. 180-211.

23. Michaelis LS: The problem of pain in paraplegia and tetraplegia. Bull N Y Acad Med 46:88-96, 1970.

24. Davis R: Pain and suffering following spinal cord injury. Clin Orthop 112:76-80, 1975.

25. Merskey H, Bogduk N: Classification of chronic pain: descriptions of chronic pain syndromes and definitions of pain terms. 2nd: Seattle, IASP Press, 1994.

26. Britell CW, Mariano AJ: Chronic pain in spinal cord injury. Physical Medicine and Rehabilitation: State of the Art Reviews 5:71-82, 1991.

27. Mariano AJ: Chronic pain and spinal cord injury. Clin J Pain 8:87-92, 1992.

28. Craig KD: Emotional aspects of pain, Textbook of Pain. Edited by Wall PD, Melzack R. Edinburgh, Churchill Livingstone, 1994, pp. 261-274.

29. Boivie J: Central pain, Textbook of Pain. Edited by Wall PD, Melzack R. Edinburgh, Churchill Livingstone, 1994, pp. 871-902.

30. Craig AD: Supraspinal pathways and mechanisms relevant to central pain, Pain and Central Nervous System Disease: The Central Pain Syndromes. Edited by Casey KL. New York, Raven Press, 1991, pp. 157-170.

31. Loeser JD, Ward AA, White LE: Chronic deafferentation of human spinal cord neurons. J Neurosurg 29:48-50, 1968.

32. Lenz FA: The thalamus and central pain syndromes: human and animal studies, Pain and Central Nervous System Disease: The Central Pain Syndromes. Edited by Casey KL. New York, Raven Press, 1991, pp. 171-182.

33. Woolf CJ, Shortland P, Coggeshall RE: Peripheral nerve injury triggers central sprouting of myelinated afferents. Nature 355:75-78, 1992.

34. Zimmerman M: Central nervous mechanisms modulating pain-related information: do they become deficient after lesions of the peripheral or central nervous system? Pain and Central Nervous System Disease: The Central Pain Syndromes. Edited by Casey KL. New York, Raven Press, 1991, pp. 183-199.

35. Sivilotti LG, Woolf CJ: The contribution of GABAA and glycine receptors to central sensitization: disinhibition and touch-evoked allodynia in the spinal cord. J Neurophysiol 72:169-179, 1994.

36. Melzack R: The John J. Bonica Distinguished Lecture: The gate control theory 25 years later: new perspectives in phantom limb pain, Pain Research and Clinical Management, Vol. 4, Proceedings of the VIth World Congress on Pain. Edited by Bond M, Charlton E, Woolf CJ. Amsterdam, Elsevier, 1991, pp. 9-21.

37. Melzack R, Loeser JD: Phantom body pain in paraplegics: evidence for a central "pattern generating mechanism" for pain. Pain 4:195-210, 1978.

38. Hao JX, Xu XJ, Aldskogius H, et al: Allodynia-like effects in rat after ischaemic spinal cord injury photochemically induced by laser irradiation. Pain 45:175-185, 1991.

39. Xu X-J, Hao JX, Aldskogius H, et al: Chronic pain-related syndrome in rats after ischemic spinal cord lesion: a possible animal model for pain in patients with spinal cord injury. Pain 48:279-290, 1992.

40. Yezierski RP, Santana M, Park SH, Madsen PW: Neuronal degeneration and spinal cavitation following intraspinal injections of quisqualic acid in the rat. J Neurotrauma 10:445-456, 1993.

41. Siddall PJ, Xu CL, Cousins MJ: Allodynia following traumatic spinal cord injury in the rat. Neuroreport 6:1241-1244, 1995.

42. Hao JX, Xu XJ, Yu YX, et al: Transient spinal cord ischaemia induces temporary hypersensitivity of dorsal horn wide dynamic range neurons to myelinated, but not unmyelinated, fiber input. J Neurophysiol 68:384-391, 1992.

43. Yezierski RP, Park SH: The mechanosensitivity of spinal sensory neurons following intraspinal injections of quisqualic acid in the rat. Neurosci Lett 157:115-119, 1993.

44. Lenz FA, Kwan HC, Martin R, et al: Characteristics of somatotopic organization and spontaneous neuronal activity in the region of the thalamic principal sensory nucleus in patients with spinal cord transection. J Neurophysiol 72:1570-1587, 1994.

45. Xu XJ, Hao JX, Seiger A, et al: Chronic pain-related behaviors in spinally injured rats—evidence for functional alterations of the

endogenous cholecystokinin and opioid systems. Pain 56:271-277, 1994.

46. Hao J-X, Xu X-J: Treatment of chronic allodynia-like response in spinally injured rats: effects of systemically administered nitric oxide synthase inhibitors. Pain 66:313-319, 1996.

47. Hao J-X, Xu X-J: Treatment of chronic allodynia-like response in spinally injured rats: effects of systemically administered excitatory amino acid receptor antagonists. Pain 66:279-285, 1996.

48. Hao JX, Yu W, Xu XJ, Wiesenfeld-Hallin Z: Effects of intrathecal vs. systemic clonidine in treating chronic allodynia-like response in spinally injured rats. Brain Res 736:28-34, 1996.

49. Zachariah SB, Borges EF, Varghese R, et al: Positive response to oral divalproex sodium (Depakote) in patients with spasticity and pain. American Journal of the Medical Sciences 308:38-40, 1994.

50. Drewes AM, Andreasen A, Poulsen LH: Valproate for treatment of chronic central pain after spinal cord injury. A double-blind cross-over study. Paraplegia 32:565-569, 1994.

51. Chiou-Tan FY, Tuel SM, Johnson JC, et al: Effect of mexiletine on spinal cord injury dysesthetic pain. Am J Phys Rehabil 75:84-87, 1996.

52. Canavero S, Bonicalzi V, Pagni CA et al: Propofol analgesia in central pain—preliminary clinical observations. J Neurol 242:561-567, 1995.

53. Eide PK, Stubhaug A, Stenehjem AE: Central dysesthesia pain after traumatic spinal cord injury is dependent on N-methyl-D-aspartate receptor activation. Neurosurgery 37:1080-1087, 1995.

54. Taira T, Kawamura H, Tanikawa T, et al: A new approach to control central deafferentation pain: spinal intrathecal baclofen. Stereotact Funct Neurosurg 65:101-105, 1995.

55. Loubser PG, Akman NM: Effects of intrathecal baclofen on chronic spinal cord injury pain. J Pain Symptom Manage 12:241-247, 1996.

56. Siddall PJ, Gray M, Rutkowski S, Cousins MJ: Intrathecal morphine and clonidine in the management of spinal cord injury pain: a case report. Pain 59:147-148, 1994.

57. Middleton JW, Siddall PJ, Walker S, et al: Intrathecal clonidine and baclofen in the management of spasticity and neuropathic pain following spinal cord injury: a case study. Arch Phys Med Rehabil 1996.

58. Cioni B, Meglio M, Pentimalli L, Visocchi M: Spinal cord stimulation in the treatment of paraplegic pain. J Neurosurg 82:35-39, 1995.

59. Friedman AH, Nashold BS: Pain of spinal origin, Neurological Surgery. Edited by Youmans J. Philadelphia, W.B. Saunders, 1989, pp. 3950-3959.

60. Sampson JH, Cashman RE, Nashold BS, Jr., Friedman AH: Dorsal root entry zone lesions for intractable pain after trauma to the conus medullaris and cauda equina. J Neurosurg 82:28-34, 1995.

61. Rath SA, Braun V, Soliman N, et al: Results of DREZ coagulations for pain related to plexus lesions, spinal cord injuries and postherpetic neuralgia. Acta Neurochirurgica 138:364-369, 1996.

62. Pagni CA, Canavero S: Cordomyelotomy in the treatment of paraplegia pain—experience in two cases with long-term results. Acta Neurologica Belgica 95:33-36, 1995.
63. Elliott TR, Wegener ST: Introduction to the special section on chronic pain and spinal cord injury. Clin J Pain 8:861992.
64. Cohen MJ: Comments on psychosocial factors in chronic spinal cord injury pain by Summers, Rapoff, Varghese, Porter and Palmer. Pain 58:280-281, 1994.
65. Cohen MJ, McArthur DL, Vulpe M, et al: Comparing chronic pain from spinal cord injury to chronic pain of other origins. Pain 35:57-63, 1988.
66. Summers JD, Rapoff MA: Comments on M.J. Cohen [letter]. Pain 58:281-282, 1994.
67. Calodney A: Pain after spinal cord injury. Pain Digest 3:112-115, 1993.
68. Ditunno JF, Formal CS: Chronic spinal cord injury. N Engl J Med 330:550-556, 1994.
69. Segatore M: Deafferentation pain after spinal cord injury. Part 1. Theoretical aspects. SCI Nursing 9:46-50, 1992.
70. Yoshida KY: Institutional impact on self concept among persons with spinal cord injury. International Journal of Rehabilitation Research 17:95-107, 1994.
71. Spencer J, Young ME, Rintala D, Bates S: Socialization to the culture of a rehabilitation hospital: an ethnographic study. American Journal of Occupational Medicine 49:53-62, 1995.
72. Craig AR, Hancock KM, Dickson HG: A longitudinal investigation into anxiety and depression in the first 2 years following a spinal cord injury. Paraplegia 32:675-679, 1994.
73. Craig AR, Hancock KM, Dickson HG: Spinal cord injury: a search for determinants of depression two years after the event. Br J Clin Psychol 33:221-230, 1994.
74. Taylor DA, Siddall PJ, Cousins MJ, Rutkowski SB: Psychological strength following spinal cord injury. 12th World Congress, International Federation of Physical Medicine and Rehabilitation, Sydney, 1995.
75. Stensman R: Adjustment to traumatic spinal cord injury—a longitudinal study of self-reported quality of life. Paraplegia 32:416-422, 1994.
76. Miller T, Eggerth D: Spinal cord injury as a stressful life event. SCI Psychosocial Process 7:3-7, 1994.
77. Maurer S: Comments on pain: self management and psychotherapy. SCI Psychosocial Process 7:81-83, 1994.
78. Cundiff G, Blair K, Puckett M: Group pain management therapy for persons with SCI. SCI Psychosocial Process 8:61-66, 1995.
79. Cairns DM, Adkins RH, Scott MD: Pain and depression in acute traumatic spinal cord injury-origins of chronic problematic pain. Arch Phys Med Rehabil 77:329-335, 1996.

PREVENTION OF POST-HERPETIC NEURALGIA

A. P. Winnie

INTRODUCTION

While the pain of herpes zoster usually disappears with or shortly after the healing of the skin lesions, the most common (and dreaded) complication of the disease is persistent pain, termed post-herpetic neuralgia. Post-herpetic neuralgia can vary in degree from a mild, bothersome discomfort to severely debilitating and agonizing pain. Severe post-herpetic neuralgia, most frequently described as a burning pain, is unique in that it may occur spontaneously and continuously without stimulation, though it is exacerbated by light tough and/or temperature changes. Post-herpetic neuralgia produces significant physical, mental, and emotional incapacitation, and is associated with a high rate of drug addiction and suicide (1).

The therapeutic benefit of sympathetic blocks in herpes zoster was discovered by coincidence by Rosenak (2), who was utilizing lumbar paravertebral sympathetic blocks to treat a patient with severe peripheral vascular disease. The patient also had developed painful, acute herpes zoster in the gluteal area two days earlier, and following the blocks the patient had dramatic relief of the zoster pain with drying and crusting of the vesicles within 48 hours. Startled by the seemingly illogical but dramatic effect of sympathetic blocks on acute herpes zoster, Rosenak undertook further trials of this therapeutic modality, and in 21 subsequent patients he obtained relief of pain in 19, with prompt drying and crusting of the vesicles. In one case the sympathetic block was incomplete on the first attempt; and when it was repeated, the patient obtained complete relief. Rosenak's only failure was a patient who had a six-year history of recurrent neuralgia which was frequently accompanied by a rash, and it may be that this patient had zosteriform herpes simplex (3) rather than repetitive episodes of acute herpes zoster. Nonetheless, Rosenak still achieved a 95% success rate in his series, an impressive finding in a disease for which there had previously been no treatment whatsoever.

T. H. Stanley et al. (eds.), Pain Management and Anesthesiology, 263–275.

Since Rosenak's original publication a multitude of reports concerning the use of sympathetic nerve blocks for the treatment of acute herpes zoster have appeared sporadically in the literature (2,4-27). Because most of these studies were uncontrolled, Tenicela (28) reconfirmed the efficacy of sympathetic blocks in terminating acute herpes zoster in a double blind, randomized study. It is important to realize that the data presented in most of the studies cited were obtained in patients treated within one month of the onset of their pain; and Colding, who has the largest series of cases in the literature (12,14), has stated that it would appear from his data that the earlier this treatment is started, the more successful it will be. In fact, in his second paper, Colding (14) reported that 90% of those patients treated before the eruption was two weeks old exhibited a dramatic response to sympathetic block, whereas only 40% of those treated more than two weeks after onset, responded to this treatment. Anyone with significant experience treating acute herpes zoster with sympathetic blocks is certainly aware that there is, indeed, a time after which the blocks cease to be effective in terminating acute herpes zoster and preventing post-herpetic neuralgia. The present study was undertaken to determine more precisely the relationship between the time of treatment of acute herpes zoster and the prevention of post-herpetic neuralgia and to utilize this clinical data to support our theory as to the mechanism by which sympathetic blocks provide their therapeutic benefit (20).

METHODS AND MATERIALS:

The charts of 122 patients treated in the University of Illinois Pain Control Center for pain related to herpes zoster were reviewed retrospectively. Only the records of patients with complete follow-up, whether by personal or telephone interview, were utilized for the study; and all patients with complete follow-up were included, regardless of their response to treatment. The technique by which sympathetic blockade was provided, of course, depended on the location of the patient's pain. Patients who had trigeminal, cervical, brachial, or high thoracic nerve involvement received stellate ganglion blocks by the anterior approach; while patients with a thoracic, lumbar, or sacral distribution received epidural blocks. In a few cases where the herpetic lesions did not extend all the way to the midline, intercostal blocks were utilized for thoracic involvement. The local anesthetic agents utilized in the epidural (and intercostal) blocks were administered in a sufficient concentration to produce sensory as well as sympathetic blockade in order to confirm that the level of the blockade was appropriate for the level of the patient's pain.

The agents utilized for the blocks included bupivacaine, mepivacaine, lidocaine, and 2-chloroprocaine, all without epinephrine.

In order to assess the importance of time of treatment on the efficacy of sympathetic blockade in terminating acute herpetic pain and in preventing post-herpetic neuralgia, great care was taken to accurately determine the duration of the patient's symptoms prior to the initial treatment and to note carefully the timing of subsequent treatments. Thus, patients were grouped according to the duration of their symptoms prior to the initiation of treatment as follows: Group A consisted of those patients whose treatment occurred less than two weeks following the onset of symptoms; Group B represents those patients treated at least 2 weeks but less than 1 month after the onset of symptoms; Group C patients were treated at least 1 month but less than 2 months after the initial onset of symptoms; the patients in Group D were treated at least 2 months but less than 6 months following their first symptoms; Group E patients were treated at least 6 months but less than 1 year after the initial symptoms; and the patients in Group F were all treated at least 1 year after the onset of their symptoms. In all cases the first sympathetic block was administered on the first visit to the Pain Control Center. The patient was told to return immediately if and when their pain returned for a second block. If a second block was carried out, again the patient was told to return if and when their pain recurred for a third block. If their pain returned after a third block, with rare exceptions, further sympathetic blocks were not administered.

Similarly, the various responses to treatment were grouped as follows: a Type I response indicates complete and permanent relief was achieved after a single block. A Type II response indicates that the first treatment provided pain relief, but though the relief outlasted the effect of the anesthetic (by as long as several days), the pain subsequently returned. However, when it returned, it was significantly less severe, and with this type of response repeated blocks (usually two or three) did provide permanent pain relief. A Type III response indicates that temporary pain relief was provided by each treatment; but the relief only lasted as long as the local anesthetic, and when the pain returned, the intensity was the same as before the block. However, in this type of response subsequent to the series of blocks these patients had a slow, gradual improvement in their pain until they were ultimately (and permanently) pain free. It is significant to note that all of those who exhibited a Type I, II, or III response ultimately became and remained pain free, unlike those exhibiting a Type IV or Type V response: A Type IV response, like the Type III response, indicates that temporary pain relief was provided by each treatment, relief which only lasted as long as the local anesthetic. But unlike the Type III response, patients exhibiting a Type IV response, though improved, still had residual pain at the time of follow-up. A Type V response indicates no apparent improvement whatsoever with treatment and residual pain at the time of follow-up. So all patients exhibiting a Type IV or V response continued to have pain in spite of the treatment.

All patients included in this study were followed up by telephone. In addition to the data concerning age, sex, distribution of lesions, duration of symptoms prior to treatment, number of treatments and response to treatment, information was obtained concerning any complications of the treatment, any co-existent diseases and any medications being taken concomitantly.

The results of this study were analyzed using a contingency table (Table 1), which gives the number of patients in each group (A-F), and within each group, the number exhibiting each type of response (I-IV). This table was then analyzed by a chi-square approximation (29).

Table 1. Number of patients of each group demonstrating each type of response.*					
	Type of Response				
	I	II	III	IV	V	I, II, III Combined
Group A n=21	7(33.3%)	11(52.4%)	3(14.3%)	-	-	100%
Group B n=13	3(23%)	7(54%)	2(15%)	1(8%)	-	92.3%
Group C n=15	-	10(67%)	2(13.3%)	1(6.7%)	2(13.3%)	80%
Group D n=28	2(7%)	2(7%)	1(4%)	9(32%)	14(50%)	18%
Group E n=19	2(10.5%)	2(10.5%)	-	4(21%)	11(58%)	21%
Group F n=26	-	1(3.5%)	-	4(15.5%)	21(81%)	4%
Combined Groups	Prevented Post-herpetic Neuralgia			Developed Post-herpetic Neuralgia		Prevented Post-herpetic Neuralgia

*Except for the combined groups (far right column) and the relationship between the type of response and the development of post-herpetic neuralgia (bottom line), this table represents a contingency table giving the numbers of patients classified into response Classes I-V and into Groups A-F (defined by time elapsed between onset of symptoms and institution of treatment). When analyzed by a chi-square approximation of 5x6 contingency table (21), chi-square = 91.24 with 20 degrees degrees of freedom (P<0.0001), demonstrating that the effect of time elapsed between onset of symptoms and institution of therapy has a highly significant effect in the type of response.

RESULTS

The results of this study are tabulated in Table 1 and presented graphically in Figure 1, which indicates dramatically the relationship between the type of response to treatment and the time interval between the initial symptoms and the initiation of treatment. Of the 21 patients in Group A, all 21 (100%) had complete relief of their pain at the time of follow-up: 7 in this Group demonstrated a Type I response, 11 demonstrated a Type II response, and 3 a Type III response.

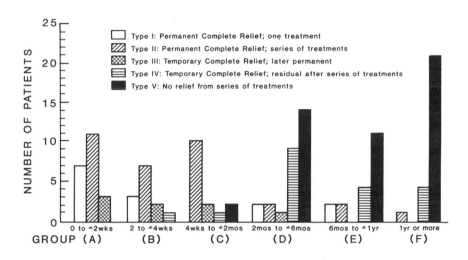

Figure 1. Graphic representation of the relationship between time of treatment and type of response (see text).

Of the thirteen patients in Group B, twelve (92.3%) were pain free at the time of follow-up, and one was improved, though he did still have some residual pain: three of the patients in this Group exhibited a Type I response, seven a Type II response, and two a Type III response, and one a Type IV response.

Of the fifteen patients in Group C, twelve (80%) were pain free at the time of follow-up, while three had residual pain; of the patients who were pain free at the time of follow-up, none exhibited a Type I response, ten exhibited a Type II response, and two a Type III response. Of those who still had pain at the time of follow-up, one represented a Type IV response, while two exhibited a Type V response.

Of the twenty-eight patients in Group D, five (18%) were pain free at the time of follow-up, while twenty-three still had pain: of the five who were pain free at the time of follow-up two had exhibited a Type I response, two a Type II response, and one a Type III response. Of those who had persistent pain at the time of follow-up, nine represented a Type IV response and fourteen a Type V response.

Of the nineteen patients in Group E, four (21%) were pain free, and fifteen had persistent pain: of the patients who were pain free at the time of follow-up, two had exhibited a Type I response and two a Type II response. Of those patients with persistent pain at the time of follow-up, four represented a Type IV response and eleven a Type V response.

Of the twenty-six patients in Group F, only one (4%) was pain free, with all of the other twenty-five complaining of persistent pain: the patient who was pain free at the time of follow-up had exhibited a Type II response, while four of the patients with persistent pain represented a Type IV response and twenty-one a Type V response.

With respect to complications specifically related to the treatment, only 3 of the 134 patients who received epidural blocks developed hypotension, and in each case the hypotension responded promptly to intravenous fluid therapy and/or small doses of ephedrine without further sequelae. In two of the patients treated with epidural injections the dura was inadvertently punctured. Of these two, one had no sequelae and went home after remaining supine several hours, while the other experienced a severe spinal headache with nausea and vomiting and ultimately required an epidural blood patch to obtain relief. Interestingly, in spite of having had such a severe headache, this patient remained enthusiastic about the treatment, because it had provided complete relief from her herpetic pain. Of the 135 stellate ganglion blocks carried out, only one resulted in undesirable side effects, which in this case consisted of hoarseness, blurred vision, and nausea, all of which resolved spontaneously without treatment.

DISCUSSION

Certainly this study corroborates Colding's impression that the earlier sympathetic blocks are initiated, the more successful they will be in terminating the acute phase of the disease and preventing post-herpetic neuralgia. As may be seen in Table 1 (I, II, III Combined column, far right), 100% of the patients in Group A were pain free at the time of follow-up. However, only 85% were pain free upon completion of their last sympathetic block. In Group B 92.3% of the patients were pain free at the time of follow-up, though again, only 77% were pain free at the time of their last block. In Group C, while the overall success rate decreased somewhat, nonetheless, 80% of the patients were pain-free at the time of follow-up,

67% of whom were free of pain following their last block. It is important to note that when the initial treatment was delayed beyond two months, as was the case in Groups D, E, and F, the overall success rate fell drastically to 18%, 21%, and 4% respectively. Interestingly enough, at six months and beyond, it is only those patients who obtained relief at the time of the last treatment that are pain free at the time of follow-up, i.e., there are no Type III responses.

From these data it would appear that while success in terminating acute herpes zoster is greatest when the patient is treated within the first few weeks, if treatment is begun within two months, the chance of preventing post-herpetic neuralgia is still almost 80%. To test statistically the difference between treatment before and after two months in terms of preventing post-herpetic neuralgia (i.e., whether 2 months is the latest that this therapy will provide a reasonable expectation of preventing post-herpetic neuralgia), the data were analyzed using a contingency table (Table 2) and applying the Fisher Exact test (30). Such analysis indicates the highest statistical significance ($P<0.000001$). Nonetheless, in spite of the low incidence of Type I and Type II responses to sympathetic blocks when they were administered more than 2 months after the initial onset of symptoms, this form of therapy should be tried no matter how late after the initial symptoms the patient is seen, since the occasional success achieved represents 100% success to that patient. And even if the treatment fails, it is innocuous in competent hands, as attested to by the fact

Table 2. Relationship between time of treatment and prevention of post-herpetic neuralgia (residual pain).*

Time Elapsed Between Initial Symptoms And Treatment	No Residual Pain	Residual Pain	Total
4 weeks to < 2 months	45	4	49
> 2 months	10	63	73
TOTAL	55	67	122

*In order to test the effect of considering 60 days as the longest elapsed time (between the onset of symptoms and the institution of therapy) which will give reasonable expectation of not having residual pain after cessation of therapy, the data was analyzed using a contingency table giving the numbers of patients classified on the basis of response (no residual pain or residual pain) and time of treatment (60 days or less or more than 60 days). This table was analyzed by the Fisher Exact Test (22), giving a P value of <0.000001. Thus, the proportion of patients treated within 60 days of onset of disease who do not have residual pain after cessation of treatment is highly significantly greater than those who are treated more than 60 days after the onset of the disease.

that we experienced no serious complications in our entire study, in spite of the fact that most of the blocks were performed by residents and fellows.

Any theory as to how sympathetic blockade terminates the acute phase of herpes zoster must also explain how sympathetic blockade prevents the development of post-herpetic neuralgia if a patient is treated early enough and why it fails to do so when treatment is delayed. It is well established that shortly after reactivation, the Varicella-Zoster virus moves rapidly out along the course of the involved nerve(s), producing an inflammatory reaction that is responsible for the initial hyperesthesia, dysesthesia, and pain, and ultimately, the characteristic vesicular eruption (31). Such an inflammatory response typically produces intense sympathetic stimulation, and Selander has recently demonstrated experimentally that sympathetic stimulation can reduce blood flow in the intraneural capillary bed by as much as 93% (32). Furthermore, Lundborg (33) has shown that when ischemia is prolonged, there is anoxic damage to the endoneurial capillary endothelium with leakage of albumen, and the formation of endoneurial edema. This edema, in and of itself, can cause increased intrafascicular pressure and result in even greater impairment of endoneurial blood flow and ultimately irreversible nerve damage (33). In addition to the production of hypoxic damage, such a reduction in blood flow results in glucose deprivation, which like hypoxia produces preferential destruction of large nerve fibers with survival and/or recovery of the less metabolically active small fibers (34).

It would appear, then, from the available laboratory data that in the acute phase of herpes zoster the virus (or its toxin) is capable of producing severe sympathetic stimulation which results in ischemia of the involved nerves; and it would appear from our clinical data that after the first few weeks the reversal of the results of the ischemia (the hypoxic, hypoglucic, and toxic damage to large fibers) takes progressively longer and requires a greater number of sympathetic blocks. And finally, also from our clinical data, it would appear that after two months the ischemic damage becomes irreversible.

Both Fink and Lundborg have demonstrated experimentally in animals that, unlike large fibers, small fibers are able to survive prolonged periods of ischemia and still recover full function (33,35). That this is also true in man is supported histologically by the work of Noordenbos (36), who many years ago compared cross-sections of post-herpetic and normal nerves under the light microscope and found that in the post-herpetic nerve, the vast majority of the large nerve fibers have been destroyed and replaced by fibrous tissue (Figure 2A and 2B). As a result, unlike the situation in a normal nerve, where the population of nerve fibers is predominately composed of large fibers, Noordenbos found that in the

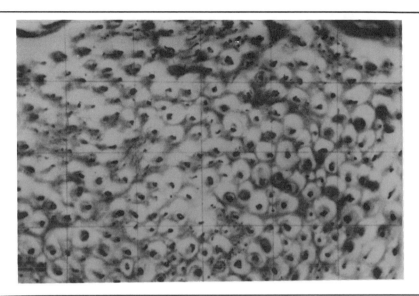

Figure 2-A: Cross-section of a normal 5th intercostal nerve from a patient with post-herpetic neuralgia. The loss of myelinated fibers in the affected nerve is obvious, and there is an increase in the number of fine, apparently unmyelinated fibers as compared to the normal nerve. The change in ratio between myelinated and unmyelinated fibers is clearly demonstrated. (From Noordenbos (26): Reproduced with permission of the publisher)

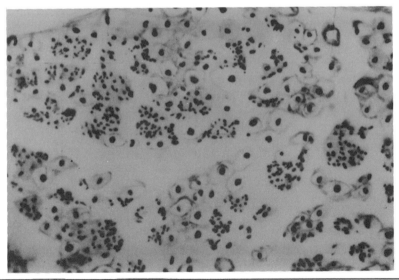

Figure 2-B: Cross-section of an affected 5th intercostal nerve from a patient with post-herpetic neuralgia. The loss of myelinated fibers in the affected nerve is obvious, and there is an increase in the number of fine, apparently unmyelinated fibers as compared to the normal nerve. The change in ratio between myelinated and unmyelinated fibers is clearly demonstrated. (From Noordenbos(26): Reproduced with permission of the publisher)

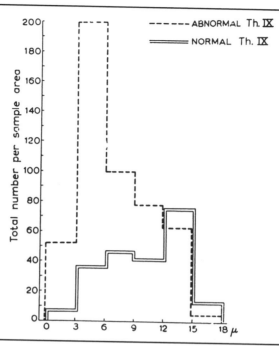

Figure 3: Superimposed fiber spectra of an abnormal nerve (dashed outline) from a patient with post-herpetic neuralgia and its normal counterpart (double outline), demonstrating the reversal of the normal ratio of myelinated and unmyelinated fibers in the post-herpetic nerve. Noordenbos termed this phenomenon "fiber dissociation" and offered it as an explanation for the spontaneous pain exhibited in post-herpetic neuralgia.

post-herpetic nerve, the vast majority of the large nerve fibers have been destroyed and replaced by fibrous tissue. As a result, unlike the situation in a normal nerve, where the population of nerve fibers is predominately composed of large fibers, Noordenbos found that in the post-herpetic nerve there was a predominance of small fibers, a phenomenon he referred to as "fiber dissociation" (Figure 3). Correlating these histological findings with the clinical picture of spontaneous pain in the post-herpetic patient, Noordenbos postulated that large fibers tend to inhibit the entry of noxious impulses into the central nervous system, while small fibers tend to enhance such entry. Therefore, in the post-herpetic nerve, "fiber dissociation" abolishes the normal inhibitory effect of large fiber predominance with the result that not only is the entry of noxious impulses into the spinal cord enhanced, many impulses that are not ordinarily noxious are interpreted as noxious by the altered large/small fiber balance.

The similarity of Noordenbos' theory to the Gate Control Theory conceptualized by Melzack and Wall six years later (37) is remarkable in itself; but more importantly, it is critical to our hypothesis as to the mechanism by which sympathetic blocks produce their therapeutic benefit. Since the characteristic lesion in post-herpetic neuralgia is the death and replacement of large nerve fibers within the nerve, clearly, if the sympathetic response responsible for the ischemic state of the nerve is interrupted before the changes in the large fibers become irreversible, the symptoms of acute herpes zoster disappear, and the development of post-herpetic neuralgia is avoided. It would appear from the data obtained in the present study that this is precisely what has happened in those patients who had a favorable response to sympathetic blocks. It would also appear from this study that if this therapy is instituted within the first few weeks of the onset of the disease, in most cases, reversal of the ischemic changes is almost immediate, whereas if treatment is delayed, the changes secondary to the ischemia become progressively more severe; and after about two months, large fiber death and fiber dissociation make the process virtually irreversible.

Interestingly, the advent of acyclovir for the "specific" treatment of herpes zoster at first appeared to represent a replacement for the nerve block therapy of this disease. However, it now has been shown that while acyclovir is effective in terminating the acute phase of herpes zoster in a high percentage of cases, it does not prevent against the development of post-herpetic neuralgia (38). As a matter of fact, it may even enhance this possibility, since in those patients in whom acyclovir fails to terminate the acute phase of the disease, the time required for a course of acyclovir only serves to delay the institution of sympathetic blocks by several weeks. Thus, because the effectiveness of sympathetic blocks in terminating the disease process is related to the time of therapy, the delay to administer acyclovir could reduce the efficacy of the sympathetic blocks, once they are administered.

REFERENCES:

1. Bonica JJ. Thoracic Segmental and Intercostal Neuralgia. Chapter 26 in "The Management of Pain," Lea & Febiger, 1953:865.
2. Rosenak S. Procaine injection treatment of herpes zoster. Lancet 1938;2:1056-1058.
3. Juel-Jensen BE, MacCalum FO. Herpes Simplex Varicella and Zoster. Clinical Manifestations and Treatment. JB Lippincott Company, Philadelphia, 1972:79-116, 44.
4. Leger L, Audoly P. Traitement du zona par l'infiltration stellaire. La Presse Med 1942;50:588.

5.   Street A. The use of sympathetic nerve block in: (1) herpes zoster; (2) Bell's palsy. Mississippi Doctor 1943;20:480-481.

6.   Verhaeghe A, Merlen J, Lagache G. Sur un cas d'algies brachiales post-zonateuses gueries par infiltration stellaire. La Presse Med 1943;51:249.

7.   Findley T, Patzer R. The treatment of herpes zoster by paravertebral procaine block. JAMA 1945;128:1217-1219.

8.   Rougues L. Traitement du zona par l'infiltration des ganglions sympathiques. La Presse Med 1945;53:716.

9.   Lovell WW. The treatment of herpes zoster. South Med J 1946; 39:777-779.

10. Ferris LM, Martin GH. The use of sympathetic nerve block in the ambulatory patient with special reference to its use in herpes zoster. Ann Intern Med 1950;32:257-260.

11. Marmer MJ. Acute herpes zoster: Successful treatment by continuous epidural analgesia. Calif Med 1965;103:277-279.

12. Colding A. The effect of regional sympathetic blocks in the treatment of herpes zoster. Acta Anaesth Scand 1969;13:133-141.

13. Tamesa T, Wakasugi B, Yuda Y, et al. Nerve block therapy in the treatment of herpes zoster. Masui 1971;20:903-905.

14. Colding A. Treatment of pain: Organization of a pain clinic: Treatment of acute herpes zoster. Proc R Soc Med 1973;66:541-543.

15. Gale DA. The management of neuralgias complicating herpes zoster. Practitioner 1973;219:794-798.

16. Motegi K, Bamba S, Shimizu M, et al. A case of topical application of rifampicin with blocks of the infraorbital nerve and stellate ganglion in the treatment of herpes zoster. J Jpn Stomatol Soc 1973;40:80-84.

17. Miyazaki T, Masaharu O. The nerve block treatment of herpes zoster. Am Soc Anesth Annual Meeting Abstracts 1974:173-174.

18. Tamesa T, Wakasugi B, Yuda Y. Nerve block therapy in the treatment of herpes zoster in the pain clinic. Masui 1974;22:333-339.

19. Masud KZ, Forster KJ. Sympathetic block in herpes zoster. Am Family Physician 1975;12:142-144.

20. Mani M, Keh L, Lee KN, Winnie AP, Salem MR, Collins VJ. Sympathetic blockade for herpes zoster and postherpetic neuralgia. Am Soc Anesth Annual Meeting Abstract 1976:469.

21. Rickles JA. Ambulatory use of sympathetic nerve blocks: Present day clinical indications. Angiology 1977;28:394-400.

22. Perkins HM, Hanlon PR. Epidural injection of local anesthetic and steroids for relief of pain secondary to herpes zoster. Arch Surg 1978;113:253-254.

23. Bauman J. Treatment of acute herpes zoster neuralgia by epidural injection or stellate ganglion block. Anesthesiology 1979;51:S223.

24. LaFlamme MY, Labrecque B, Mignault G. Zona ophthalmique: Traitement de la nevralgie zonateuse par infiltrations stellaires repetees. Can J Ophthalmol 1979;14:99-101.

25. Schreuder M, Fothergill WT. Shingles: a belt of roses from hell. Br Med J 1979;1:5.

26. Bettinger R, Patrick L, Thompson R. Outpatient therapy prevents or relieves herpes zoster pain. Anesth News 1981;7:1.

27. Riopelle JM, Naraghi M, Grush KP. Chronic neuralgia incidence following local anesthetic therapy for herpes zoster. Arch Dermatol 1984;120:747-750.

28. Tenicela R, Lovasik D, Eaglstein W. Treatment of herpes zoster with sympathetic blocks. Clin J Pain 1985;1:63-67.

29. Brownlee KA. Statistical Theory and Methodology in Science and Engineering. John Wiley & Sons, New York, 1960:155.

30. Conover WJ. Practical Nonparametric Statistics. John Wiley & Sons, New York, 1971:140-149.

31. Burgoon CF, Jr, Burgoon JS. The natural history of herpes zoster. JAMA 1957;164:265-269.

32. Selander D, Mansson LG, Karlsson L, Svanvic J. Adrenergic vasoconstriction in peripheral nerves of the rabbit. Anesthesiology 1985;62:6-10.

33. Lundborg G. Structure and function of the intraneural microvessels as related to trauma, edema formation, and nerve function. J Bone & Joint Surg 1975;57-A:938-948.

34. Fink BR, Cairns AM. A bioenergetic basis for peripheral nerve fiber dissociation. Pain 1982;12:307-317.

35. Fink BR, Cairns AM. Differential tolerance of mammalian myelinated and unmyelinated nerve fibers to oxygen lack. Reg Anes 1982;7:2-6.

36. Noordenbos W. Pain. Elsevier, Amsterdam, 1959.

37. Melzack R, Wall PD. Pain mechanisms: New theory. Science 1965;150:971-979.

38. McKendrick MD, McGill JI, Wood MJ: Lack of effect of acyclovir on postherpetic neuralgia. Br Med J 1989;298:431.

UPDATE ON ANATOMY, PHYSIOLOGY AND PHARMACOLOGY OF EPIDURAL NEURAL BLOCKADE

M. J. Cousins and B. T. Veering

Although techniques of epidural anesthesia do not offer the economy of drug dosage or degrees of blockade of spinal anesthesia, they are currently more versatile and better studied. No other neural blockade techniques are used as extensively in each of the fields of surgical anesthesia, obstetric anesthesia, and diagnosis and management of acute and chronic pain. Epidural blockade is also unique because of special features of the anatomic site of injection and the resultant diverse sites of action of the local anesthetic solution.

The most practical and widely used continuous method of neural blockade is spinal epidural blockade; pharmacokinetic data have helped to increase the efficacy and safety of epidural infusion techniques. New developments in the understanding of pain conduction have extended the use of continuous epidural blockade to the administration of drugs that selectively block pain conduction, while leaving sensation, motor power, and sympathetic function essentially unchanged. The safety and the reliability of spinal epidural catheter techniques with the addition of bacterial filters, have permitted relief of acute pain and chronic pain for many days, often with patients remaining ambulatory. This has heralded an even more vigorous and fruitful era of investigation and clinical application of epidural blockade than did the unprecedented development of the past 20 years.

APPLIED ANATOMY OF EPIDURAL BLOCKADE: AN UPDATE

The reader should review the description of the anatomy of bony spine, ligaments, meninges, cerebrospinal fluid (CSF), and spinal arteries since this is directly applicable to epidural blockade.

T. H. Stanley et al. (eds.), Pain Management and Anesthesiology, 277–294.
© 1998 *Kluwer Academic Publishers. Printed in the Netherlands.*

THE POSTERIOR EPIDURAL SPACE

During the previous years new techniques have been used to investigate the anatomy of the epidural space, in particular the lumbar region. These developments include endoscopic examination, computed tomography, magnetic resonance and cryomicrotome section (1-6).

Cryomicrotome sectioning of cadavers, in which the spine is frozen in situ allows examination of the epidural anatomy less distorted by artefact (6). Using this technique, segmentally distributed compartments in the epidural space were observed posteriorly, laterally and anteriorly, being partly occupied with nerves, fat and fibrous tissue. Fat appeared to be the principal epidural tissue. Basically posterior and lateral compartments were found to be discontinuous circumferentially, with a repeated metameric segmentation of the epidural contents in the longitudinal axis (Figure 1). Posterior compartments were formed between the middle of one lamina and the cranial edge of the next lower lamina, limited dorsally by the flaval ligaments. These posterior compartments were separated by areas, where the dura is attached directly to the cranial part of the vertebral lamina and the vertebral arches. The contents of the posterior epidural compartment are separated from the lateral contents by an intervening area where the dura is against the lamina with no tissue between. In

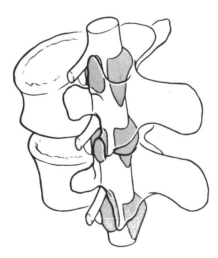

Figire.1.   Posterior Epidural Space (see text). Reproduced with permission from Cousins MJ, Veering B. Epidural Neural Blockade. In Cousins MJ, Bridenbaugh PO (Eds), Neural Blockade in Clinical Anesthesia and Management of Pain, 3rd Edition, J.B. Lippincott, Philadelphia, 1998, pp 243-321

normal conditions the respective subcompartments usually show a mutu-
ally free communication as can be demonstrated on epidurograms
(canalgrams) (7). Injected solutions can pass from compartment to compartment, since the dura is not adherent to the canal wall. The compart-
mentalization of the epidural space is supported by observations using
computed tomographic and magnetic resonance imaging (3-5).

Various studies have demonstrated a fold in the posterior dura
along the midline (1,8,2). This fold has been termed the *plica mediana
dorsalis* and is formed as the dura is prevented from collapsing by fibrous
strands going from the ligamentum flavum to the medial portion of the
dura (Figure 2). This is the matter which is demonstrated when a considerable quantity of air or fluid is injected in the lumbosacral epidural space,

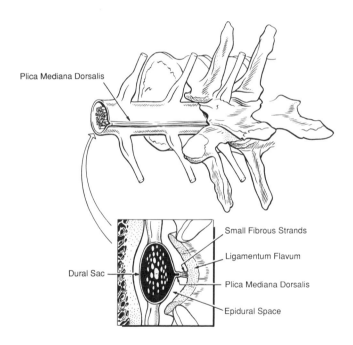

Figure.2. The dural sac after removal of an arch of a vertebra. The dorsal plica mediana is seen as a dural fold. Enlarged view shows median fibrous strands going
from the ligamentum flavum to the median portion of the dura. Consequently
these strands will give rise to a dorsomedian fold of the dura mater, i.e., the
plica mediana dorsalis. Reproduced with permission from Cousins MJ, Veering
B. Epidural Neural Blockade. In Cousins MJ, Bridenbaugh PO (Eds), Neural
Blockade in Clinical Anesthesia and Management of Pain, 3rd Edition, J.B.
Lippincott, Philadelphia, 1998, pp 243-321

compressing the dural sac and distorting the anatomy. During epiduroscopy Blomberg (1) observed in cadavers a dorsomedian connective tissue band between the dura and the flaval ligaments, which fixed the dura and caused a dorsomedian fold. However conclusions derived from examination of cadavers should be applied with care to the situation of clinical epidural anesthesia. The pressure of the cerebrospinal space in cadavers is very low or completely equalized with atmospheric pressure, causing the dura to collapse. The observed dorsomedian fold is thereby accentuated. In living humans a dorsomedian connective tissue band causing a dorsomedian fold of the dura mater was also seen by epiduroscopy, but not as prominent as that seen in cadavers (2). In this study, the epidural space was found to be present as a potential space, that opened up only temporarily as small increments of air were injected. A distinction should however be made between the substantial fold of the dura mater itself and the dorsomedian ligamentous strands connecting the lumbar sac to the ventral side of the vertebral arches (9). The clinical relevance of the dorsomedian connective tissue band of the dura mater has been related to the possibility of developing unilateral epidural blockade (10). Probably it is not the dorsomedian tissue band that causes problems but the technique used. Most likely other factors, such as the position of the catheter and injection of small volumes of local anesthetic solution are more frequently responsible for the development of a unilateral block.

EPIDURAL PRESSURES

The epidural space is identified traditionally by the negative pressure in the space believed to be created by tenting of the dura by the advancing needle, (11-14). Blunt needles with side openings produce the greatest negative pressures: they produce a good "coning" effect of the dura without puncturing it and transmit the negative pressure well because of their side opening.

By using a manometer attached to the advancing needle Usubiaga et al. (15) found negative epidural entry pressures measured at cervical, thoracic, lumbar and sacral levels. Also a relationship was demonstrated between the pressure generated at injection into the epidural space and the extent of block that developed. However in these early reports the instantaneous entry epidural pressures were only obtained. Using a closed measurement system which permitted continuous measurement of positive and negative pressure, Telford and Hollway (16) studied the pressures generated during deliberate dural puncture with a Tuohy needle. Such a closed measurement system facilitates the development of large transdural pressure gradients because of the inability of the epidural space pressure to equilibrate with subatmospheric pressure. Epidural space pressures were always positive with the needle stationary in the epidural space, except when the subarachnoid space was to be entered. The negative pressure that then developed was stated to be artificial and caused by tenting of the dura by the blunt Tuohy needle. The authors reported that spontaneous respiration with its associated negative intrapleural pressure would be insufficient to cause negative lumbar epidural pressure. A similar device was used to measure thoracic epidural pressure continuously at the time of insertion a Tuohy needle at the T7-8 intervertebral level using a loss of resistance technique (17). High negative epidural pressures up to -60mmHg were only observed at the moment of epidural puncture, equilibrating to a positive value within 90 seconds in both expiratory and inspiratory phases. This suggests that subsequent adaptation of the surrounding tissue results in restoration of the normal positive epidural pressure.

Shah (18) demonstrated with Macintosh balloon indicators attached to Tuohy needles that the lumbar epidural pressure increased with stimuli known to increase CSF pressure like jugular venous compression, ventilation with carbon dioxide and positive end expiratory pressure. The increase in epidural pressure produced by jugular venous compression agreed with those of Usubiaga (15). This suggests that the lumbar epidural pressure is in equilibrium with the prevailing spinal CSF pressure.

Paul and Wildsmith (19) investigated the influence of the pressure generated by low lumbar epidural injection of two different volumes of bupivacaine upon epidural pressure and showed that the epidural pressure stabilized within 60 seconds, irrespective of the pressure applied by the local anesthetic injection. The same plateau pressure in both groups at the upper limit of normal for CSF pressure suggests a pressure-limiting feature in the epidural space; displacement of CSF may be the main safety valve limiting epidural pressure. In addition no significant correlation was found between the individual level of analgesia and the epidural pressure at any time or with patient characteristics. The authors suggest that a relationship might exist between the height of the pressure and an increase in the escape of injected fluid from the space through the intervertebral foramina to the paravertebral space.

If one routinely uses a *negative pressure test* for epidural puncture, it is important to be aware of factors that result in marked changes in epidural pressure. In severe lung diseases such as emphysema, epidural negative pressure may be abolished, particularly if the patient is lying down (20,21). Any factor that increases abdominal pressure and/or occlusion of the inferior vena cava may distend the epidural veins and increase pressure in the lumbar epidural space. This results in only slight changes in the thoracic epidural space, particularly if the patient is sitting (15). During labor, baseline lumbar epidural pressures are higher in women in the supine position compared with those in the lateral position. As labour progresses, baseline pressures increase to as high as +10cm water at full dilatation (22). Also, there are peaks of epidural pressure during each uterine contraction, with increases of 8-15cm of water (23).

Coughing or a Valsalva maneuver increases both intrathoracic and intra-abdominal pressure, so that pressure in thoracic and lumbar epidural space increases (15), resulting in high positive pressures being recorded throughout the epidural space.

Comparison of patients having prior lumbar surgery, to those who did not, revealed a higher baseline lumbar epidural space in patients with previous lumbar surgery (24). However additional pressure from epidural injections decays at a similar rate to that in patients who did not undergo operations. This suggests that the alteration induced by surgery is one of different initial condition, rather than a change in distensibility. On the other hand the resistance to fluid injection in the epidural space was higher in patients with a diseased space as the result of epiduro-arachnoiditis compared with that of the normal space (25). Therefore one should be careful with the injection of fluid into parts of the epidural space that do not communicate freely with the surroundings.

Studies by Usubiaga (15) have helped to explain why successful entry into the epidural space is sometimes followed by 'drip back' when local anesthetic is subsequently injected; classic pressure-volume compliance studies showed that compliance decreased with increasing age and that residual pressure after injection of 10ml of solution at a standard rate had a positive correlation with age. Thus, some patients with a low compliance in the epidural space will be unable to accommodate a large volume of solution if it is injected rapidly; 'drip back' will be less common in young patients and if injection is made slowly because, although there was a transient increase in epidural pressure in young patients, Usubiaga found that pressure was essentially back to baseline in 30 seconds.

PHARMACOLOGIC ASPECTS OF EPIDURAL BLOCKADE: AN UPDATE

EFFECT OF AGE

Over the past several years the anesthesiologist has been faced with a growing number of elderly patients presenting for surgery. Epidural anesthesia has enjoyed a resurgence of popularity for elderly patients undergoing surgery in areas amenable to conduction anesthesia. With advancing age anatomic changes do occur in the epidural space (26). In the young individual the areolar tissue around the intervertebral foramina is soft and loose. In the elderly, this areolar tissue becomes dense and firm, partially sealing the intervertebral foramina (27). With aging the dura becomes more permeable to local anesthetic, because of significant increase in the size of the arachnoid villi (28).

Discrepancies exist between studies in which the influence of age on epidural anesthesia has been assessed. The classical study of Bromage regarding the influence of age on epidural spread reported a strong relationship between age and the epidural segmental dose requirement. [E.S.D.R.]; i.e., the amount (dose) of local anesthetic required to block one spinal segment (29). Assuming a linear dose-relationship, Bromage demonstrated that with age the E.S.D.R. decreased in a linear way. In contrast to Bromage's assumption others have found no direct linear relationship between volume and anesthetic spread (30-33). The greater the total amount used , the greater the E.S.D.R. calculated.

From this it can be concluded that the results of Bromage's study concerning the linear decrease of E.S.D.R. with age are questionable, because he assumed a direct linear relationship between the amount (dose) of local anesthetic and extent of anesthesia and because he used variable total anesthetic amounts (29). Using a given dose (fixed volume and concentration) other investigators have found a significantly greater number of spinal segments blocked in older patients. However, the magnitude of this effect was small: only 1-3 segments more in the elderly patients compared to younger adult patients (30-37). When using different volumes the dose-effect relationship varied with these volumes (1,38).

Age has also been shown to be associated with a higher upper level of analgesia following thoracic epidural administration of a fixed dose of mepivacaine (39).

Increases in longitudinal spread of analgesia with increasing age have been attributed to reduced leakage of local anesthetic solution, because of progressive sclerotic closure of intervertebral foramina (26,27). Also the cephalad spread of radioactivity after epidural injection of iodine-131 mixed in 2 per cent lidocaine was higher in patients older than 50 years compared to younger ones (40). Radiological studies have however failed to show a relationship between age and spread in the epidural space (41). It is possible that radio-opaque material and local anesthetic do not spread in an identical manner. On the other hand the increased permeability of the dura with aging as described by Shantha and Evans (28) may contribute to the higher levels of the analgesic spread in the elderly. Usubiaga et al. (15) reported that older patients have a higher residual pressure and that there is a positive relationship between residual epidural pressure and the extent of analgesic spread. Also increased epidural compliance and decreased epidural resistance with advancing age may contribute to this enhanced spread in the elderly (42).

The onset time to maximal caudad spread has been reported to decrease with advancing age following epidural administration of bupivacaine, allowing surgery in areas innervated by these segments to be started sooner in older compared with younger patients (35,36). In addition a more rapid onset and enhanced intensity of motor blockade has been shown in older patients (36). With aging the neural population declines steadily within the spinal cord and peripheral nerves show a linear reduction in conduction velocity, especially in motor nerves (43). This could make older patients more sensitive to local anesthetics, which is probably (partially) the cause of the shorter onset time of analgesia in the caudad segments and the altered motor block profile. Nydahl et al. (37) reported a shorter duration of motor blockade, as assessed by electromyographic recordings, following epidural administration of epinephrine containing bupivacaine solutions. This may be attributed to a stronger reaction of younger subjects to epinephrine (44).

Epidural anesthesia carries some problems in elderly patients. The technique is technically more difficult, so there is always a chance of a failure. This is partially attributed to the fact that the ligamentum flavum probably changes into a form that is easily ossified (45).

The more extensive spread of analgesia is likely to be accompanied by more extensive sympathetic blockade. Therefore prevention of hypotension, by intravenous administration of crystalloid fluids, will be very important in older patients. It should be emphasized however that rapid volume preloading constitutes a potential risk in elderly patients with poor cardiac function, in whom there is a risk of pulmonary edema and cardiac failure. With epidural anesthesia there is a decline in the thermoregulatory response with age, as has been shown by the decrease in core temperature (46). Consequently the postoperative rewarming process will occur slower in older patients. Lumbar epidural anesthesia with lidocaine did not affect the resting ventilation parameters such as minute ventilation and tidal volume in older patients and stimulated the ventilatory response to hypercapnia to the same degree as in young patients (47). Therefore lumbar epidural anesthesia appears to be a safe technique in elderly patients.

ALTERATIONS OF ABSORPTION AND DISPOSITION:

EFFECT OF AGE

After a single epidural administration of lidocaine, the peak plasma concentrations are unaffected by age (48). The peak plasma concentrations and corresponding peak times of bupivacaine after epidural administration do not seem to change with age (35,36). In order to evaluate the role of the pharmacokinetics i.e., the rate of systemic absorption in the observed age related change in the clinical profile of epidural anesthesia with bupivacaine a stable isotope method has been used (49,36). Bupivacaine shows a biphasic absorption profile; a rapid initial phase, followed by a much slower phase. The systemic absorption is unchanged with age.

Increasing age has shown to be associated with a decrease in the clearance of lidocaine (48) and bupivacaine after epidural administration (35,36). Consequently plasma concentrations will rise to higher levels with prolonged epidural infusion or with intermittent multiple administrations in older patients. The observed age-related decline in clearance of bupivacaine cannot be explained on the basis of changes in serum protein binding, but probably reflects a concomitant decline in hepatic enzyme activity.

PHYSIOLOGICAL EFFECTS OF EPIDURAL BLOCKADE: AN UPDATE

LUMBAR EPIDURAL BLOCK AND GENERAL ANESTHESIA

Lumbar epidural anesthesia combined with general anesthesia is commonly used for prolonged major lower abdominal and pelvic surgery. Combined epidural and general anesthesia offers the advantage of a rapid and less painful recovery. This combination technique may result in a greater degree of hypotension than with each technique alone. The cardiovascular effects of combined lumbar epidural and general anesthesia have received relatively little attention in the literature to date.

Stephen (50) and colleagues studied the combination of lumbar epidural block administered approximately 20 minutes after the induction of light anesthesia consisting of thiopentone-nitrous oxide-oxygen. Unfortunately, the level of blockade could not be recorded in this study, although it was likely to be in the region of T5, considering the dose of local anesthetic used (30ml of 2% plain lidocaine). Decreased venous return associated with this level of analgesia will result in increased vagal activity (51). This combination produced large reductions in arterial blood pressure up to 30%. Elevation of legs (to simulate a head down tilt) resulted in increased mean arterial pressure, central venous pressure and peripheral resistance, but no change in cardiac output, whereas intravenous bolus administration of ephedrine (10mg) increased both cardiac output and mean arterial pressure. Further reductions in arterial pressure were observed when epinephrine was added to the epidurally administered local anesthetic solution. The absorbed epinephrine stimulates β-adrenergic receptors in peripheral vascular beds, leading to vasodilatation and hypotension.

Nancarrow (52) and associates compared the cardiovascular effects of epidural block to T5 level, given before nitrous oxide-halothane (0.35% end-tidal) general anesthesia, with the same general anesthesia minus epidural block. Decreases in mean arterial pressure were significantly greater (up to 58%) in the epidural group whereas no changes were observed in the general anesthesia group. However decreases in liver blood flow and reductive metabolism of halothane were similar in both groups, despite the occurrence of significant decreases in arterial pressure. Wright and Fee (53) examined the effect of prophylactic treatment with intravenous fluid, 1000ml, ephedrine or methoxamine on cardiovascular responses to combined lumbar epidural anesthesia and general isoflurane anesthesia. Systolic arterial pressure was significantly greater after ephedrine than after preloading or methoxamine. The reduction in arterial blood pressure after induction of general anesthesia was associated with a decrease in vascular resistance after methoxamine. A decrease in venous return, resulting mostly in hypotension during epidural block, is less likely to occur following prophylactic administration of ephedrine, since the systemic vascular resistance is maintained at pre-block values. Goertz et al. (54) demonstrated that administration of phenylephrine boluses effectively restored mean arterial pressure in patients who were moderately hypotensive during lumbar epidural anesthesia combined with general anesthesia. The range of the level of analgesia was T8-T11. In addition the left ventricular function assessed by transesophageal echocardiography was unaltered. In summary it appears that light general anesthesia can be safely combined with epidural block to the level of T5 in healthy patients. Use of a slight head-down tilt to maintain venous return, small incremental doses of atropine to maintain heart rate of approximately 90 beats per minute are recommended to treat moderate hypotension during combined lumbar epidural and general anesthesia. If additional cardiovascular support is required ephedrine should be used depending on each patient's cardiovascular status.

EFFECTS OF THORACIC EPIDURAL BLOCKADE ON THE ISCHEMIC HEART

During experimentally induced myocardial ischemia in anesthetized dogs it has been shown that thoracic epidural anesthesia (TEA), with a selective blockade of cardiac sympathetic segments, favorably alters the myocardial oxygen supply/demand ration (55,56). Furthermore during coronary occlusion TEA improved the transmural distribution of regional myocardial blood flow by increasing the endocardial to epicardial blood flow ratio with maintenance of the coronary perfusion pressure (55). The altered distribution of myocardial blood flow is most likely to occur by the decreased inotropy, heart rate and impedance to left ventricular injection. Using a similar model, Davis et al. (56) confirmed these observations. The authors discovered that not only did thoracic sympathetic blockade enhance regional myocardial blood flow, but it also reduced the anatomic extent of the experimentally induced infarction. The most likely mechanism for this reduction in tissue injury was the pronounced reduction of heart rate and inotropy with little effect on coronary perfusion pressure observed in dogs with high TEA compared to control animals. In addition the incidence of ischemia-induced malignant arrhythmias in anesthetized rats was reduced by high TEA (57). Thus high TEA exerts a cardioprotective effect during experimental myocardial ischemia by improving the myocardial oxygen supply/demand ratio.

The influence of high thoracic epidural anesthesia with a plain solution of bupivacaine on central hemodynamics has been studied in patients with severe coronary artery disease and unstable angina pectoris (2,58). During basal conditions, i.e., during rest without ischemic pain, high TEA did not change the central hemodynamic variables. However, TEA achieved during ischemic chest pain, was associated with significantly reduced indices of myocardial oxygen demand, such as systolic arterial

288

blood pressure, heart rate and pulmonary capillary wedge pressure, accompanied in some patients by less pronounced S-T segment depression. The main variable regulating myocardial oxygen availability, coronary perfusion pressure, remained unchanged, as well as stroke volume, cardiac output and systemic vascular resistance. Significant arterial hypotension did not occur, possibly due to limited spread of the small volumes of bupivacaine injected. On the other hand a more extended TEA (from T1-T12) caused pronounced arterial hypotension to the detriment of coronary perfusion in similar patients (59). High TEA in association with physical stress also reduced ischemic chest pain and decreased heart rate in patients with unstable angina pectoris, in spite of maximal beta-adrenergic blockade, to a greater degree than in patients with beta-adrenergic blockers at rest (2). Thus depending on the prevailing cardiac sympathetic tone, high TEA may cause a greater or lesser number of changes in central hemodynamics in patients with coronary artery disease (CAD) who are being treated with beta adrenergic blockers. Furthermore it has been reported that high TEA improves ischemia induced left ventricular global and regional wall motion abnormalities, while diminishing associated changes in ST-segments in patients with CAD during physical stress (60). This is probably related to the decrease in left ventricular afterload per se, improving regional wall motion.

Regional cardiac sympathetic blockade with high TEA has been shown to increase the diameter of the lumina of diseased portions of epicardial coronary arteries in patients with severe coronary artery disease treated with beta blockers (61). However the diameter of non-stenotic epicardial coronary artery segments remained unchanged. These results indicate that there is a resting cardiac sympathetic alpha constrictor tone of the atherosclerotic epicardial coronary arteries.

Regional cardiac sympathetic blockade caused no changes in coronary perfusion pressure, myocardial blood flow, or coronary venous oxygen content, indicating a lack of effect on coronary resistance vessels. High TEA had probably no influence upon the autoregulation of coronary resistance vessels and should therefore not adversely affect regional blood flow distribution in patients with coronary artery disease, which provides a basis for coronary steal (i.e., maldistribution of coronary blood flow) (62,63).

THORACIC EPIDURAL ANESTHESIA AND GENERAL ANESTHESIA

Thoracic epidural anesthesia (TEA) associated with light general anesthesia is increasingly used for upper abdominal surgery and for major vascular surgery. Light general anesthesia with mechanical ventilation added to thoracic epidural anesthesia may induce substantial hypotension. Such hypotension arises mainly from a decrease in venous return and is also due to attenuation of the compensatory vasoconstriction of nonanesthetized sympathetic tone via central depressant effects on vasomotor center. So a combined technique of TEA plus light general anesthesia may alter hemodynamics, principally by a decrease in the loading conditions of the heart and by a negative inotropic effect resulting from both the cardiac sympathetic blockade and the direct myocardial depressant effect of general anesthesia (64,65).

Obviously the greatest concern for the consequences of hypotension is in patients with coronary artery disease. Coronary artery disease is common in patients undergoing major vascular surgery. Therefore these patients are prone to develop cardiac complications (66). Several studies have demonstrated a beneficial effect of TEA on the heart and coronary circulation in patients with coronary artery disease (37,58-61), This beneficial effect however cannot be extrapolated to patients receiving TEA combined with light general anesthesia. The fall in blood pressure induced by such a technique may compromise coronary blood flow and so myocardial oxygen supply, despite a decrease in myocardial oxygen consumption. In this context, Saada et al. (67) examined the effect of TEA, induced during light general anesthesia, on segmental ventricular wall motion (SWM) as monitored by transesophageal echocardiography. In patients with coronary artery disease scheduled for major vascular surgery, lidocaine 2%, 12.5ml was injected through an epidural catheter placed at T6-7 or T7-8, 30 minutes after induction of general anesthesia. TEA induced a decrease in heart rate, mean arterial pressure, cardiac index and estimated coronary perfusion pressure due to sympathetic blockade. Pulmonary occlusion pressure remained constant owing to colloid infusion. Despite these reductions, TEA plus light general anesthesia did not worsen (or improve) ventricular wall motion or induce myocardial ischemia, suggesting that myocardial oxygen balance was maintained. In an earlier almost identical study by the same group it was shown that lumbar epidural anesthesia may cause impairment of SWM, indicating myocardial ischemia (68). In comparing these two studies it would seem that block of the efferent sympathetic innervation to the heart that occurs with TEA but not with lumbar epidural blockade has beneficial effects. Despite prophylactic intravenous hydration, TEA plus general anesthesia may cause hypotension requiring vasopressor therapy. In clinical practice ephedrine and phenylephrine are the two agents that are commonly recommended to treat hypotension during epidural anesthesia associated with general anesthesia (53). Ideally the vasopressor agent should restore blood pressure without increasing heart rate or impairing left ventricular function. Ephedrine and phenylephrine may differently affect left ventricular (LV) function in high risk patients. Accordingly Samain et al.(69) determined the effects of ephedrine versus phenylephrine on LV function in high risk patients who developed arterial hypotension during high thoracic epidural anesthesia combined with general anesthesia. Level of analgesia extended to T3 in these patients who received epidural block before general anesthesia. LV function was assessed by transesophageal echocardiography. Both cardiac index and ejection fraction area were significantly compromised when phenylephrine was given. This is consistent with the results of Goertz (54) who determined the effect of phenylephrine bolus administration on LV function during TEA combined with general anesthesia in patients without cardiovascular disease. When ephedrine was given no acceleration of heart rate was noted. In addition the rise in blood pressure did not compromise LV emptying. Thus ephedrine appears to be the drug of choice to restore blood pressure under TEA associated with general anesthesia.

The evidence in animals and humans now points strongly to a beneficial effect of <u>restricted</u> thoracic epidural neural blockade on cardiac performance in patients with compromised cardiac function (70).

There is an emerging role for <u>adjunctive</u> high thoracic epidural block (restricted T1-T4 block) during and after coronary artery bypass surgery. Tunnelled epidural catheters and "Portacath" systems are also being used for palliation of intractable angina in patients awaiting, or unsuitable for, coronary revascularization. These applications in acute and chronic pain management have arisen from meticulous basic and clinical research.

ACKNOWLEDGMENT

The material in this chapter is largely drawn from: Cousins M.J., Veering, B. Epidural Neural Blockade. <u>In</u>: Cousins M.J. Bridenbaugh P.O. (Eds) Neural Blockade in Clinical Anesthesia and Pain Management. 3rd Edition J.B. Lippincott Philadelphia pp 243-321, 1998.

References
1. Blomberg R: The dorsomedian connective tissue band in the lumbar epidural space of humans. Anesth Analg 65:747, 1986.
2. Blomberg RG, Olsson SS: The lumbar epidural space in patients examined with epiduroscopy. Anesth Analg 68:157, 1989.

3. Savolaine ER, Pandya JB, Greenblatt SH, Conover SR: Anatomy of the human lumbar epidural space: New insights using CT-. Anesthesiology 68:217, 1988.

4. Ho PS, Yu S, Sether L, et al: Ligamentum flavum: appearance on sagittal and coronal MR images. Radiology 168:469, 1988.

5. Westbrook JL, Renowden SA, Carrie LES: Study of the anatomy of the extradural region using magnetic resonance imaging. Br J Anaesth, 71:495, 1993.

6. Hogan QH: Lumbar epidural anatomy: A new look by cryomicrotome section. Anesthesiology 75:767, 1991.

7. Luyendyk W, van Voorthuisen AE: Contrast examination of the spinal epidural space. Acta Radio 5:1051, 1966.

8. Luyendyk W: The plica mediana dorsalis of the dura mater and its relation to lumbar peridurography (canalography). Neuroradiology 11: 147, 1976.

9. Huson A, Luyendyk W, Tielbeek A, Van Zundert A: CT-Epidurography and the anatomy of the human epidural space. Anesthesiology 69:797, 1988.

10. McCrae AF, Whitfield A, McClure JH: Repeated unilateral epidural blockade. Anaesthesia, 47:859, 1992.

11. Bromage PR: The "hanging-drop" sign. Anaesthesia, 8:237, 1953.

12. Janzen E: Der Negative Vorschlag bei Lumbalpunktion: Dtsch. Z Nervenheilk, 94:280, 1926.

13. Eaton LM: Observations on the negative pressure in the epidural space. Mayo Clin, Proc, 14:566, 1939.

14. Usubiaga JE, Dos Reis A, Usubiaga LE: Epidural misplacement of catheters and mechanisms of unilateral blockade. Anesthesiology, 32: 158, 1970.

15. Usubiaga JE, Moya F, Usubiaga LE: Effect of thoracic and abdominal pressure changes on the epidural space pressure. Br J Anaesth 39:612, 1967.

16. Telford RJ, Hollway TE: Observations on deliberate dural puncture with a Tuohy needle: pressure measurement. Anaesthesia 46:725, 1991.

17. Okutomi T, Watanabe S, Goto F: Time course in thoracic epidural pressure measurement. Can J Anaesth 40:1044, 1993.

18 Shah JL: Positive lumbar extradural space pressure. Br J Anaesth 73:309, 1994.

19. Paul D, Wildsmith JAW: Extradural pressure following the injection of two volumes of bupivacaine. Br J Anaesth 62:368, 1989.

20. Frank NR, Mead J, Ferris BG: The mechanical behaviour of the lungs in healthy elderly persons. J Clin Invest 36:1680, 1957.

21. Pierce, JA Ebert RV: The elastic properties of the lungs of the aged. J Lab Clin Me, 51:63, 1958.

22. Galbert MW, Marx GF: Extradural pressures in the parturient patient. Anesthesiology 40:499, 1974.

23. Bromage PR: Epidural needle. Anesthesiology, 22:1018, 1961.

24. Thomas PS, Gerson JI, Strong G: Analysis of human epidural pressures. Reg Anesth 17:212, 1992.
25. Rocco AG, Scott DA, Boas RA, Philip HH: Epidural space behaves as a Starling resistor and inflow resistance is higher in spinal stenosis than in disc disease. Anesthesiology 73:A816, 1990.
26. Bromage PR: Mechanism of action of extradural analgesia. Br J Anaesth 47:199, 1975.
27. Bromage PR: Epidural analgesia. Philadelphia, W.B. Saunders, 1978.
28. Shantha TR, Evans JA: The relationship of epidural anesthesia to neural membranes and arachnoid villi. Anesthesiology 37:543, 1972.
29. Bromage PR: Ageing and epidural dose requirements. Segmental spread and predictability of epidural analgesia in youth and extreme age. Br J Anaesth 41:1016, 1969.
30. Grundy EM, et al: Extradural analgesia revisited. A statistical study. Br J Anaesth 50:805, 1978.
31. Park WY, Hagins FM, Rivat EL, MacNamara TE: Age and epidural dose response in adult men. Anesthesiology 56:318, 1982.
32. Park WY, Massengale M, Kin SI, et al: Age and the spread of local anesthetic solutions in the epidural space. Anesth Analg (Cleve), 59:768, 1980.
33. Sharrock NE: Epidural anesthetic dose responses in patients 20-80 years old. Anesthesiology, 49:425, 1978.
34. Rosenberg PH, Saramies L, Alila A: Lumbar epidural anaesthetic with bupivacaine in old patients: Effect of speed and direction of injection. Acta Anaesth Scand, 25:270, 1981.
35. Veering BT, Burm AGL, Van Kleef JW, et al: Epidural anesthesia with bupivacaine: effects of age on neural blockade and pharmacokinetics. Anesth Analg 66:589, 1987.
36. Veering BT, Burm AGL, Vletter AA, et al: The effect of age on the systemic absorption and systemic disposition of bupivacaine after epidural administration. Clin Pharmacokinet 22:75, 1992.
37. Nydahl PA, Philipson L, Axelsson K, Johansson JE: Epidural anesthesia with 0.5% bupivacaine: influence of age on sensory and motor blockade. Anesth Analg, 73:780, 1991.
38. Anderson S, Cold GE: Dose response studies in elderly patients subjected to epidural analgesia. Acta Anaesthesiol Scand 25:279, 1981.
39. Hirabayashi Y, Shimozu R: Effect of age on extradural dose requirement in thoracic extradural anaesthesia. Br J Anaesth 71:445, 1993.
40. Nishimura N, Kitahara T, Kusakabe T: The spread of lidocaine and 1-131 solution in the epidural space. Anesthesiology 20:785, 1959.
41. Burn JM, Guyer PB, Langdon L: The spread of solutions injected into the epidural space: A study using epidurograms in patients with the lumbosciatic syndrome. Br J Anaesth 45:338, 1973.
42. Hirabayashi Y, Shimizu R, Matsuda I, Inoue S: Effect of extradural compliance and resistance on spread of extradural analgesia. Br J Anaesth 65:508, 1990.

43. Dorfman L J, Bosley TM: Age-related changes in peripheral and central nerve conduction in man. Neurology 29:38, 1979.

44. Vestal RE, Wood AJJ, Shand DG: Reduced beta-adrenoceptor sensitivity in the elderly. Clin Pharmacol Ther 26:181, 1979.

45. Okada A, Harata S, Takeda Y, et al: Age-related changes in proteoglycans of human ligamentum flavum. Spine 18:2261, 1993.

46. Frank SM, Shir Y, Raja SN, Fleisher LA, Beattie C: Core hypothermia and skin surface temperature gradients. Epidural versus general anesthesia and the effects of age. Anesthesiology 80:502, 1994.

47. Sakura S, Saito Y, Kosaka Y: Effect of extradural anaesthesia on the ventilatory response to hypoxaemia. Anaesthesia 48:205, 1993.

48. Bowdle TA, Freund PR, Slattery JT: Age dependent lidocaine pharmacokinetics during lumbar peridural anesthesia with lidocaine hydrocarbonate or lidocaine hydrochloride. Reg Anesth, 11: 123, 1986.

49. Burm AGL: Clinical pharmacokinetics of epidural and spinal anaesthesia. Clin Pharmacokinet 16:283, 1989.

50. Stephen GW, Lees MM, Scott DB: Cardiovascular effects of epidural block combined with general anaesthesia. Br J Anaesth 41:933, 1969.

51. Baron JF, Decaux-Jacolot A, Edouard A, et al: Influence of venous return on baroreflex control of heart rate during lumbar epidural anesthesia in humans. Anesthesiology 64:188, 1986.

52. Nancarrow C, Plummer JL, Isley AH, McLean CF, et al: Effects of combined extradural blockade and general anaesthesia on indocyanine green clearance and halothane metabolism. Br J Anaesth 58:29, 1986.

53. Wright PMC, Fee JPH: Cardiovascular support during combined extradural and general anesthesia. Br J Anaesth 68:585, 1992.

54. Goertz AW, Seeling W, Heinriech H, et al: Effect of phenylephrine bolus administration on left ventricular function during high thoracic and lumbar epidural anesthesia combined with general anesthesia. Anesth Analg 76:541, 1993.

55. Klassen GA, Bramwell RS, Bromage PR, Zborowska-Sluis DT: The effect of acute sympathectomy by epidural anesthesia on the canine coronary circulation. Anesthesiology 52:8, 1980.

56. Davis, RF DeBoer WV, Maroko PR: Thoracic epidural anesthesia reduces myocardial infarct size after coronary artery occlusion in dogs. Anesth Analg, 65:711 1986.

57. Blomberg S, Ricksten SE: Thoracic epidural anesthesia decreases the incidence of ventricular arrhythmias during acute myocardial ischemia in anaesthetised rats. Acta Anaesthesiol Scand 32:173, 1988.

58. Blomberg S, Curelaru J, Emanuelsson H, et al: Thoracic epidural anaesthesia in patients with unstable angina pectoris. Eur Heart J 10:437, 1989.

59. Reiz S, Nath S, Rais O: Effects of thoracic block and prenalterol on coronary vascular resistance and myocardial metabolism in patients with coronary artery disease. Acta Anaesthesiol Scand 24:11, 1980.

60. Koch M, Blomberg S, Emanuelsson H, et al: Thoracic epidural anesthesia improves global and regional left ventricular function during

stress induced myocardial ischemia in patients with coronary artery disease. Anesth Analg 71:625, 1990.

61. Blomberg S, Emanuelsson H, Kvist H, et al: Effects of thoracic epidural anesthesia on coronary arteries and arterioles in patients with coronary artery disease. Anesthesiology 73:840, 1990.

62. Heusch G, Deussen A, Thamer V: Cardiac sympathetic nerve activity and progressive vasoconstriction distal to coronary stenosis: feedback aggravation of myocardial ischemia. J Auton Nerve Syst 13:311, 1985.

63. Buffington CW, Davis, KB, Gillispie S: The prevalence of steal prone-coronary anatomy in patients with coronary artery disease: an analysis of the coronary artery surgery study registry. Anesthesiology 69:721, 1988.

64. Reiz S, Balfors E, Sorensen MB, et al: Coronary hemodynamic effects of general anesthesia and surgery: Modification by epidural analgesia in patients with ischemic heart disease. Reg Anaesth 7[Suppl]:S8, 1982.

65. Wattwil M, Sundberg A, Arvill, Lennquist C: Circulatory changes during high thoracic epidural anesthesia—influence of sympathetic block and of systemic effect of the local anaesthetic. Acta Anaesthesiol Scand 29:849, 1985.

66. Tuman KJ, McCarthy RJ, March RJ, et al: Effects of epidural anesthesia and analgesia on coagulation and outcome after major vascular surgery. Anesth Analg 73:696, 1991.

67. Saada M, Catoire P, Bonnet F, et al: Effects of thoracic epidural anesthesia with general anesthesia on segmental wall motion assessed by transesophageal echocardiography. Anesth Analg 75:329, 1992.

68. Saada M, Duval AM, Bonnet F, et al: Abnormalities in myocardial segmental wall motion during lumbar epidural anesthesia. Anesthesiology 71:26, 1989.

69. Samain C, Coriat P, Le Bret F, et al: Ephedrine vs phenylephrine for hypotension due to thoracic epidural anesthesia associated with general anesthesia: effects on left ventricular function. Anesthesiology 73:A82, 1989.

70. Meibner A, Rolf N, Van Aken H: Thoracic epidural anesthesia and the patient with heart disease: benefits, risks and controversies. Anesth Analg (In press 1997).

THE INTERFACE BETWEEN ACUTE AND
CHRONIC PAIN MANAGEMENT

L. B. Ready

INTRODUCTION

There is widespread interest among anesthesiologists in the management of acute and postoperative pain (1) and many have focused attention on development of in-hospital services to improve care in these areas. Many acute pain services are designed primarily to address management of well defined pain of short duration. The treatment offered is primarily pharmacologic and is provided by such modalities as patient-controlled analgesia, neuraxial opioids or opioid/local anesthetic mixtures, and local anesthetic blockade. Treatment objectives are typically to alleviate pain, preserve function (e.g., ambulation, effective coughing), and to prevent complications of surgery that cause morbidity and increase medical costs.

By contrast, only a small proportion of anesthesiologists wish to participate in the treatment of chronic pain—a pattern also seen among primary care physicians and other medical specialties. Although anesthesiologists who manage chronic pain are a dedicated minority, many facilities have been described for its evaluation and treatment. The frequently used multidisciplinary approach often includes a focus on the importance of psychosocial influences, and on including behavioral change and increased function as treatment goals (2).

Those who choose to manage acute pain should recognize that it is not possible to completely isolate this task while avoiding all involvement with chronic main management. Patients with underlying cancer pain commonly experience acute pain following surgical procedures. The patient with chronic low back pain will require control of surgical pain following a laminectomy. And patients with sickle cell disease are likely to experience pain problems that are both acute and chronic in nature. These

T. H. Stanley et al. (eds.), Pain Management and Anesthesiology, 295–301.

and many other examples represent some of the most complex and difficult challenges that the acute pain therapist will encounter.

DEFINITIONS

A clear understanding of common terminology and correct use of these terms is essential in making appropriate treatment decisions for patients in both acute and chronic pain. Lack of this understanding is a common reason for therapeutic problems.

1. NOCICEPTION

Nociception is defined as potentially tissue-damaging thermal or mechanical energy acting on the specialized nerve endings of A-delta and C fibers. Nociception usually leads to pain after it is perceived.

2. PAIN

A simple definition of pain is the perception of nociceptive input. Two important features about pain should be emphasized. First, nociceptive input must be perceived to become pain. Second, it is possible to perceive a nociceptive event when no tissue-damaging energy has been imparted to the body. This type of pain reflects alterations within the nervous system so that centrally conducting axons and their synapses are activated as if there had been a peripheral stimulus (e.g., phantom limb pain).

3. SUFFERING

Suffering is a negative affective response generated in higher centers by pain and other emotional situations (e.g., stress, anxiety, depression, loss of a loved one). It is essential to recognize that suffering is not uniquely related to pain in spite of the fact that the language of pain is extensively utilized to refer to suffering.

4. PAIN BEHAVIOR

Suffering usually leads to pain behavior which can be defined as any output from an individual that is commonly understood to suggest the existence of a tissue-damaging stimulus. Common examples include verbal expressions (e.g., moaning), posture (e.g., grimace, limp), seeking of health care, or refusing to work. Although all pain behavior is real, it does not necessarily indicate nociception. The proper question is not, "Does this patient hurt?" but "What factors lead to this patient's pain behavior?" It is rare to find a patient with chronic pain whose pain does not have multiple etiologic factors.

5. DEFINITIONS RELATED TO OPIOID THERAPY

A number of terms in this category are also commonly used as though they are interchangeable. This practice frequently leads to misunderstanding and inappropriate treatment decisions. The following definitions should be familiar to all therapists managing pain, particularly with opioids.

A. PHARMACOLOGIC TOLERANCE

Tolerance can be defined to indicate that a patient is less susceptible to the effect of a drug as a consequence of it prior administration. Clinically, in relation to the treatment of pain with opioids, it is manifested as a pattern of increasing dose requirement to maintain a given level of analgesia.

B. PHYSICAL DEPENDENCE

Physical dependence is a pharmacologic property of opioids characterized by the occurrence of an abstinence syndrome after abrupt discontinuation of the drug or administration of an antagonist. Although often associated with signs of tolerance, the emergence of a withdrawal syndrome alone is considered sufficient to use this term. The label does not imply the aberrant psychological state or behaviors of the addicted patient.

C. ADDICTION

Addiction is a chronic disorder characterized by the compulsive use of a substance resulting in physical, psychological, or social harm to the user, and continued use despite that harm. The term implies "psychological and physical need for opioid intake, coexisting with the craving of opioids and drug-seeking behavior" (3). Addiction often results in illegal or dishonest behavior such as prescription forgery or theft, tampering with drug-related devices such as PCA machines or "sharps" containers, and obtaining controlled substances from multiple prescribers without disclosure.

In general, management of acute pain will become progressively more complex and more difficult for the therapist to treat as one moves from opioid-naive patients to those with tolerance, dependence, and addiction.

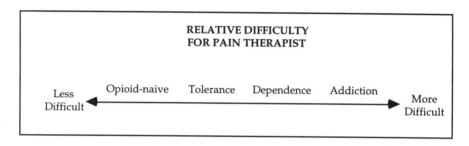

Table. Differences between acute and chronic pain.	
Acute Pain	*Chronic Pain*
Signals an organic disease process.	No useful function served.
Cause is usually obvious.	Cause is often unclear.
Disappears with treatment of the cause.	Often unresponsive to many forms of therapy.
Opioids typically indicated and effective.	Opioids only indicated and effective in highly selected cases.
No secondary gains.	Secondary gains commonly present.

PAIN ASSESSMENT

It can be very challenging to correctly assess acute pain and the effectiveness of its treatment in patients with chronic pain and/or chronic opioid use. The emphatic expression of pain is commonly a deeply ingrained part of the daily human interactions of this population. As a result pain assessment tools and treatment goals well suited for "normal" patients may not be appropriate for this group. The language used to report pain can be a clue to the type of individual being treated. For example, when asked to describe their pain after surgery, most patients use words such as sharp, cutting, cramping, pulling, or throbbing. By contrast, the patient whose dominant problem is anxiety or fear may choose words like buzzing, funny, strange, or "don't know". The drug-seeking patient is more likely to choose words such as terrible, excruciating, horrible, unbearable, "can't stand it", "you've got to do something".

Patients with chronic opioid use may or may not be clinically obvious. It has been reported that patients with chronic pain markedly underestimate their actual drug use during medical history-taking (4). Certain observations, however, suggest that regular opioid use has occurred. Consider the possibility of previously unrecognized tolerance, dependence, or addiction when the following clinical triad is seen:

1. High pain scores compared to other patients having the same procedure.
2. High opioid use compared with other patients having the same procedure (5-7).
3. Absence of opioid-related side effects.

TREATING ACUTE PAIN IN PATIENTS WITH CHRONIC PAIN ± CHRONIC OPIOID USE

Although each patient is a unique human being, it is possible to define a number of general principles that can be applied to the treatment of acute pain in patients with underlying chronic pain:

1. Expect high self-reported pain scores. These are common in chronic pain patients.
2. Base treatment of the pain on objective findings (ability to deep breath, cough, ambulate, etc.).
3. Recognize and treat non-nociceptive sources of suffering (e.g., an anxiolytic for anxiety).
4. Use appropriate measures for as long as is appropriate for acute pain. Avoid extended therapy if it is not appropriate for a chronic condition.

Consider the following principles of management of acute pain in patients who have chronic pain and/or have chronic opioid use:

1. Recognize the need to identify and treat two major problems:
   a. Replacement of basal opioid requirement (protection from withdrawal syndrome).

      b.   Control of acute pain.

2. Provide the basal opioid unconditionally i.e.. independent of reported pain. Make it clear to the patient that the need for opioid replacement is recognized.

3. Add short-term therapy for acute pain. A nonopioid-based approach (local anesthetic, NSAID, etc.) to treat the acute pain is preferred whenever possible.

4. Expect high subjective pain scores. Do not rely on them exclusively to guide therapy. Make decisions based on objective findings—overall appearance of the patient, ability to cough and move, physiologic variables, etc.

5. Detoxification is usually not an appropriate goal in the perioperative period.

6. Discuss the treatment plan with the patient early; repeat it often.

Is there a role for PCA in the Patient with Chronic Opioid Use?

Probably not for the purpose of providing basal requirement. This may better be given by the oral route or by a fixed IV infusion controlled by the therapist.

Probably in selected patients for the extra opioids needed on a short-term basis to treat acute pain The following selection criteria should be considered:

1. Patients in whom cooperation and agreement has been demonstrated when a treatment plan is presented.

2. In particular, patients who agree to short-term therapy only.

3. Patients who show an appropriate pattern of use once therapy has begun.

It is worth recalling that the central premise for PCA is based on an assumption that a simple feedback loop exists such that when pain is present, the patient will self-administer an opioid; when pain is relieved, self administration will cease. It is worth considering on a patient-by-patient basis whether this loop is likely to be intact. If not, PCA should probably be avoided. All the advantages of placing "control" in the hands of opioid-naive patients with acute pain become liabilities if the basic loop does not exist. Under such conditions, a patient with chronic opioid use is likely to consume as much narcotic as the PCA pump settings permit while still reporting uncontrolled pain.

Discontinuing a PCA pump in a patient who is not demonstrating appropriate use can give rise to a great deal of conflict and hostility. At such times, it is helpful to emphasize that the PCA is being discontinued because it has failed to meet therapeutic goals; not because the pattern of use was inappropriate. By defining a therapeutic failure of PCA as the reason for stopping it, the patient is not made to feel that their own behavior is in question. Rather, the therapist is seen as accepting responsibility for finding an alternative form of therapy for the purpose of improving comfort.

REFERENCES

1. Ready LB: How many acute pain services are there in the United States and who is managing patient-controlled analgesia? (letter). Anesthesiology 82:322, 1995
2. Loeser JD: What is chronic pain? Theoretical Medicine 12:213-225, 1991
3. Hord AH: Postoperative analgesia in the opioid-dependent patient. Acute Pain: Mechanisms & Management. Edited by Sinatra, RS, Hord, AH, Ginsberg, B, Preble, LM. St. Louis: Mosby-Year Book Inc., 1992, pp 390-398
4. Ready LB, Sarkis E, Turner JA: Self-reported vs. actual use of medications in chronic pain patients. Pain 12:285-294, 1982
5. Pillow KJ, Moote CA, Komar WE, Lampe KM: Postoperative pain management in patients with inflammatory bowel disease. Can J Anaesth 37:S63, 1990
6. Brody MC, Wheeler DS, Stacey BR, Burke DF, Dunwoody C: Increased analgesia requirements in patients using PCA narcotics for postoperative analgesia. Anesth Analg 72:S27, 1991
7. Rapp SE, Ready LB, Nessly ML: Acute pain management in patients with prior opioid consumption: a case-controlled retrospective study. Pain 61:195-201, 1995

RADIATION SAFETY FOR THE PAIN PHYSICIAN AND THE USE OF A LASER GUIDED C-ARM TO FACILITATE PAIN BLOCK PLACEMENTS

L. M. Broadman

Thirty-five years ago this author was sitting in a military classroom and receiving basic indoctrination in the fine art of self protection against the effects of gamma radiation and nuclear fallout. I learned that I could be exposed to 100 rads of gamma radiation with little or no effect. If however I were to receive 300 rads, I might develop bleeding gums and transiently slough the lining of my small and large bowel one or two weeks after the exposure, but I would recover. If I were unfortunate enough to be exposed to 600 or more rads of total body irradiation, I would not survive the insult. This was fine with me. The Cuban missile crises had come and gone, and the cold war had become very cold. Moreover, I was young, invincible and had no idea what one rad was other than a unit of measure for gamma rays or other forms of ionizing radiation.

Fortunately, I now know that exposure to even minuscule amounts of ionizing radiation can be harmful. All practical steps should be taken to limit your own personal exposure and that of your patients and co-workers. During the next 30 minutes you will learn how a C-arm works and how you can protect yourself and those around you from the harmful effects of ionizing radiation while still being able to reap the benefits of C-arm guided block placements.

WHAT IS A RAD AND IS IT BAD?

A rad (radiation absorbed dose) is an older and now obsolete unit for the measure of deposited energy in tissue from ionizing radiation such as x-rays and gamma radiation. The newer unit is the Gray (Gy). One Gy is equal to 100 rads (1 Gy=100 rads), and is better defined as the deposition of energy (absorbed dose) in tissue equivalent to one joule/kg of tissue. There are 1000 mGy in one Gy. There are also several other traditional and Systems Internationale des Units (SI) used to describe radiation dosages. The Roentgen (R) or coulomb/kilogram (C/kg) is equal to 2.58 X 10^{-4} C/kg. Two units, the rem (radiation equivalent man) and the sievert

T. H. Stanley et al. (eds.), Pain Management and Anesthesiology, 303–309.
© *1998 Kluwer Academic Publishers. Printed in the Netherlands.*

(Sv), are used to express the quantity of radiation received by radiation workers. One Sv is equal to one Gy which equals 100 rem (1 Sv=1 Gy=100 rem). Finally, one Roentgen (R) is equal to one rad, which is equal to one rem (1 R=1 rem=1 rad).

To place this all in proper perspective the United States Food and Drug Administration (FDA) has limited incidental occupational exposure to 50 mGy/calendar year. The FDA policy states "no occupational exposed person may receive an effective whole-body dose of more than 50 mGy (5 rads) per calendar year as a result of incidental exposure to radiation in the workplace. This is equivalent to your performing one four-minute fluoroscopic study per day without the benefit of a protective lead apron. So much for 100 rads being an insignificant exposure.

GUNS, TARGETS AND RICOCHET ROUNDS

How does fluoroscopy work? The function of the fluoroscope is quite analogous to a gun and a target. A gun fires bullets through a barrel, an X-ray tube fires a beam of electrons through a high voltage vacuum tube, and X-rays are formed and emitted through a tinny opening. Some of the particles leaving the gun strike the patient and are absorbed, while others pass through the subject and go on to strike the target. In this case the target is an image intensifier, a device which collects the electro-magnetic particles (X-rays) and translates them into a usable picture which can be viewed on a television monitor. Unfortunately, some of the X-ray particles strike bone, muscle and organs of differing density and scatter. It is these scattering particles like ricocheting bullets (rounds) that can cause injury to you and your co-workers.

How does one adjust the C-arm to give the best picture possible with the least amount of potential tissue damage to your patient and yourself? There are two key adjustments on all fluoroscopy units: tube voltage (kVp) and tube current (mA). The high voltage through which the electron beam passes in the X-ray vacuum tube is referred to as kilovolt peak (kVp). If we once again use our gun analogy we can liken kVp to muzzle velocity. Shoot a high muzzle velocity bullet and it will most certainly pass through most human beings. Unfortunately, if all of the fired X-rays pass through our hypothetical patient and hit the image intensifier, we would have no contrast. To get an image with contrast (gray-scale ordering) some of the particles must become absorbed or refracted by more dense tissues while other pass virtually unimpeded through air filled cavities and less dense tissues. It is this gray-scale ordering which allows us to interpret the fluoroscopic image. Bones always appear as the whitest tissue on x-ray and fluoroscopic images, followed by muscle and fat, and air always appears black. A good place to begin on a normal sized adult is with the kilovolt peak (kVp) set at about 75. Larger patients like larger animals require bullets with higher muzzle velocity in order to get the round to pass through all tissue and hit the target. It may be necessary to use as much as 125 kVp on large subjects to obtain more penetration or as little as 65 kVp on small women. One size does not fit all and one should always attempt to use the highest possible kVp setting which still produces adequate contrast or gray-scale ordering. This will minimize the total X-ray exposure by your patient and potential exposure for you and your co-workers as the result of scattering.

If we once again return to our gun analogy we can liken tube current (mA) to the number of bullets our gun can fire per minute. Turn up the tube current and you fire more electrons through the high voltage vacuum tube and more X-rays are produced and emitted. But, like bullets the more you fire per unit of time the better the chance that some of them will hit rocks and ricochet. It is these ricocheting rounds (scattered X-rays) which are harmful to you and your co-workers. The tube current may be set between 1 and 5 mA, but the lower setting (1 mA) is usually adequate for most situations.

The proper adjustment of picture contrast on the monitor is obtained by balancing kVp against mA for any given patient and study. By using higher kVp settings one can reduce the number of X-rays emitted by the fluoroscopy unit and allow for a lower mA setting. But, unfortunately higher kVp settings reduce contrast because each X-ray is imparted with more penetrating power. Modern machines contain a computer controlled system called automatic brightness control (ABC). With this system in place all one needs to do is turn on the machine, enter an initial kVp setting, activate the ABC system and begin the fluoroscopic study. The computer will automatically analyze picture contrast and make appropriate mA adjustments in order to give you the best balance between picture contrast and patient safety. Patient safety is paramount and it must be remembered that it is the balance between kVp and mA which controls patient dose.

PROTECTING YOUR PATIENT

The best way to protect your patient is minimize beam on time. Picture what needs to be done from the stored image on the monitor and make the necessary corrections in needle position. Then briefly activate the fluoroscopy unit to update your monitor picture. Do not think and plan with the beam activated.

Keep the X-ray tube as far away from your patient as possible. All modern fluoroscopy units have a separator cone. This is a plastic device which surrounds the X-ray tube orifice and maintains a minimum safe distance between the source and the patients skin. Increasing the distance form the X-ray source to the patient improves picture quality and at the same time reduces the risk of skin burns.

The use of tight collimation reduces patient tissue exposure. The collimator on your fluoroscopy unit is similar to firing our imaginary gun at a target. This time our gun is a shot gun and the shell contains 100 pellets. The pellets disperse evenly over the whole target at perhaps 10 pellets per sq. inch of target area. However, if we cover the target with a thin metal shield and allow pellets to only impact on the "bulls-eye", we will still have 10 pellets per sq. inch impacting on the one sq. inch of exposed target. But, we will have reduced by 90 the total number of pellets hitting the rest of the target. Similarly, collimation, the placing of a thin metal shield over the X-ray tube opening, prevents the emission of electromagnetic particles into unwanted fields and thereby reduces the amount of X-ray exposure received by your patient by simply reducing the total area which is irradiated. There is no reason to monitor a full screen view of a patients lumbar spine and both flanks while making fine adjustments in needle placement over a single lumbar facet joint. One simply needs to tightly collimate over the area in question and allow X-rays to only impact on the facet joint and a small area of surrounding tissue. This will improve the quality of the image by reducing scatter and in turn will reduce the occupational exposure risks to you and your staff. Remember, it is scattered radiation that is the major health risk to you and your staff. If one doubles the area exposed to X-rays in any given patient one increases the volume of exposed tissue by a factor of four. This in turn will increase scattered X-ray particles by a factor of four.

Positioning the image intensifier as close to the patient as possible will improve the quality of the image and reduce the dose of radiation administered to your patient. Remember, the image intensifier is a passive unit. It omits no radiation and poses no threat to either you or your patient. By selecting needles of the most appropriate length one can optimize image intensifier to patient distance. Do not use 8 inch (20 cm) needles when 3.5 in (9 cm) ones will get the job done. If a work gap of more than 25 cm is required between the image intensifier head and the surface of your patient, remove the grid from the fluoroscopy unit. The grid is a devise that filters scattered X-rays and thereby improves image contrast. However, only negligible interference is caused by scattered particles at a distance of more than 25 cm from your patient and removal of the grid can significantly reduce patent exposure. More energy and X-ray particles are required with the grid in place. Have your technologist help you remove and protect the grid. It is very expensive and easily damaged.

Finally, limit the use of magnification. The dose per unit area delivered to your patient increases when you elect to magnify the image. This in turn increases the amount of scatter to which you and your co-workers become exposed.

PROTECTING YOURSELF AND YOUR CO-WORKERS?

When asked how can one best protect themselves against the harmful effect of X-rays, the first response that comes to the mind of most health care professionals is the wearing of a protective lead apron. This is true, but there is a great deal more you can do to protect yourself and your associates. You already know that you can reduce total patient dose and subsequent scatter by reducing X-ray tube mA to the lowest possible level while optimizing contrast with the appropriate kVp setting. You also know to keep beam on-time to a minimum. Finally, you are aware that it is the scattered radiation from your patient that poses the greatest health risk to you and your associates, and it is relatively easy to reduce this risk by simply imposing some distance between your patient and yourself. Step back from the field whenever possible before activating the beam. The intensity of this scattered ionizing radiation decrease in an exponential manner as one increases the distance from the source. So, a small increase in distance can dramatically reduce exposure. If 100 scattered X-ray particles are available to impact upon you at one meter from the patient, only 25 will still be a threat to you at two meters and just 4 at five meters. However, be careful when stepping back from the source so that you do not inadvertently turn your unshielded back toward the beam.

Lead aprons only provide protection when they are properly worn and have received proper care and storage. Do not fold lead aprons or worse yet throw them on the floor as these flawed storage techniques may produce creases which may in turn form breaks in the protective barrier. When not in use, hang your lead apron on a hook. Most lead aprons have a shielding equivalent equal to that of a 0.5 mm lead barrier. This will reduce your exposure to scattered radiation by about 90%. The shielding characteristics of your personal apron can be found on the tag sewn into a corner seam of the lining. Scooped or plunging neck-lines may be in vogue with certain sports attire but this is to be avoided when wearing a lead apron. Your thyroid tissue is at significant risk from the carcinogenic effects of ionizing radiation. Protect your thyroid by covering it with your apron and a thyroid shield. Finally, two other types of personal protective equipment are worthy of mention: leaded glasses with side shields and "leaded" surgical gloves. The former reduce the risk of cataract formation and are relatively inexpensive. The later may afford some protection against radiation induced dermatitis. However, the best protection for your hands is to use tight collimation and to keep your hands out of the beam. In fact, X-ray attenuating surgical gloves may increase your occupational exposure. If you are operating your fluoroscopic unit in the ABC mode, the fluoroscopic unit will sense that there is poor contrast between the bones of your inadvertently exposed hand and the surrounding soft tissue. The ABC system will automatically adjust the mA to produce a higher dose rate and better contrast, thereby increasing your exposure.

One can not feel the effects of moderate radiation exposure. The only way one can ascertain their personal exposure is by wearing a film badge. The badge should be worn on the outside of your apron or thyroid shield. It should be changed monthly and the results of all exposures should be reviewed by the radiation safety officer and promptly shared with you.

Dosing and scattering can be quite variable depending upon the size of your patient, the study being performed and the duration of beam on-time. Fluoroscopic doses can range from as little as 10 to as much as 500 mGy/minute. At the upper limit of 500 mGy/minute just a four minute exposure can produce transient tissue erythema in your patient (2.0 Gy total exposure). This latter fact points out that the five-minute timer found on all fluoroscopic units is just a reminder and that even brief periods of exposure can be harmful to your patient.

Finally, there is a substantial risk of direct beam exposure to you when you are operating your C-arm unit in the lateral position. In this position it is possible to interpose your hands between the X-ray tube and the patient. With inadvertent activation of your unit you will be exposed to 100% of the dose. To avoid this scenario always place the X-ray tube away form the side upon which you are working. This also holds true for oblique projections. Moreover, the exposure to your head and chest from scattered radiation will be higher when you are working on the X-ray tube side. On the other hand, with conventional positioning where the X-ray tube is placed some distance beneath your patient and all radiation first passes through your patient, less than 1.0% of the total dose will still be available to impact upon your hands after passing through your patients torso.

FDA WARNING OF PATIENT INJURIES FROM FLUOROSCOPY

You have now completed a basic course in C-arm function, operation and safety, and are in compliance with the FDA letter of 9 September

1994. This letter warns of serious X-ray induced skin injuries which have recently occurred during fluoroscopically guided invasive procedures. The letter suggests that physician training and credentialing in the safe operation of fluoroscopic equipment are the most crucial ingredients in preventing the occurrence of such unfortunate mishaps. As captain of the ship, you and only you are responsible for the safety of your patient, the safety of your co-workers, and the safe operation of the portable fluoroscopy equipment which you are using.

Now that you know how to properly operate portable C-arm equipment, what can you do with it and how can it help you help your patients? The author will spend the final few minutes of the lecture sharing with you his experience in how to use the laser guided C-arm to facilitate placement of lumbar sympathetic, facet joint and sacroiliac joint blocks. He will correlate the X-ray pictures with corresponding C-arm X-ray tube and image intensifier positions and the laser pattern on a human skeleton.

SUGGESTED READING AND VIEWING

C-ARM FUNCTION AND SAFETY:

1. Boshong SC. Radiologic Science for the Technologist (physics, biology and protection) 6th edition. Mosby. St. Louis, MO. 1997.
2. Selman J. The Fundamentals of X-ray and Radium Physics. 8th edition. Charles C. Thomas. Springfield, IL. 1994
3. Thompson MA, Hattaway MP, Hall JD, Dowd SB. Principles of Imaging Science and Protection. W.B. Saunders Co. Philadelphia, PA. 1994.
4. Wagner LK, Archer BR. Minimizing risks from fluoroscopic X-rays. Partners in Radiation Management. Houston, TX. 1996
5. Series 9600 System Operation Overview. OEC Medical Systems. Salt Lake City, UT. Available by calling 1-800-874-7378.

C-ARM GUIDED BLOCK PLACEMENT:

1. Kline MT. Stereotactic radiofrequency lesions as part of the management of pain. St. Lucie Press. Delray Beach, FL. 1996.
2. Waldman SD, Winnie AP. Interventional pain management. W.B. Saunders Co. Philadelphia, PA. 1996.

DEVELOPMENTS IN
CRITICAL CARE MEDICINE AND ANESTHESIOLOGY

1. O. Prakash (ed.): *Applied Physiology in Clinical Respiratory Care.* 1982
ISBN 90-247-2662-X

2. M.G. McGeown: *Clinical Management of Electrolyte Disorders.* 1983
ISBN 0-89838-559-8

3. T.H. Stanley and W.C. Petty (eds.): *New Anesthetic Agents, Devices and Monitoring Techniques.* Annual Utah Postgraduate Course in Anesthesiology. 1983
ISBN 0-89838-566-0

4. P.A. Scheck, U.H. Sjöstrand and R.B. Smith (eds.): *Perspectives in High Frequency Ventilation.* 1983
ISBN 0-89838-571-7

5. O. Prakash (ed.): *Computing in Anesthesia and Intensive Care.* 1983
ISBN 0-89838-602-0

6. T.H. Stanley and W.C. Petty (eds.): *Anesthesia and the Cardiovascular System.* Annual Utah Postgraduate Course in Anesthesiology. 1984
ISBN 0-89838-626-8

7. J.W. van Kleef, A.G.L. Burm and J. Spierdijk (eds.): *Current Concepts in Regional Anaesthesia.* 1984
ISBN 0-89838-644-6

8. O. Prakash (ed.): *Critical Care of the Child.* 1984
ISBN 0-89838-661-6

9. T.H. Stanley and W.C. Petty (eds.): *Anesthesiology: Today and Tomorrow.* Annual Utah Postgraduate Course in Anesthesiology. 1985
ISBN 0-89838-705-1

10. H. Rahn and O. Prakash (eds.): *Acid-base Regulation and Body Temperature.* 1985
ISBN 0-89838-708-6

11. T.H. Stanley and W.C. Petty (eds.): *Anesthesiology 1986.* Annual Utah Postgraduate Course in Anesthesiology. 1986
ISBN 0-89838-779-5

12. S. de Lange, P.J. Hennis and D. Kettler (eds.): *Cardiac Anaesthesia.* Problems and Innovations. 1986
ISBN 0-89838-794-9

13. N.P. de Bruijn and F.M. Clements: *Transesophageal Echocardiography.* With a contribution by R. Hill. 1987
ISBN 0-89838-821-X

14. G.B. Graybar and L.L. Bready (eds.): *Anesthesia for Renal Transplantation.* 1987
ISBN 0-89838-837-6

15. T.H. Stanley and W.C. Petty (eds.): *Anesthesia, the Heart and the Vascular System.* Annual Utah Postgraduate Course in Anesthesiology. 1987
ISBN 0-89838-851-1

16. D. Reis Miranda, A. Williams and Ph. Loirat (eds.): *Management of Intensive Care.* Guidelines for Better Use of Resources. 1990
ISBN 0-7923-0754-2

17. T.H. Stanley (ed.): *What's New in Anesthesiology.* Annual Utah Postgraduate Course in Anesthesiology. 1988
ISBN 0-89838-367-6

18. G.M. Woerlee: *Common Perioperative Problems and the Anaesthetist.* 1988
ISBN 0-89838-402-8

19. T.H. Stanley and R.J. Sperry (eds.): *Anesthesia and the Lung.* Annual Utah Postgraduate Course in Anesthesiology. 1989
ISBN 0-7923-0075-0

20. J. De Castro, J. Meynadier and M. Zenz: *Regional Opioid Analgesia.* Physiopharmacological Basis, Drugs, Equipment and Clinical Application. 1990
ISBN 0-7923-0162-5

21. J.F. Crul (ed.): *Legal Aspects of Anaesthesia.* 1989
ISBN 0-7923-0393-8

DEVELOPMENTS IN
CRITICAL CARE MEDICINE AND ANESTHESIOLOGY

KLUWER ACADEMIC PUBLISHERS – DORDRECHT / BOSTON / LONDON